Microneuroanatomy and Lab

Feres Chaddad-Neto
Marcos Devanir Silva da Costa

Microneuroanatomy and Lab

A Step-by-Step Guide to Dissection

Springer

Feres Chaddad-Neto
Department of Neurology and Neurosurgery
Universidade Federal de São Paulo
São Paulo, São Paulo, Brazil

Marcos Devanir Silva da Costa
Department of Neurology and Neurosurgery
Universidade Federal de São Paulo
São Paulo, São Paulo, Brazil

ISBN 978-3-031-91025-8 ISBN 978-3-031-91026-5 (eBook)
https://doi.org/10.1007/978-3-031-91026-5

This Springer imprint is published by the registered company Springer Nature Switzerland AG
The registered company address is: Gewerbestrasse 11, 6330 Cham, Switzerland

To my wife, Patricia, for her unconditional love and support that drive me to reach new horizons.

To my daughter, Marina, who brings light and meaning to my life and reminds me daily of the value of small joys.

To my parents, Arlindo Chaddad (in memoriam) and Neide Gomes Chaddad, who, with love and wisdom, taught me that there are no limits to what can be achieved with dedication and courage.

To Dr. Evandro de Oliveira (in memoriam), whose brilliance, teaching, and legacy shaped not only my neurosurgical training but also how I view the art of microsurgery.

To all neurosurgery students (undergraduates, postgraduates, residents, and fellows), whose enthusiasm and dedication were key elements in the realization of this work. You represent the future and the continuity of the quest for knowledge.

To the patients, whose trust inspires us to overcome challenges and to relentlessly pursue advancements in care and treatment, recognizing that each story is a reminder of the importance of our work.

To the specimens that silently contributed to the advancement to neuroanatomical knowledge. May their scientific legacy Always be treated with the utmost respect and gratitude.

May this book inspire its readers to explore the complexity and beauty of neuroanatomy, for it is in the details that science becomes art and art, transformation.

Feres Chaddad-Neto, MD, PhD – *Editor of the Book*

To God for life.

To my wife, Vanessa, and my children Augusto, Julia, and Vitor for their daily support and for being my joy.

To my parents Devanir (in Memoriam) and Eponina and all my family who have always supported me and encouraged me to go further.

To my professors and mentors for their dedication and commitment to passing on knowledge.

To my students, residents, and fellows who encourage us to break down the current barriers to knowledge.

To the neurosurgeons who will use this book as a source of knowledge.

Marcos Devanir Silva da Costa, MD, PhD – *Editor of the Book*

Preface

Mastering the microneurosurgery and the microneuroanatomy requires extensive study, dedication, and hours of training; the place for training in both Anatomy and Surgery is the Laboratory of Microneuroanatomy. It is ultimately important to understand the philosophy of the Lab training as a place not just for memorizing the anatomy but rather a place for training microsurgery techniques, a place to translate the knowledge from the LAB to the Operating Room. In the lab, the neurosurgeon can train to gain the ability necessary to perform a world-class microsurgery.

This book aims to introduce the Microneuroanatomy Lab to medical students, neurosurgical residents, and neurosurgeons. It addresses all the basic tenets of the laboratory routine, specimen preparations, and a guide for all types of brain dissections. Therefore, it presents a step-by-step guide from basic to advanced dissection for all the important anatomical regions.

São Paulo, São Paulo, Brazil — Feres Chaddad-Neto
São Paulo, São Paulo, Brazil — Marcos Devanir Silva da Costa

Acknowledgments

This book would never be possible without the commendable work of our valuable collaborators that have helped by writing, dissecting specimens, producing and editing pictures/figures, and editing videos. We are grateful for their collaboration, enthusiasm, and commitment. Their names and institutions are listed below:

Alexander Feliciano Vilcahuamán Paitán – Fellow of Vascular Neurosurgery at Universidade Federal de São Paulo – São Paulo, SP, Brazil.

Alice Giotta Lucifero – Fellow of Vascular Neurosurgery at Universidade Federal de São Paulo – São Paulo, SP, Brazil.

Edgar David Tenelema Aguaisa – Fellow of Vascular Neurosurgery at Universidade Federal de São Paulo – São Paulo, SP, Brazil.

Erica Antunes Effgen – Fellow of Vascular Neurosurgery at Universidade Federal de São Paulo – São Paulo, SP, Brazil.

Érico Samuel Gomes Galvão da Trindade – Fellow of Vascular Neurosurgery at Universidade Federal de São Paulo – São Paulo, SP, Brazil.

Felipe Ostermann Magalhães – Neurosurgery Resident at Universidade Federal de São Paulo – São Paulo, SP, Brazil.

Felipe Salvagni Pereira – Fellow of Vascular Neurosurgery at Universidade Federal de São Paulo – São Paulo, SP, Brazil.

Glaucia Suzanna Jong A Liem – PhD Student and Fellow of Vascular Neurosurgery at Universidade Federal de São Paulo – São Paulo, SP, Brazil.

Guilherme Salemi Riechelmann – Fellow of Vascular Neurosurgery at Universidade Federal de São Paulo – São Paulo, SP, Brazil.

Joao Vitor Lima Fernandes - Neurosurgery Resident at Universidade Federal de São Paulo – São Paulo, SP, Brazil.

José Maria Campos Filho – Neurosurgeon at Hospital BP Paulista, São Paulo, SP, Brazil.

Juan Carlos Ahumada Vizcaíno – PhD Student and Fellow of Vascular Neurosurgery at Universidade Federal de São Paulo – São Paulo, SP, Brazil.

Juan Leonardo Serrato Avila – Neurosurgeon at Neurosurgery Department, Hospital General Dr. Agustín O'Horan. Merida, Yucatán, Mexico.

Liezel Ulloque Caamaño – Fellow of Vascular Neurosurgery at Universidade Federal de São Paulo – São Paulo, SP, Brazil.

Luis Ángel Canache Jiménez – PhD student and Fellow of Vascular Neurosurgery at Universidade Federal de São Paulo – São Paulo, SP, Brazil.

Luís Gustavo Biondi Soares – PhD student and Fellow of Vascular Neurosurgery at Universidade Federal de São Paulo – São Paulo, SP, Brazil.

Mariano Teyssandier – Fellow of Vascular Neurosurgery at Universidade Federal de São Paulo – São Paulo, SP, Brazil.

Manuel Moreno Hernández – Fellow of Vascular Neurosurgery at Universidade Federal de São Paulo – São Paulo, SP, Brazil.

Pedro José Ramiro Muiños –Neurosurgery Resident at Universidade Federal de São Paulo – São Paulo, SP, Brazil.

Rene Alejandro Apaza Tintaya – Fellow of Vascular Neurosurgery at Universidade Federal de São Paulo – São Paulo, SP, Brazil.

Ricardo Chmelnitsky Wainberg – Neurosurgeon at Hospital São Lucas da PUC-RS - Pontifícia Universidade Católica do Rio Grande do Sul, Porto Alegre, Brazil.

Richard Gonzalo Párra – Director of the Institute of Neurosurgery of Bolivia (INEB), Cochabamba, Bolivia.

Roberto Duprat Oberg – Former Fellow of Vascular Neurosurgery at Universidade Federal de São Paulo – São Paulo, SP, Brazil.

Rodrigo Akira Watanabe – Neurosurgery Resident at Universidade Federal de São Paulo – São Paulo, SP, Brazil.

Victor Camara Della Betta – Medical Student at Universidade Federal de São Paulo – São Paulo, SP, Brazil.

Vinicius Santos Baptista - Medical Student at Universidade Federal de São Paulo – São Paulo, SP, Brazil.

Talita Helena Martins Sarti – PhD Student and Fellow of Vascular Neurosurgery at Universidade Federal de São Paulo – São Paulo, SP, Brazil.

Contents

Chapter 1
Journey from the Laboratory to the Operating Room

The microscope was introduced by Theodore Kurze in 1957, pioneering the concept of augmented visualization in the field of surgery. The application of microsurgery to neurosurgical procedures has paved the way for advancements in microneuroanatomy. Establishing a dedicated training environment for neurosurgeons and residents to develop microsurgical skills and study microneuroanatomy is a top priority in neurosurgical education. Adequate training must be conducted in controlled environments, using laboratory microscopes for the application of microsurgical techniques on specimens and other simulators. For neurosurgeons, anatomical knowledge is only valuable when applied to surgical practice. However, microsurgery is inadequate if the surgeon lacks anatomical knowledge and the ability to identify anatomical landmarks. Neuroanatomical knowledge and technical microsurgical skills should be integrated to provide adequate surgical treatment for specific pathologies, thereby reducing the risk of damage to the uninvolved structures.

The laboratory serves as a training ground where surgeons acquire surgical skills, refine their hand movements for surgery, enhance the accuracy and dexterity of their techniques, and deepen their understanding of neuroanatomy. Finally, although mistakes are permissible in this controlled environment, they are not acceptable in actual patient care.

An increasing number of neurosurgical training models are introduced annually in neurosurgical literature. These models can be broadly categorized into those that focus on the acquisition of anatomical or technical knowledge and the practice of technical skills and those that allow for skill acquisition in anatomically and clinically relevant contexts. Various skills can be trained and perfected in the laboratory, ranging from ergonomics to the dissection of vessels. These topics will be discussed in the following sections.

F. Chaddad-Neto, M. D. S. da Costa, *Microneuroanatomy and Lab*,
https://doi.org/10.1007/978-3-031-91026-5_1

1.1 Ergonomics

Ergonomics involves establishing a position that ensures task effectiveness, which is essential for neurosurgical procedures that often involve prolonged durations and require sustained focus and attention. The key aspects of ergonomics in neurosurgical procedures include proper posture and hand positioning, achieved by maintaining spine alignment and providing support for the arms and hands. This approach enhances comfort for the surgeon and lessens exertion during the procedure. Therefore, ergonomics should be incorporated into laboratory training to optimize the reproducibility of the operating room (OR) environment (Figs. 1.1 and 1.2).

Neurosurgical procedures often involve prolonged use of the microscope. Therefore, ergonomics is crucial for preventing fatigue and reducing the risk of inattention due to discomfort in the neck, arms, or back of the surgeon. It also diminishes the occurrence of tremors. Adopting a seated position is recommended whenever possible; additionally, the chair height should be adjusted to fit the surgeon's position, further supporting ergonomic practices.

Resting the hands reduces the effort required to use instruments (Fig. 1.3), which enhances the accuracy and dexterity of movements. Hand support is typically achieved using the ulnar surface, both in the laboratory, where the ulnar surfaces rest on compresses, and in the OR, where the ulnar surfaces rest on the bone and edges of the craniotomy.

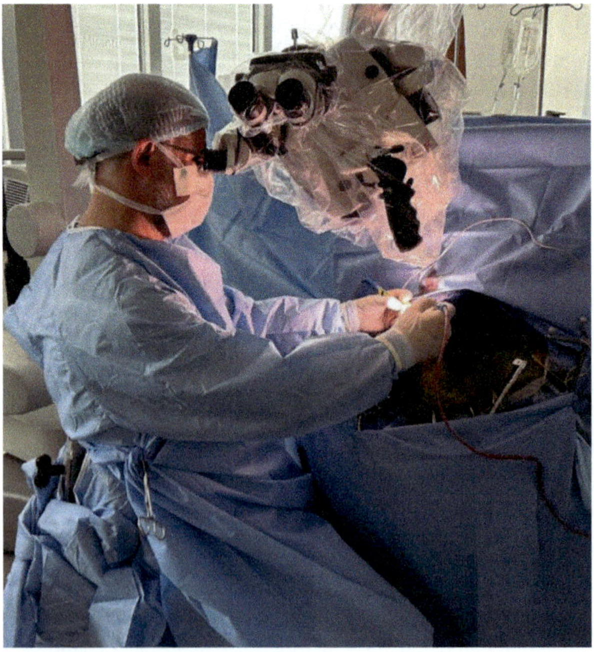

Fig. 1.1 Observe the ergonomic posture, aligned spine, and hand support around the craniotomy

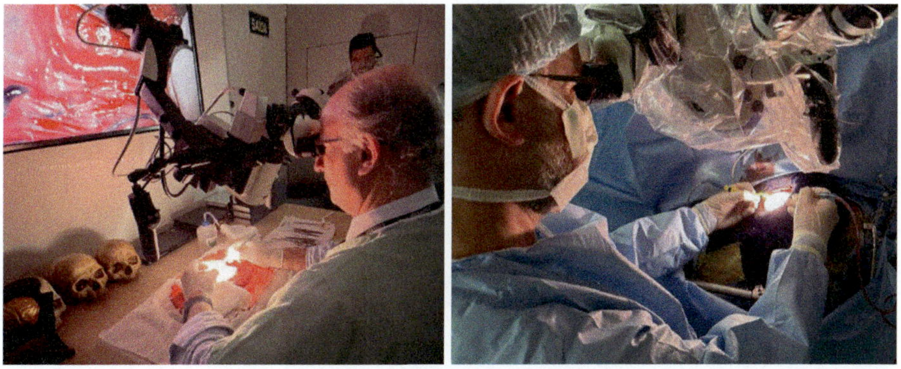

Fig. 1.2 Note the consistent posture in the laboratory (left image) and operating room (right image). Proper hand placement in the operative field optimizes instrument use

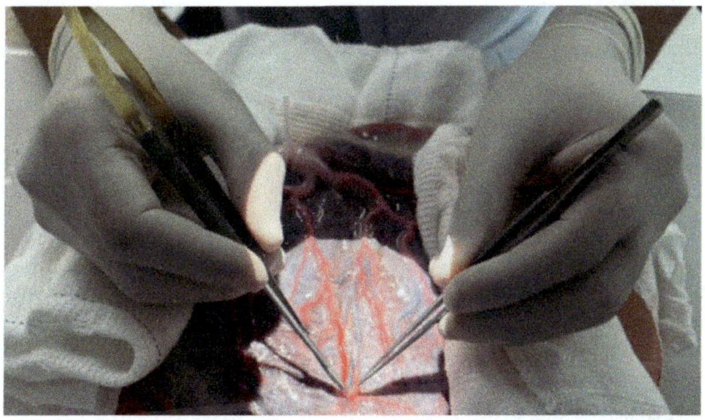

Fig. 1.3 In the laboratory, the ulnar surface of the hands is supported by compresses

1.2 Instruments

During microsurgical and neurosurgical procedures, it is common for surgery to progress from a more superficial plane to a deeper plane. This requires the use of different sizes and types of instruments that can be reproduced in the laboratory. During the approach, before the beginning of the microsurgical stage of the surgery, straight forceps (such as anatomical and rat tooth forceps) are predominantly used. As the procedure advances to the microsurgical stage, bayonet forceps are preferred as they facilitate access to deeper structures. Similarly, straight microsurgical scissors are often used during superficial microdissection at the beginning of the microsurgical stage. As the dissection proceeds, bayonet microscissors are more suitable for reaching deeper structures and preventing obstruction of the microscope's light. Different instrument sizes and lengths are appropriate for various depths, with microscissors, suction surgical tubes, bipolar forceps, dissectors, and bayonet forceps becoming necessary as the procedure progresses (Fig. 1.4). Additionally, the diameter of the suction surgical tubes is also crucial, depending on the specific situation. Finally, various types of surgical instruments available in the laboratory are essential for training and preparation for the actual procedure (Fig. 1.5).

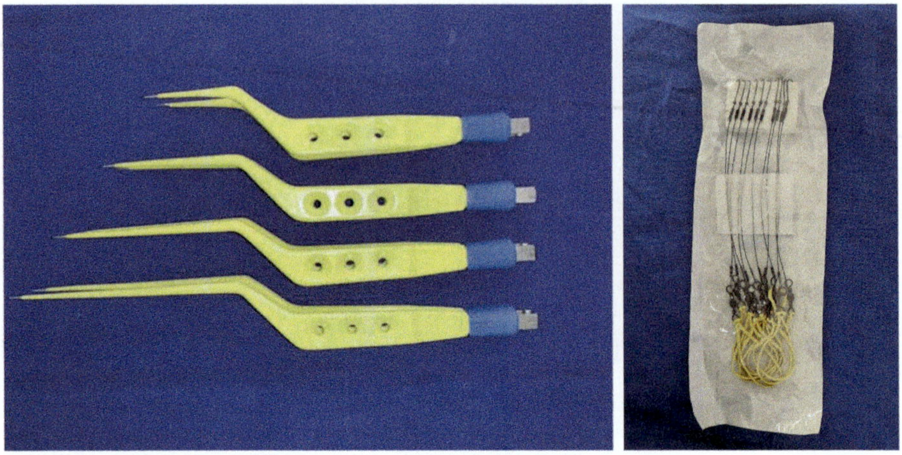

Fig. 1.4 The left image shows bipolar forceps of various lengths available for training in the laboratory. The right image displays an instrument table arranged with different sizes of several different surgical instruments

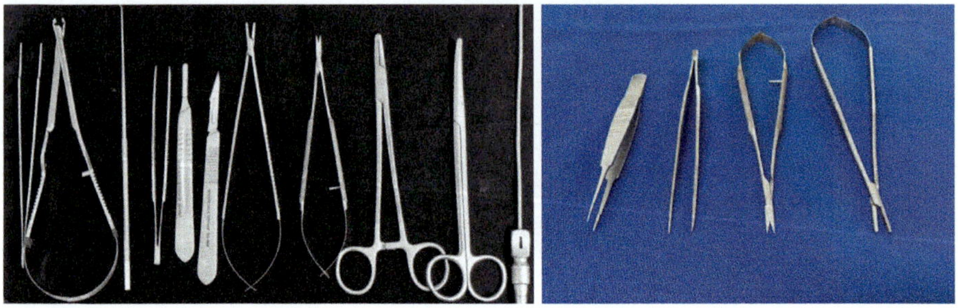

Fig. 1.5 The images demonstrate a variety of surgical instruments that should be included in the laboratory for training to closely replicate real surgery in the OR

During laboratory training, each hand should hold a surgical instrument so that the surgeon can become accustomed to working with both hands. This optimizes the use of instruments, improves surgical performance, and is an efficient method for rehearsing tasks.

1.3 Practicing Resources

Hand-eye coordination under the surgical microscope and the maneuvering of the microsurgical instruments improved after frequent training and repeated movements. Laboratory practice facilitates and accelerates the learning curve associated with mastering the techniques under a microscope. In addition, preparatory steps

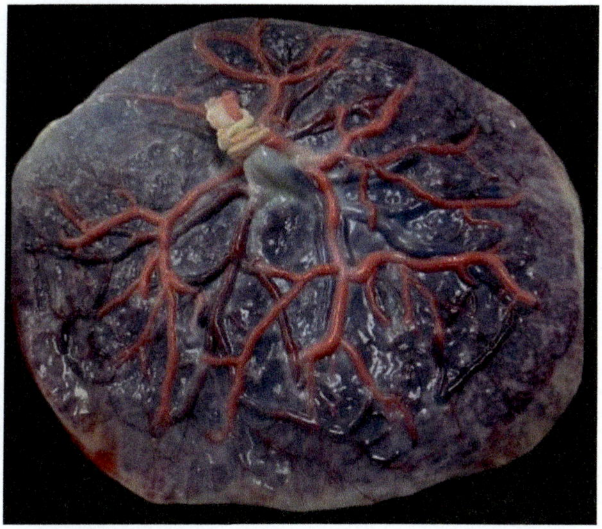

Fig. 1.6 A human placenta injected with color dye

before the microsurgical stage of the procedure, such as positioning and approach, are essential for effective training and skill refinement. Therefore, specific practice specimens can be used for this purpose, each designed to provide training at different steps.

Human placentas are a cost-effective and readily available resource for practicing vascular dissection. The chorioamniotic membrane of the placental fetal surface closely resembles the arachnoid membrane, and the placental vessels are similar in caliber to the cerebral arteries (Fig. 1.6). Different calibers of placenta vessels (e.g., the smaller caliber of more distal vessels) enable simulations that closely mimic those encountered in living patients (Fig. 1.7). Additionally, the presence of intersections between the arteries and veins, with veins being incompletely covered and in close proximity to the pia mater, presents varying levels of difficulty for the microsurgical technique (Fig. 1.7). Folding the placenta, placing a compress beneath it, or working on a placenta inside a container enhances its resemblance to the brain tissue, owing to the variations in depth and the presence of surface irregularities. Moreover, inflating a balloon catheter can create aneurysm-like structures in the placental arteries. Consequently, using color-dyed placentas for practice facilitates the simulation of subarachnoid space dissection in surgeries for the treatment of aneurysms and arteriovenous malformations, or when bypasses are required (Fig. 1.8).

Using anatomical pieces for dissection aids in developing a three-dimensional understanding of anatomical relationships and landmarks along with step-by-step dissection, which supports the practice of microsurgical techniques. Structures such as the gyri, sulci, arteries, and ventricles can be studied anatomically. The important anatomical relationships of these structures can be learned; for example, understanding the limits, contents, and components of the ceiling and floor of the ventricles can be achieved. Practicing with a microscope further enhances this knowledge (Fig. 1.9).

Fig. 1.7 The intersections between arteries and veins and the variety of calibers increase the resemblance to live patient dissection and provide different levels of difficulties for microsurgical training

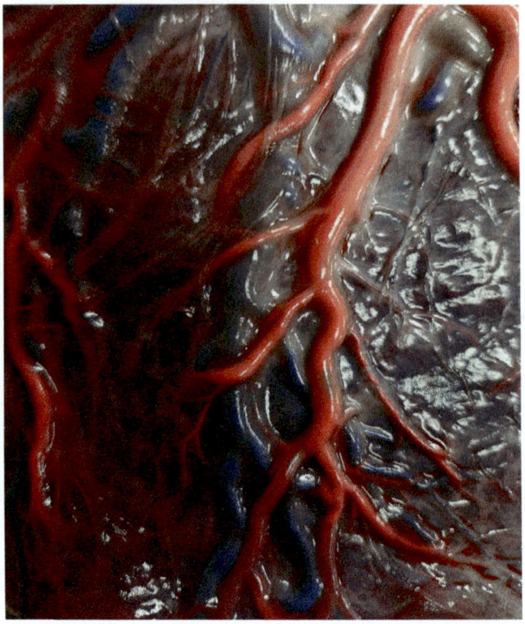

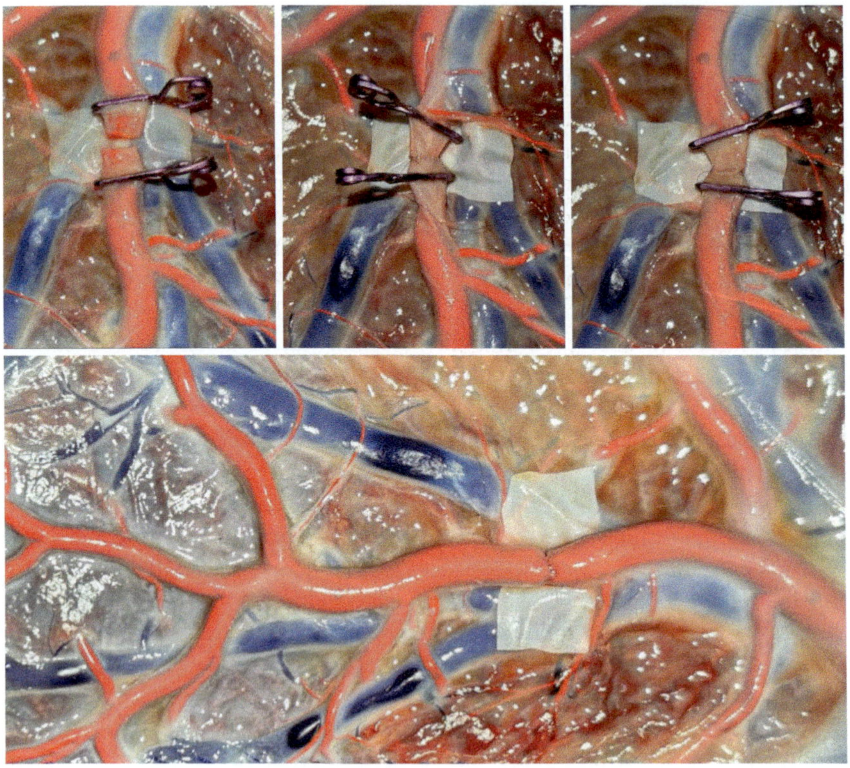

Fig. 1.8 Vascular dissection, clipping, and anastomosis can be practiced on placentas. The figure demonstrates an end-to-end arterial anastomosis using a 10–0 nylon suture in a placental artery

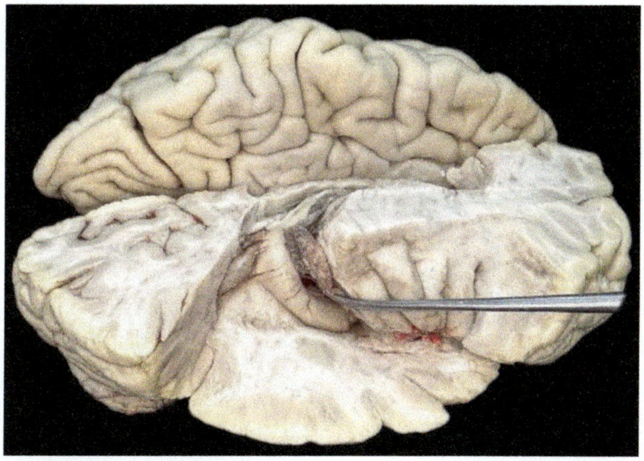

Fig. 1.9 Anatomical piece demonstrating the relationships of the atrium and temporal horn of the lateral ventricle. The dissector is holding the choroid plexus and exposing the choroidal fissure. Other identifiable structures include the bulb of the corpus callosum, collateral trigone, hippocampus, and insula

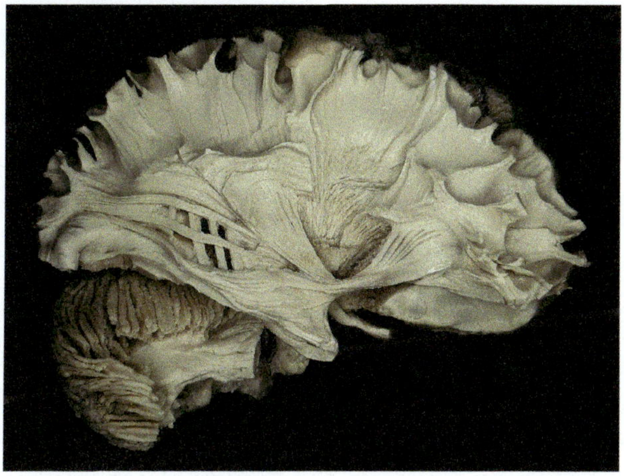

Fig. 1.10 An anatomical piece demonstrating some of the main white matter tracts after dissection using the Klingler's technique

The dissection of white matter fibers, although not performed on living patients, is crucial for studying the position and anatomical relationships of the main tracts and fasciculus. This knowledge is essential during microsurgical procedures, as identifying the white matter tracts with a microscope not feasible. This dissection is usually performed on frozen anatomical pieces using the Klingler technique (Fig. 1.10).

Cadaveric heads can be used for practicing surgical positioning and the execution of different approaches (Figs. 1.11 and 1.12). Furthermore, similar to anatomical specimens, the dissection of cadaveric heads enables a three-dimensional study and a deeper understanding of anatomical relationships. However, cadaveric heads provide the added benefit of allowing detailed examination of specific structures, such as veins (Fig. 1.13).

Therefore, to facilitate microsurgical practice and neuroanatomical studies, the laboratory can replicate many aspects of the OR, making it a vital environment for practicing and mastering surgical techniques.

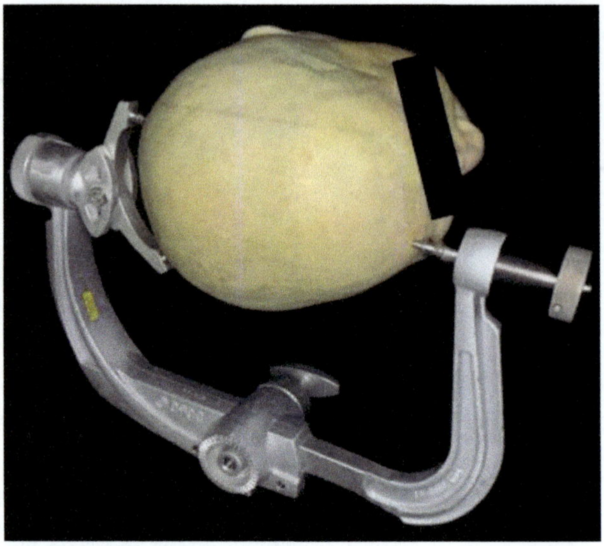

Fig. 1.11 Cadaveric heads can be used for practicing the positioning in a three-point skull clamp system with pins. This setup simulates the position typically adopted for performing a subtemporal approach, where the head is aligned paralleled to the floor

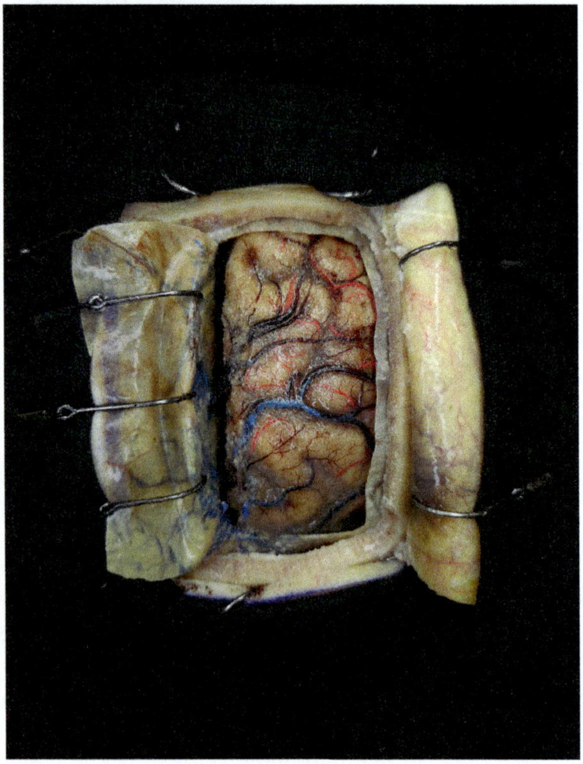

Fig. 1.12 Cadaveric head with a demonstration of a frontal craniotomy for the interhemispheric approach. The image clearly shows the falx cerebri and a bridging vein from the frontal lobe draining to the superior sagittal sinus

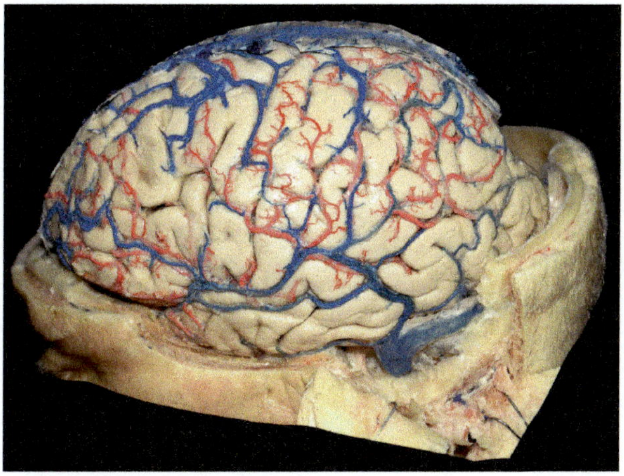

Fig. 1.13 Cadaveric heads provide superior study of cerebral veins compared with anatomical specimens. This cadaveric head shows the superficial Sylvian vein, the vein of Labbé, the transverse sinus, and several parasagittal bridging veins

Bibliography

1. Romero FR, Fernandes ST, Chaddad-Neto F, Ramos JG, Campos JM, Oliveira, editors. Microsurgical techniques using human placenta. Arq Neuropsiquiatr. 2008;66(4):876–8.
2. Ahumada-Vizcaino JC, Wuo-Silva R, Hernández MM, Chaddad-Neto F. The art of combining neuroanatomy and microsurgical skills in modern neurosurgery. Front Neurol. 2023;12(13):1076778.
3. Mastorakos P, McGavern D. The anatomy and immunology of vasculature in the central nervous system. Sci Immunol. 2019;4(37):eaav0492.
4. Jiménez LÁC, Salvagni FP, Biondi-Soares LG, Apaza-Tintaya RA, Aguaisa EDT, de Almeida IR, Wuo-Silva R, da Costa MDS, Sarti THM, Chaddad-Neto F. Model of arteriovenous malformation created in human placenta for training in vascular microneurosurgery. In: Operative neurosurgery (Hagerstown, Md.); 2024. https://doi.org/10.1227/ons.0000000000001305.
5. Apaza-Tintaya RA, Canache Jiménez LÁ, Salvagni Pereira F, Biondi Soares LG, Tenelema Aguaisa ED, Vilcahuamán Paitán AF, Wuo-Silva R, Chaddad-Neto F. Topographical systematization of human placenta model for training in microneurosurgery. World Neurosurg. 2024;182:e471–7.
6. Korotkov D, Rodrigues de Almeida I, Wuo-Silva R, Vilcahuamán Paitán AF, Chaddad-Neto F. Enhancing the microneurosurgical training: development of the folded placenta model for simulation of the deep operative field challenges of cranial procedures. World Neurosurg. 2024;187:29–34.
7. Klingler J. Erleichterung der makroskopischen Praeparation des Gehirns durch den Gefrierprozess. Schweiz Arch Neurol Psychiatr. 1935;36:247–56.
8. Pereira FS, Jiménez LÁC, Aguaisa EDT, Apaza-Tintaya RA, Biondi-Soares LG, Paitán AFV, Soto PHT, Wuo-Silva R, Chaddad-Neto F. Superior frontal sulcus: a non-eloquent corridor for cavernomas of the internal capsule. Front Neurol. 2024;15:1355338.
9. Costa M, Braga VL, Yağmurlu K, Centeno RS, Cavalheiro S, Chaddad-Neto F. A Technical guide for fiber tract dissection of the internal capsule. Turk Neurosurg. 2018;28(6):934–9.
10. Goiri MAA, de Amorim BL, Sarti THM, da Costa MDS, Chaddad-Neto F. Building a microneurosurgical laboratory in Latin America: challenges and possibilities. Surg Neurol Int. 2021;12:573.
11. Chaddad-Neto F, Silva da Costa MD. Microneuroanatomy and surgery. Cham: Springer; 2022.

Chapter 2
Laboratory Setup

The microneuroanatomy laboratory is a space reserved for practicing neuroanatomy and also for microsurgery. It is in the laboratory that we gain manual skills and anatomical knowledge, so it is necessary to have a minimum structure with some equipment and instruments to carry out this practice. In this chapter, we will explore some basic equipment and instruments, as well as aspects related to ethics and safety.

2.1 Types of Microscopes

The microscope was the paramount tool added to the surgical armamentarium in the last century for neurosurgeons. The microscope magnifies brain structures and vessels during surgery, allowing for precise dissection and detailed visualization. As a result, mastering the use of microscopes has become essential for the entire generation of neurosurgeons. Although the widespread use of microscopes in neurosurgery is evident today, many senior neurosurgeons have faced challenges in adapting to this technology. Yasargil was one of the first neurosurgeons to use a microscope, paving the way for its global acceptance. Professor Rhoton introduced the concept of microneuroanatomy, which involved studying the neuroanatomical details in the context of microsurgery and applying this knowledge to surgical practice. In today's neurosurgical landscape, proficiency with the microscope is fundamental. Aspiring neurosurgeons must acquire skills in microscope usage, especially given the integral role of microsurgery in neurosurgery. Hands-on training in an anatomy laboratory is considered the most effective method for learning microscope techniques. Although various microscope brands are available, they typically share common features, such as a light source, body, and structure. Microscopes are categorized into four main types according to their settings: on-caster, wall-mounted, tabletop (Fig. 2.1), and ceiling-mounted.

F. Chaddad-Neto, M. D. S. da Costa, *Microneuroanatomy and Lab*,
https://doi.org/10.1007/978-3-031-91026-5_2

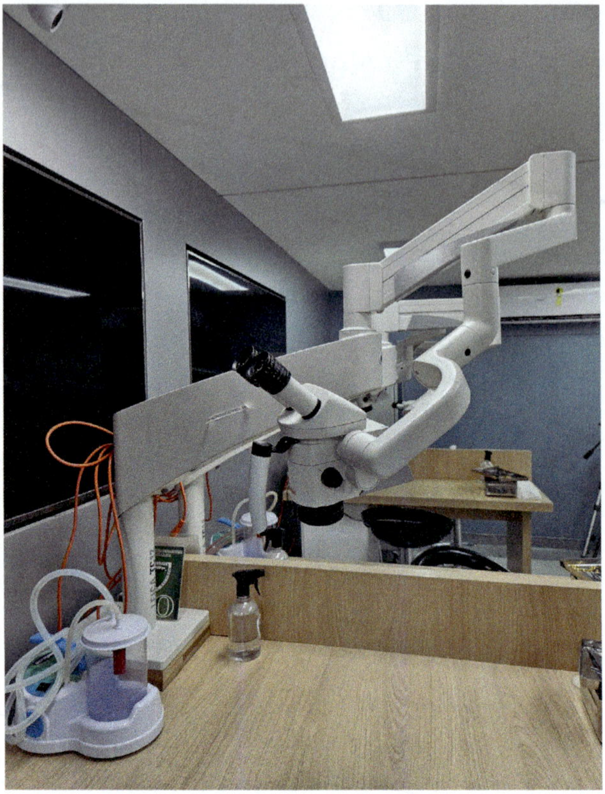

Fig. 2.1 Model of tabletop microscopes, with magnification ranging from 6.4x to 40x

Depending on the brand and availability, various filters can be placed. For example, in aneurysm surgery, an indocyanine filter can be used to perform intraoperative angiography. In brain tumor surgeries, a fluorescein filter can aid in visualizing lesions.

The point here is to ensure comfort while sitting in the laboratory chair, adjusting the interpupillary distance in the microscope objectives, and initiating dissections in the arachnoid or placentas using 11 blades and microscissors. The lesser zoom should be initiated, with magnification progressively applied thereafter. This approach allows for improved surgical movements during surgery.

2.2 Types of Instruments

A wide range of instruments are available for performing the dissection technique. They can be divided mainly into cutting instruments (scalpel and macro- and microsurgical scissors), dissection tools (dissectors), and hemostatic instruments (Kelly and bipolar forceps).

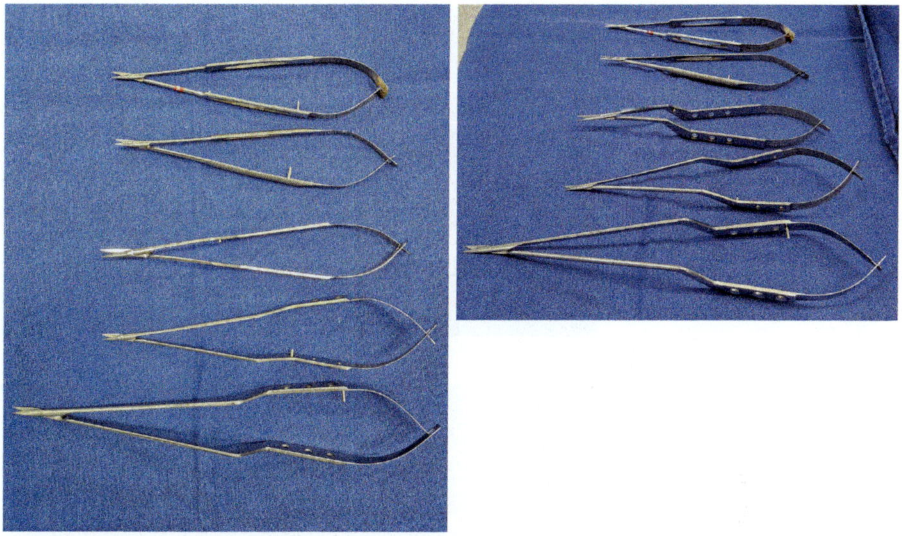

Fig. 2.2 Types of bayonet microcissors

These bayonet microscissors have a distinctive design with thin elongated blades that taper to a fine point, resembling the shape of a bayonet. They are used to cut delicate tissues or structures with minimal damage to the surrounding areas (Fig. 2.2).

The microdissection forceps (Fig. 2.3) are specialized surgical instruments used for delicate tissue manipulation and dissection.

Aspiration and microaspiration cannulas (Fig. 2.4) are typically small in diameter, often ranging from less than a millimeter to a few millimeters. They may be designed as straight or curved to facilitate access to different areas during the performance of procedures.

Dissectors and microdissectors (Fig. 2.5) have various shapes and sizes but typically consist of fine, sharp tips that allow surgeons to precisely cut or separate tissues under high magnification. These instruments were designed to be lightweight and delicately balanced to minimize hand fatigue and enable precise manipulation during the performance of procedures.

Kerrison and Goiva forceps (Fig. 2.6) are designed to remove bone or soft tissue during procedures, requiring precision and control. Meanwhile, self-retaining retractor (Fig. 2.6) locks in place once positioned, maintaining constant tension to keep the tissues or organs retracted throughout the procedure. Handheld retractors require constant manual manipulation.

Kelly forceps (Fig. 2.7) have interlocking teeth along the full length of the jaw and are commonly used for clamping blood vessels or grasping tissues. Mayo scissors (Fig. 2.7) have robust blunt-ended blades with equally sized finger holes. The blades are typically straight or curved and can vary in length, with longer blades

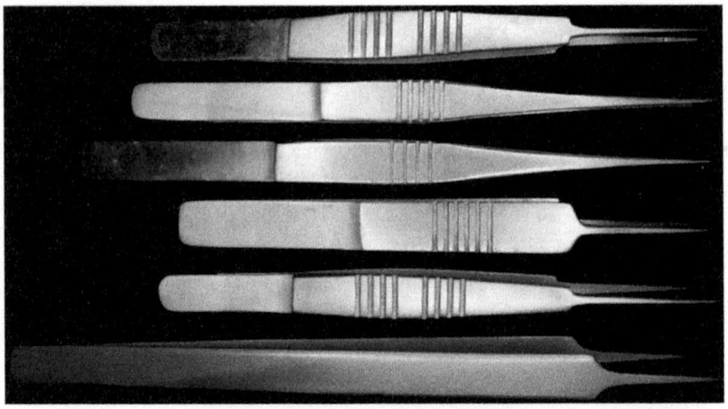

Fig. 2.3 Different types of tweezers for microsurgery and bypass in the lab

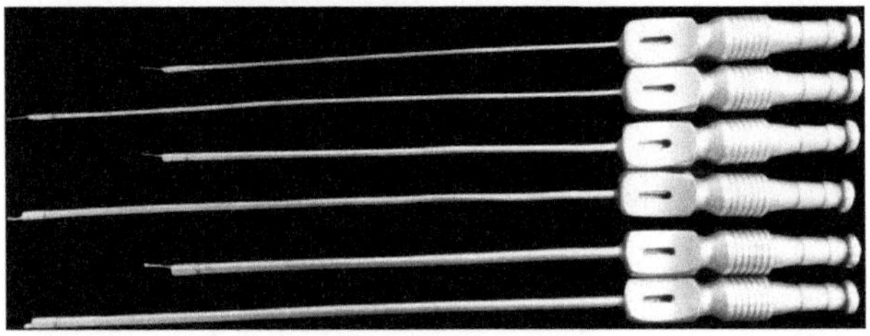

Fig. 2.4 Microaspiration cannulas of different sizes and diameter

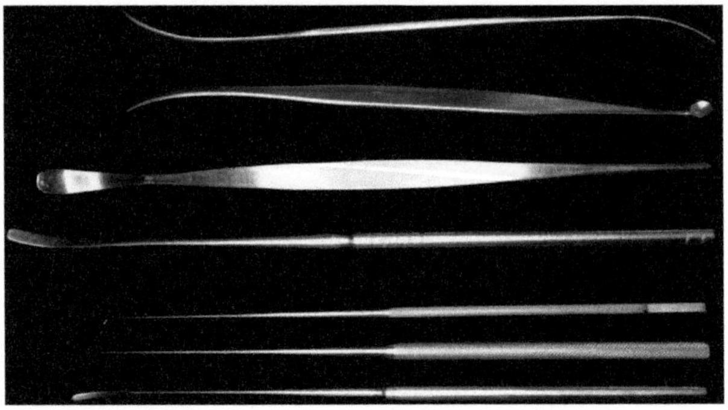

Fig. 2.5 Dissectors and microdissectors. The superior four instruments are dissector, and the inferior three instruments are microdissectors

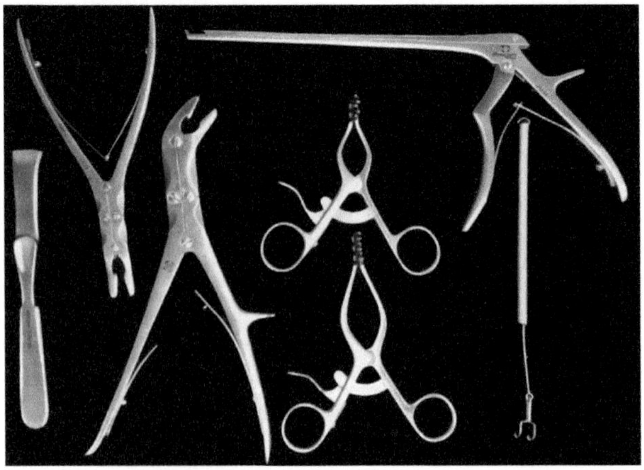

Fig. 2.6 Farabeuf raspatoy, Goiva forceps, self-retaining, Kerrison, retractor

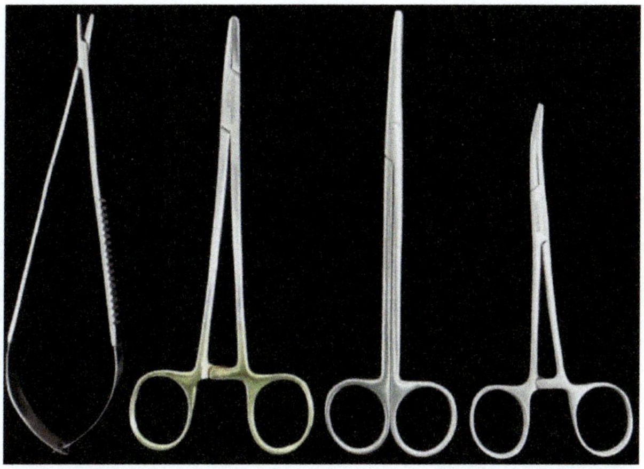

Fig. 2.7 From left to right—straight micro needle holder, straight Mayo scissor, Curved Kelly

used for deeper dissections and shorter blades used for more superficial cutting. A needle holder (Fig. 2.7) is a surgical instrument used to grasp and manipulate a suture needle during a surgical procedure. Needle holders are essential training tools.

2.3 International Laboratory Regulations

As in any neuroanatomy laboratory, adherence to international safety regulations is paramount. Ensuring good coexistence necessitates maintaining a clean environment and educate colleagues and local employees. Proper attire, such as lab coats or personal protective clothing, must be worn when entering the laboratory. Adornments should be removed, and masks, caps, and gloves should be worn. Smoking, eating, drinking, and excessive noise are strictly prohibited in the work environment.

Photographing cadavers or anatomical parts and publicizing them on any unauthorized platforms are strictly prohibited. In addition, disclosing the identities of the deceased is forbidden.

2.4 Preserving the Specimens

According to Brazilian regulations, bodies available for study or dissection must not have been claimed within the last 30 days. It is extremely important to avoid identifying and addressing these bodies. Various substances, including alcohol, formaldehyde, and glycerin, can be used for preserving specimens. Maintaining a cold temperature, ideally around 4 degrees Celsius, is essential for optimal preservation of corpses (Fig. 2.8).

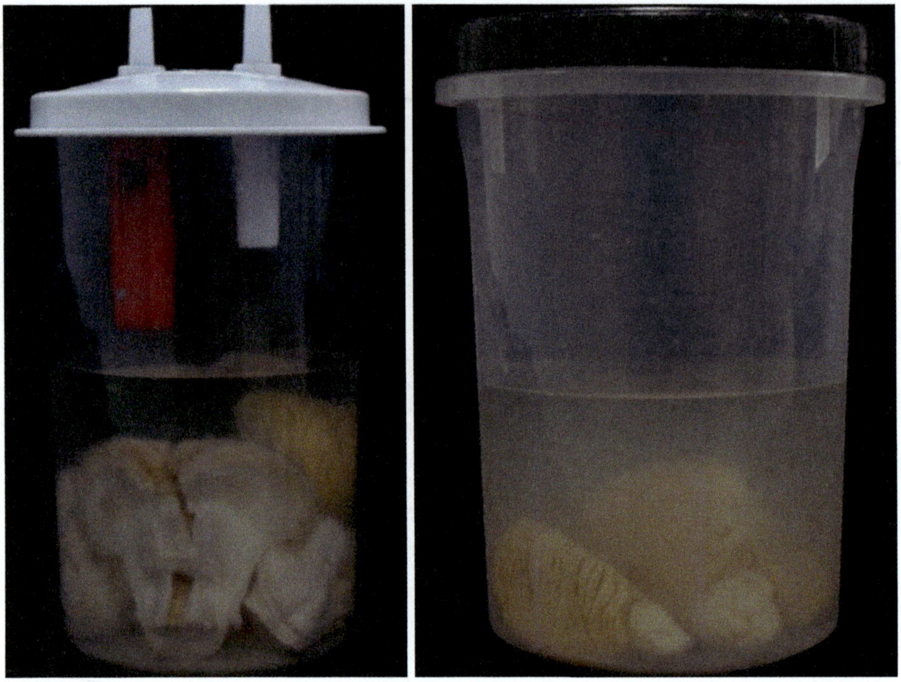

Fig. 2.8 Specimens stored in buckets with alcohol 70%

2.5 Head Holders

In a laboratory setting, a head holder is used to stabilize and immobilize the head of a specimen or animal during various procedures or training sessions.

The design of these head holders can vary depending on the specific training needs and type of specimen used.

Typically, a head holder consists of a rigid frame attached to a laboratory table. This frame is equipped with three or four fixation pins or clamps that are gently inserted into the skull of the specimen, providing stable support and preventing movement during training. Pins or clamps are typically placed on the outer table of the skull away from the critical structures to minimize the risk of damage to the species.

The specific manufacturers and models of head holders may vary, and different laboratories might use different devices based on their research requirements. Therefore, there is no standardized head holder across all laboratory settings.

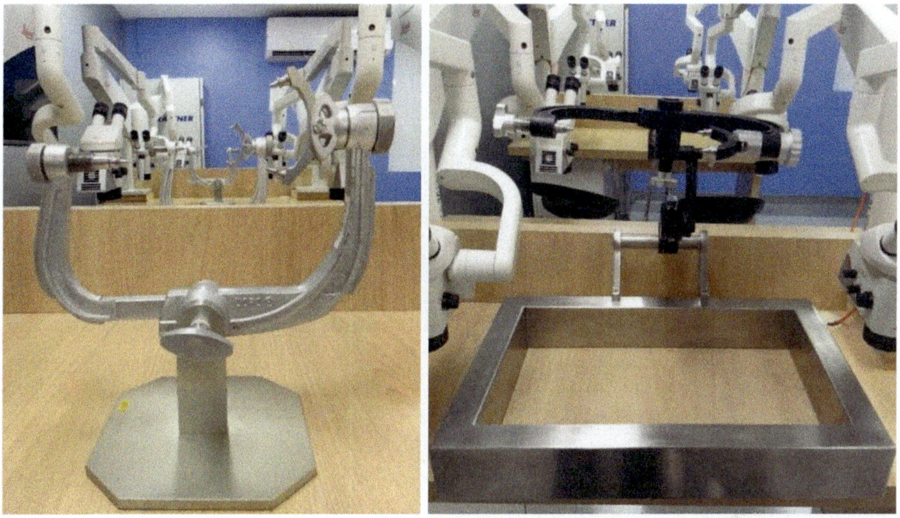

Fig. 2.9 Different types of table head holders

Specifically, the term "Mayfield head holder" refers to the head fixation system produced by Mayfield Surgical Instruments, a company specializing in neurosurgical equipment (Fig. 2.9). Other manufacturers may produce head fixation systems similar to their own proprietary names. Nonetheless, the term "Mayfield head holder" is often used generically to refer to any head fixation system based on the design principles introduced by Mayfield Surgical Instruments.

2.6 Chairs

In anatomical laboratories, chairs play a crucial role in facilitating comfortable learning and collaborative activities for students, researchers, and instructors. The specific types of chairs used in an anatomy laboratory may vary based on institutional preferences and specific spatial requirements. The common types of chairs found in anatomical laboratories are as follows:

Stools: Stools are commonly used in anatomical laboratories due to their versatility and ease of movement. They often feature adjustable heights, allowing users to customize the chair's position according to their preferences and specific tasks. Stools with swivel bases are particularly useful for maneuvering around dissection tables or workstations (Fig. 2.10).

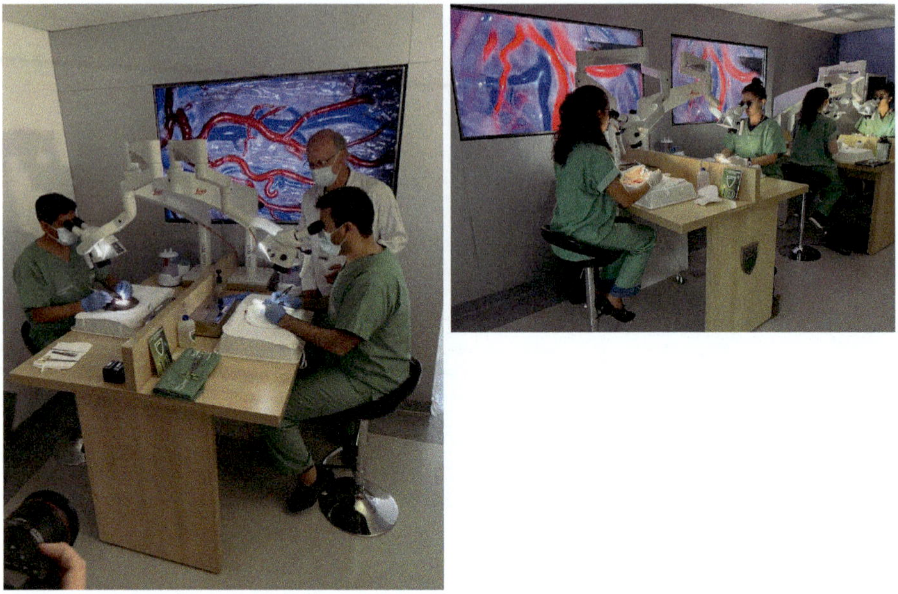

Fig. 2.10 Different types of lab stools

Task chairs: Task chairs are designed for comfort and functionality, provide ergonomic support, and are suitable for tasks involving prolonged sitting.

Drafting chairs: Drafting chairs, also known as laboratory chairs, are similar to task chairs but feature an extended height adjustment range. These chairs are suitable for use on higher work surfaces, such as microscope stations. Their taller gas-lift mechanism enables users to adjust the chair to a comfortable height while working in an upright position.

Lecture hall chairs: In larger anatomy laboratories or teaching spaces, lecture hall chairs may be installed to accommodate a larger number of students, are designed for comfort during extended sitting periods, and are often arranged in rows or tiers to facilitate clear sightlines during presentations and demonstrations.

Conference chairs: Conference chairs may be used in areas designated for group discussions, presentations, or collaborative work. These chairs typically have a cushioned seat and backrest, along with armrests, for enhanced comfort during prolonged use.

When selecting chairs for an anatomy laboratory, factors such as ergonomic support, durability, ease of cleaning, and compliance with safety and hygiene standards must be considered. Additionally, chairs should be chosen based on the specific activities and needs of the laboratory to ensure optimal comfort and functionality for all users.

2.7 Stations

Anatomical laboratories typically comprise various stations or areas designed to facilitate the study and examination of anatomical specimens. The specific stations may vary depending on factors such as the laboratory's size, available resources, and focus. Some common stations found in an anatomy laboratory are as follows:

Dissection tables: Dissection tables are central to anatomical laboratories. These large, sturdy tables provide a workspace for the examination and dissection of cadavers and anatomical models. They are equipped with sinks, drainage systems, and adjustable height options for convenience.

Specimen storage: This area is dedicated to the storage and preservation of anatomical specimens. It typically includes cabinets, refrigerators, freezers, or specialized storage units designed to maintain the integrity and quality of the specimens. The storage area may be organized according to anatomical regions or categories.

Anatomical models and skeletons: A separate station or display area can be allocated for the storage and examination of anatomical models, skeletons, and other teaching aids. These models can be used to study anatomical structures, demonstrate relationships, and provide hands-on learning experiences.

Microscopes and imaging stations: Equipped with microscopes or imaging devices, these stations facilitate the detailed examination of tissue samples, slides, or radiographic images for studying cellular structures and microscopic anatomy.

Multimedia and technology: With increasing integration of technology in education, some anatomical laboratories have multimedia stations. These stations include computer workstations with access to digital anatomical atlases, anatomical software, or virtual dissection tools. They enhance the learning experience and provide additional resources for anatomical studies.

Teaching and presentation area: Designated for lectures, presentations, or group discussions, this area typically includes audiovisual equipment, whiteboards, and seating arrangements to facilitate teaching and learning activities.

Washing and cleaning areas: An essential part of anatomy laboratories is the washing and cleaning area. This is where the equipment, dissection tools, and work surfaces can be thoroughly cleaned and disinfected after use. This may include sinks, sterilization equipment, and storage for cleaning supplies.

Personal protective equipment (PPE) stations: Safety is paramount in anatomical laboratories. PPE stations provide designated areas for donning and doffing PPE, such as gloves, laboratory coats, goggles, and masks. These stations may also include waste disposal containers for proper disposal of contaminated materials.

The specific stations and layout of an anatomy laboratory can vary depending on the resources available and institutional preferences and needs. The objective is to create a functional and organized workspace that supports the study and exploration of anatomy while maintaining a safe and efficient learning environment (Fig. 2.11).

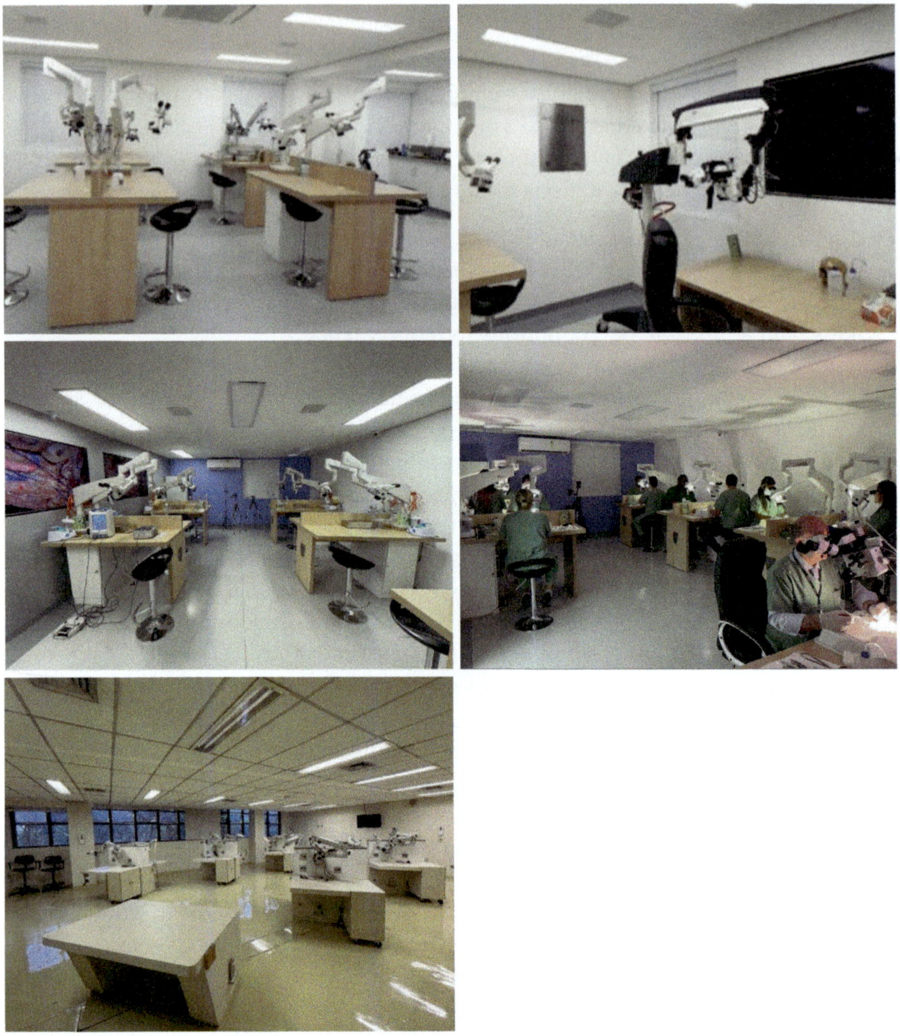

Fig. 2.11 Laboratory stations. Superior photo is the present stations at Microneuroanatomy Lab in the Universidade Federal de São Paulo. Inferior photo is the Dr. Evandro de Oliveira's past Lab at Hospital Beneficencia Portuguesa

2.8 Ethics

Ethics in the anatomy laboratory are essential to ensure that research and educational activities involving human or animal cadavers are conducted with integrity and adherence to ethical standards. Some key considerations related to ethics in the anatomy laboratory are as follows:

Informed consent: In human cadavers, informed consent should be obtained from the donors or their legal representatives before using human cadavers for research or educational purposes. The consent process involves providing clear information about the nature and purpose of the research, procedures involved, and any potential risks or benefits.

Respect for donors: Human cadavers used in anatomical laboratories should be treated with utmost respect and dignity. Proper handling and storage procedures should be followed to protect the donors' privacy and confidentiality. Identifying information should be kept confidential, and the bodies should be stored, preserved, and disposed of appropriately.

Ethical sourcing of cadavers: The human cadavers should be sourced ethically and legally. Cadavers should be obtained through donation programs, where individuals willingly consent to the use of their bodies for educational or research purposes. The acquisition of cadavers through illegal or unethical means, such as unauthorized body trafficking, must be strictly avoided.

Animal welfare: Ethical considerations regarding animal welfare emerge in laboratories where animal cadavers are used for anatomical studies or research. Animal subjects were obtained and handled in accordance with ethical guidelines and regulations. The use of animals should be justified based on scientific and educational objectives, and efforts should be made to minimize pain, distress, and unnecessary suffering.

Ethical conduct of research: Researchers should adhere to ethical guidelines and standards when conducting research in an anatomical laboratory. This includes ensuring humane treatment of subjects, maintaining integrity in data collection and analysis, obtaining appropriate ethical approval, and protecting the rights and welfare of the participants.

Education and consent: Students and researchers involved in anatomical laboratories should receive appropriate education and training on ethical principles, respect for human and animal donors, and professional laboratory conduct. Informed consent and privacy considerations should be emphasized to promote ethical awareness and responsible behavior.

Ethical review and oversight: Institutional review boards or ethics committees should oversee anatomy laboratories to ensure that research and educational activities comply with ethical guidelines and regulations. These bodies review and approve the research protocols, provide guidance on ethical considerations, and monitor ongoing projects to safeguard ethical standards.

Ethical considerations in anatomical laboratories are vital for upholding the rights and dignity of donors, promoting responsible research practices, and maintaining public trust in scientific endeavors. Researchers, educators, and institutions should prioritize ethical conduct and strive to enhance ethical awareness and practices in anatomical research and education.

2.9 Biological Hazards

Neuroanatomical laboratories are essential for studying brain structures. However, they also pose potential biological hazards that must be addressed to ensure the safety of students, instructors, and other individuals in the laboratory. The common biological hazards found in anatomical laboratories are as follows:

Chemical agents: Anatomy laboratories often use various chemical agents, such as fixatives, preservatives, and disinfectants, to preserve and prepare anatomical specimens. These chemicals can be toxic, corrosive, or irritating if not handled properly. It is crucial to follow safety protocols, wear appropriate PPE, and ensure proper ventilation in the laboratory.

Biological specimens: Handling and dissecting biological specimens, such as human or animal cadavers, can expose individuals to various pathogens. These pathogens include bacteria, viruses, fungi, and parasites. Strict adherence to standard precautions, including wearing gloves, laboratory coats, and face shields, can minimize the risk of exposure.

Blood-borne pathogens: Anatomical laboratories working with blood or blood-contaminated materials must take precautions to prevent the transmission of blood-borne pathogens, such as hepatitis B virus, hepatitis C virus, and human immunodeficiency virus. This includes handling sharps (e.g., scalpels and needles) with caution and providing readily available sharps containers for safe disposal.

Allergens: Some individuals may be allergic to certain materials used in the laboratory such as latex gloves or chemicals. It is important to identify and address any known allergies among laboratory personnel and provide suitable alternatives or precautions to prevent allergic reactions.

Zoonotic diseases: Anatomical laboratories that work with animal specimens carry the risk of zoonotic diseases, which can be transmitted from animals to humans. Precautions, including proper handling and disposal of animal tissues and wastes, should be taken to prevent exposure to potential zoonotic pathogens.

Inhalation hazards: Airborne hazards such as formaldehyde fumes used for specimen preservation pose a risk to personnel. Implementing adequate ventilation systems, installing fume hoods, and providing respiratory protection can minimize exposure to such hazards.

Contaminated surfaces: Biological materials, such as dissecting tables, countertops, and equipment, can contaminate surfaces in the laboratory. Regular cleaning and disinfection protocols should be implemented to maintain a clean and safe working environment.

To ensure safety in anatomical laboratories, it is important to have comprehensive safety protocols, provide appropriate training to laboratory personnel, promote good hygiene practices, and regularly inspect and maintain safety equipment and facilities. Additionally, staying informed about relevant safety guidelines and regulations is essential for maintaining a safe learning environment.

2.10 Security

Ensuring security in an anatomical laboratory is essential to protect the integrity of the facility, specimens, and the privacy of donors. Important considerations for maintaining security in an anatomical laboratory are as follows:

Restricted access: Access to the laboratory is controlled by implementing measures such as locked doors, key card systems, or biometric access controls. Limit entry only to authorized personnel, such as researchers, educators, and students who have received appropriate training and have a legitimate need to be in the laboratory.

Surveillance systems: Surveillance cameras are installed strategically throughout the laboratory to monitor activities and deter unauthorized access. The camera coverage should include entrances, exits, specimen storage areas, and other critical areas. Signage prominently displayed in the laboratory indicates that the area is under surveillance.

Specimen inventory and tracking: An inventory system is implemented to keep track of all specimens in the laboratory. Unique identifiers are assigned to each specimen, and accurate records of its location, use, and disposal are maintained. Audits are regularly conducted to ensure that the specimens are accounted for and that there are no unauthorized removals.

Secure storage: Store specimens are placed in secure and lockable cabinets, freezers, or other appropriate storage units. Access to these storage areas should be restricted, and these areas should be kept locked when not in use. Temperature and humidity monitoring systems are installed to ensure optimal storage conditions for the specimens.

Data security: If laboratory collects or stores sensitive data related to donors or research subjects, such as personal information or medical records, appropriate data security measures should be in place. This may include encryption, password protection, firewalls, or regular data backups. Relevant data protection laws and regulations should be followed.

Confidentiality: The importance of maintaining donor confidentiality and privacy should be emphasized to all personnel working in the laboratory. All individuals involved in anatomical research or education should be aware of the legal and ethical obligations to protect donor privacy and the sensitive nature of the information they handle.

Training and awareness: Comprehensive training on security protocols, ethical guidelines, and the importance of maintaining security and privacy should be provided to all laboratory personnel. Regular updates and reinforcement of security policies and procedures are essential. Fostering a culture of security awareness and encouraging personnel to report suspicious or unauthorized activities are crucial.

Emergency preparedness: Emergency response plans specific to the anatomical laboratory should be developed and communicated. This includes procedures for handling incidents, such as theft, unauthorized access, natural disasters, or accidents. The personnel should be trained in emergency procedures, and emergency contact information must be readily available.

Compliance with regulations: Familiarity with relevant regulations, guidelines, and legal requirements that apply to anatomical research and education should be ensured. The laboratory complies must comply with all applicable laws and regulations related to the security, privacy, and handling of specimens.

By implementing these security measures and maintaining a culture of vigilance and responsibility, the anatomy laboratory, its specimens, and the privacy of donors or research subjects can be safeguarded.

Bibliography

1. Ghosh SK. Cadaveric dissection as an educational tool for anatomical sciences in the 21st century. Anat Sci Educ. 2017;10(3):286–99. https://doi.org/10.1002/ase.1649. Epub 2016 Aug 30. PMID: 27574911
2. Leonel LCP, Carlstrom LP, Graffeo CS, Perry A, Pinheiro-Neto CD, Sorenson J, Link MJ, Peris-Celda M. Foundations of advanced neuroanatomy: technical guidelines for specimen preparation, dissection, and 3D-photodocumentation in a surgical anatomy laboratory. J Neurol Surg B Skull Base. 2021;82(3):e248–58. https://doi.org/10.1055/s-0039-3399590. Epub 2019 Nov 28. PMID: 34306946; PMCID: PMC8289531
3. Goiri MAA, de Amorim BL, Sarti THM, da Costa MDS, Chaddad-Neto F. Building a microneurosurgical laboratory in Latin America: challenges and possibilities. Surg Neurol Int. 2021;23(12):573. https://doi.org/10.25259/SNI_978_2021. PMID: 34877059; PMCID: PMC8645469
4. Dutkiewicz J. Biologiczne czynniki zagrozenia zawodowego—aktualne problemy [Occupational biohazards: current issues]. Med Pr. 2004;55(1):31–40. Polis PMID: 15156765.
5. Dutkiewicz J, Górny RL. Biologiczne czynniki szkodliwe dla zdrowia—klasyfikacja i kryteria oceny narazenia [Biologic factors hazardous to health: classification and criteria of exposure assessment]. Med Pr. 2002;53(1):29–39. Polis PMID: 12051150
6. Hoffman PN, Healing TD. Guide to infection control in the healthcare setting the infection hazards of human cadavers. Brookline, MA, USA: Published by the International Society for Infectious Diseases 9 Babcock St, Unit 3; 2021.
7. Zdilla MJ. Local exhaust ventilation systems for the gross anatomy laboratory. Morphologie. 2021;105(350):237–46. https://doi.org/10.1016/j.morpho.2020.11.002. Epub 2020 Dec 2. PMID: 33279395; PMCID: PMC8169711
8. Raja DS, Sultana B. Potential health hazards for students exposed to formaldehyde in the gross anatomy laboratory. J Environ Health. 2012;74(6):36–40. PMID: 22329207
9. Gundreddy P, Gaurkar SS. Presence of contagious bacterial flora in formalin-fixed cadavers: a potential health hazard to medical professionals. Cureus. 2022;14(10):e30684. https://doi.org/10.7759/cureus.30684. PMID: 36439597; PMCID: PMC9691388
10. Demiryürek D, Bayramoğlu A, Ustaçelebi S. Infective agents in fixed human cadavers: a brief review and suggested guidelines. Anat Rec. 2002;269(4):194–7. https://doi.org/10.1002/ar.10143. PMID: 12209557

11. Healing TD, Hoffman PN, Young SE. The infection hazards of human cadavers. Commun Dis Rep CDR Rev. 1995;5(5):R61–8. Erratum in: Commun Dis Rep CDR Rev. 1995;5(6):R92. PMID: 7749455
12. Owolabi JO, Tijani AA, Ihunwo AO. A need to protect the health and rights of anatomists working in dissection laboratories. Risk Manag Healthc Policy. 2022;15:889–93. https://doi.org/10.2147/RMHP.S362305.
13. Patterson JL. Building biosafety laboratories. Science. 2003;300(5622):1092. https://doi.org/10.1126/science.300.5622.1092a. PMID: 12750501
14. Balta JY, Cronin M, Cryan JF, O'Mahony SM. The utility of cadaver-based approaches for the teaching of human anatomy: a survey of British and Irish anatomy teachers. Anat Sci Educ. 2017;10(2):137–43. https://doi.org/10.1002/ase.1629. Epub 2016 Jun 28. PMID: 27352048
15. Jones DG, King MR. Maintaining the anonymity of cadavers in medical education: historic relic or educational and ethical necessity? Anat Sci Educ. 2017;10(1):87–97. https://doi.org/10.1002/ase.1618. Epub 2016 Apr 28. PMID: 27123986
16. Kahn PA, Gardin TM. A student proposal for ethical guidelines in anatomical education: Ethical and policy considerations. Clin Anat. 2016;29(1):60–4. https://doi.org/10.1002/ca.22649. Epub 2015 Nov 19. PMID: 26475436
17. Hildebrandt S. The role of history and ethics of anatomy in medical education. Anat Sci Educ. 2019;12(4):425–31. https://doi.org/10.1002/ase.1852. Epub 2019 Jan 22. PMID: 30580499
18. Goel A, Muzumdar DP, Phalke U. Head holder for microsurgical dissection. J Clin Neurosci. 2004;11(3):300–1. https://doi.org/10.1016/j.jocn.2003.09.009. PMID: 14975422
19. Salma A, Chow A, Ammirati M. Setting up a microneurosurgical skull base lab: technical and operational considerations. Neurosurg Rev. 2011;34(3):317–26. Discussion 326. https://doi.org/10.1007/s10143-011-0317-6. Epub 2011 May 26. PMID: 21614429
20. Zdilla MJ. Creating a human gross anatomy laboratory: the experience at a primarily undergraduate institution. Anat Sci Educ. 2020;13(5):636–47. https://doi.org/10.1002/ase.1946. Epub 2020 Mar 10. PMID: 31990441
21. Goldman E. Building a low-cost gross anatomy laboratory: a big step for a small university. Anat Sci Educ. 2010;3(4):195–201. https://doi.org/10.1002/ase.160. PMID: 20568286
22. Ahumada-Vizcaino JC, Wuo-Silva R, Hernández MM, Chaddad-Neto F. The art of combining neuroanatomy and microsurgical skills in modern neurosurgery. Front Neurol. 2023;13:1076778.
23. Jiménez LÁC, Salvagni FP, Biondi-Soares LG, et al. Model of Arteriovenous Malformation Created in Human Placenta for Training in Vascular Microneurosurgery. Oper Neurosurg (Hagerstown). 2025;28(3):418-426.

Chapter 3
Types of Training Models and Preparation Strategies

Microsurgery training facilitates the development of skills and abilities in performing surgical techniques with high precision. Microsurgery involves performing surgical procedures on small anatomical structures, such as the blood vessels, nerves, and delicate tissues. Therefore, it requires extensive laboratory time and various training models. Different microsurgical training models can be used in different laboratories.

Therefore, it is important to recognize the diversity of tools available for laboratory training, considering factors such as dynamics, flow, reproducibility, cost, accessibility, similarity with surgery, and anatomy.

3.1 Training Models

Synthetic These models simulate human tissue characteristics: consistency and texture. They are ideal for practicing suturing, tissue manipulation, bypass, and aneurysm clipping.

Animal A wide variety of models can be used for training, including rats, pigs, chickens, rams, and humans. These models provide characteristics that are similar to those of real human tissues and allow the practice of suturing, anastomosis, aneurysm clipping, and membrane dissection. Depending on the animal and the availability of anesthesia, live animals can be used to simulate a situation involving bleeding.

Virtual Reality Simulators Simulators offer interactive and virtual trainings in microsurgery. These models allow the development of surgical techniques using haptic manipulation devices that simulate the sensation of working in the surgical environment.

F. Chaddad-Neto, M. D. S. da Costa, *Microneuroanatomy and Lab*,
https://doi.org/10.1007/978-3-031-91026-5_3

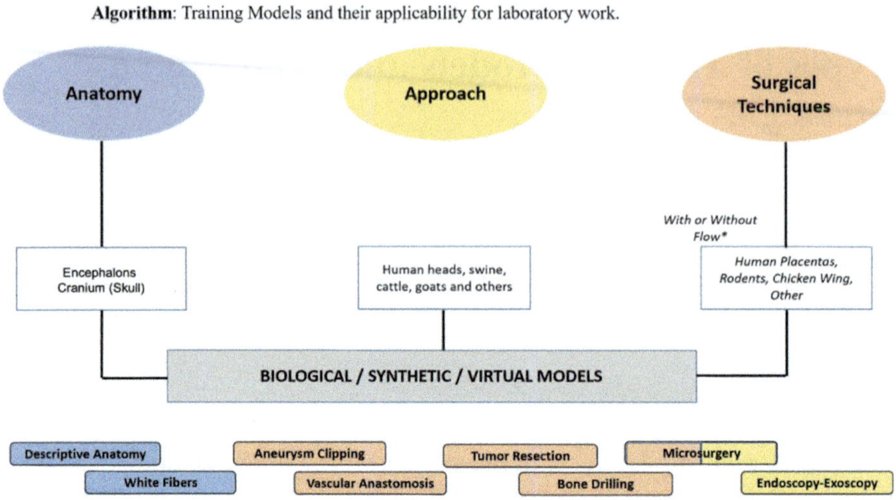

Fig. 3.1 Algorithm—Laboratory training structured based on three dimensions, anatomy, surgical technique, and approach. Various models and conditions are categorized based on their biological or synthetic origin and dynamic properties in relation to flow

Three-Dimensional Printing These models provide accurate and tangible representations of specific anatomical structures. They can be used to practice suturing and dissection techniques in controlled environments, including simulations of blood flow in the blood vessels and bone-drilling procedures.

Each type of model has advantages and limitations. Choosing the right training model involves considering several factors such as applicability in various training phases, achievement of learning objectives, availability of resources, and suitability for specific needs. In addition, combining different types of models can provide a comprehensive and varied training experience (Fig. 3.1).

3.2 Human Placenta

The human placenta serves as an effective biological training model due to its realistic tissue characteristics and anatomical structures. In laboratory settings, it allows for the practice of various techniques such as suturing, dissection simulating arachnoid dissection, aneurysm clipping, tumor resection, and anastomosis.

Limitations: Although the use of human placenta can provide valuable training experience, it has limitations in terms of durability. Thus, proper placental storage and replacement every 7 days are necessary to maintain its effectiveness. Additionally, artificial flow can be induced within the placental vessels using pumps.

Vascular injection of human placenta is performed during microsurgical training in the laboratory. This technique enables the simulation of blood circulation in a structure similar to that of cerebral vessels.

3.3 Fresh, Preserved Human Placenta, Preparation

Contrast agent (e.g., colored latex, dye, or liquid silicone).
With 15–20 ml for veins and 20–25 ml for arteries.
When considering the use of silicone, the dynamic flow is different from that of other dyes.

Syringes of adequate caliber (10–20 ml) "preferably with thread."
Hemostatic forceps and microsurgical scissors.
Cannulas or catheters 3–5 FR for vascular injection.
Saline or formalin solution for irrigation and preservation.

3.3.1 Preparation of the Placenta

The placenta needs to be washed with water and/or saline solution to remove clots and attachments, both on the maternal and fetal sides.

After cutting the umbilical cord on the fetal side to a length of 5–10 cm, the umbilical vein (1) and artery (2) are cannulated with a no. 5 feeding catheter for the vein and a no. 3 or 4 feeding catheter for the arteries. Continuous irrigation is performed until the entire placental vascular tree is adequately cleaned (Fig. 3.2).

Subsequently, the placenta is injected in an organized manner with blue (vein) and red (arteries) dyes. The silicone is diluted to 20–25 ml for arteries and 15–20 ml for veins to ensure proper identification of the model. Vascular injection procedures can be modified depending on the type of training required. Colored silicone can be used to simulate tumor resection, vascular anastomosis, and aneurysm clipping (Figs. 3.2 and 3.3).

One notable advantage of the placenta as a training model is its ability to simulate blood flow, which we performed in the laboratory using flow pumps.

Similarly, to optimize the use of the placental model, we organized the placenta topographically to facilitate the execution of various training modalities, including membrane dissection, aneurysm formation and clipping, vascular anastomosis and their variants, or resection of tumors and other lesions (Fig. 3.4).

In our laboratory, we developed a model of arteriovenous malformation in the human placenta. This model accurately reproduced the three-dimensional (3D) appearance, size, dynamic flow, and application of both arterial and venous flow testing techniques (Fig. 3.5). It serves as an effective tool for training in and applying vascular microsurgical techniques for arteriovenous malformation resection.

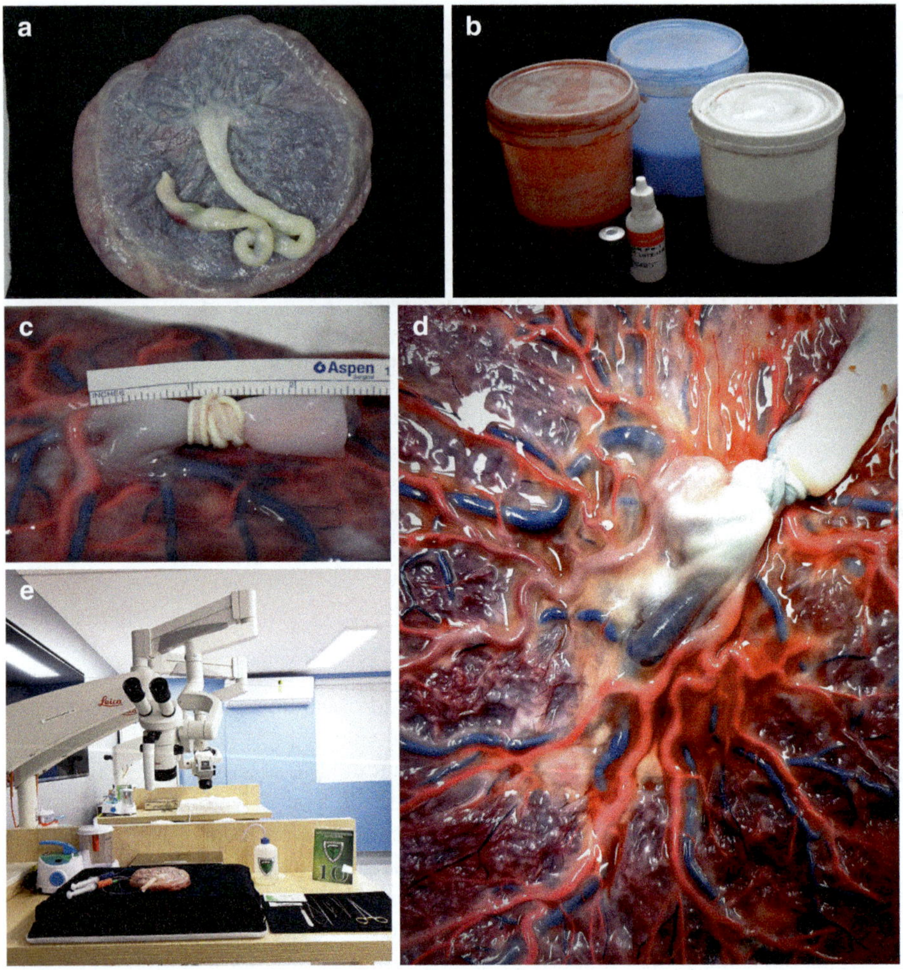

Fig. 3.2 Materials needed for preparing a human placenta for microsurgical training. (**a**): Human placenta after the removal of clots and adherent tissues. Intravascular lavage. (**b**) Dyes and catalysts used for vascular injection. (**c–d**) Human placenta with the umbilical cord cut and occluded. Note the dimensions of the umbilical cord after vascular injection of the placental tree. Peripheral view of the placenta injected with red (arteries) and blue dyes (veins). E: Laboratory training station, including magnification (microscope), microsurgical set, chair, and other conditions simulating those found during actual surgery

The methods of preserving the placenta during its period of use may vary, depending on its purpose. Typically, it is stored in a sealed container with water in a refrigeration system or in a container without water or supplements. The latter method is particularly beneficial when the placenta is utilized for performing tumor resection techniques.

The different training techniques that can be performed on the placenta as a model are listed in Table 3.1.

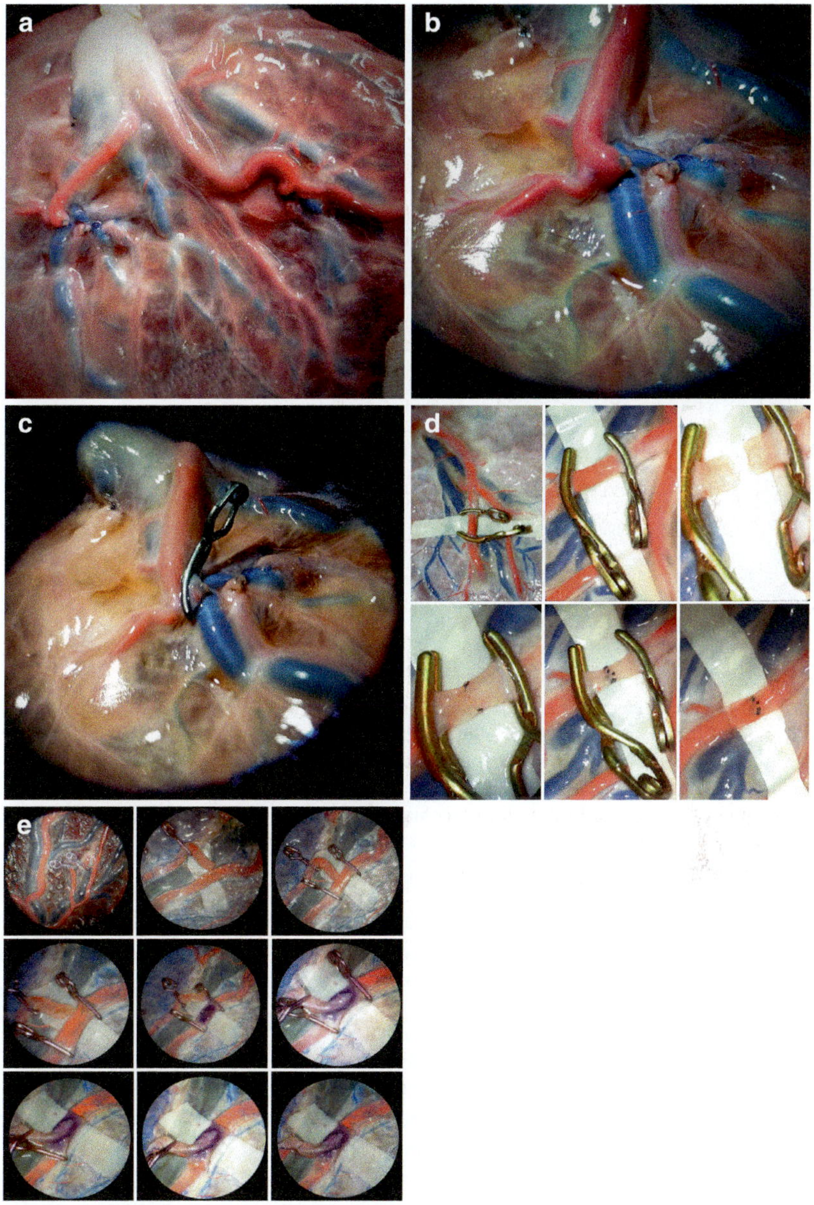

Fig. 3.3 Human placenta as a training model for aneurysm formation, clipping techniques, and bypass. (**a**) Placental model after washing the vascular tree and cutting the umbilical cord; (**b**) peripheral view of the human placenta with aneurysm formation for training; (**c**) saccular aneurysm was formed and occluded with a semi-curved clip. Note the occlusion of the aneurysm. (**d–e**) Step-by-step end-to-end and side-to-side anastomoses (bypass) in the placental model, noting the technical aspects of each anastomosis. Vascular injection is key to the visualization and representation of the arteries. In the laboratory, we were able to maintain a continuous flow within the placental model during training

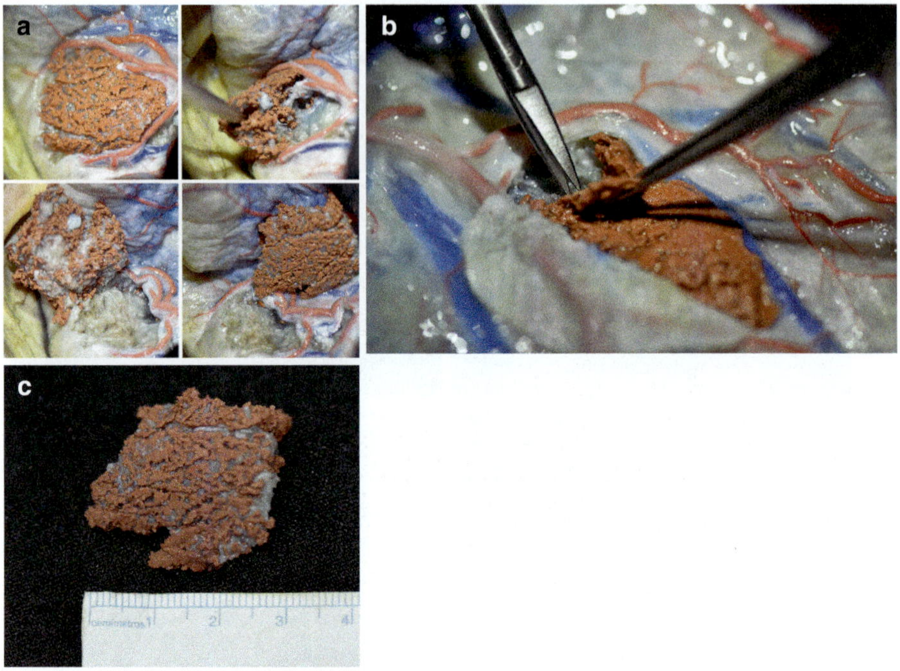

Fig. 3.4 (a–c) Placental preparation for the reproduction of microsurgical techniques applied to the resection of tumor lesions created with synthetic material. Note the arterial (red) and venous (blue) vascular injection. During microsurgical training for the resection of tumor lesions, vessel skeletonization and fragmented or en bloc resection of the tumors were performed, due to the invasive nature of tumors infiltrating the placental stroma

3.3.2 Human Brain

The human encephalon serves as an exceptional biological model for studying the descriptive and microsurgical anatomy of the sulci, gyri, and ventricles to landmark points; vascular anatomy; and white fiber dissection (Figs. 3.6 and 3.7).

However, to utilize it effectively as a model in the laboratory, certain conditions must be met to ensure proper maintenance and preservation of the specimen.

The initial step is the careful extraction of the encephalon from the cranial cavity, followed by the removal of the hematic content and/or surface clots.

The brain is suspended in a vessel containing 70% formalin for 3–4 weeks. Both carotid arteries are cannulated with a feeding catheter (6–8 FR), and a physiological solution alternating with intravascular formalin is exhaustively injected under controlled pressure or by an infusion pump for intra-arterial elimination and removal of the clot. This procedure is performed twice a day with an injection volume ranging from 2 to 3 liters for the first 3 days, followed by daily intravascular flushing until the end of the week (Fig. 3.6).

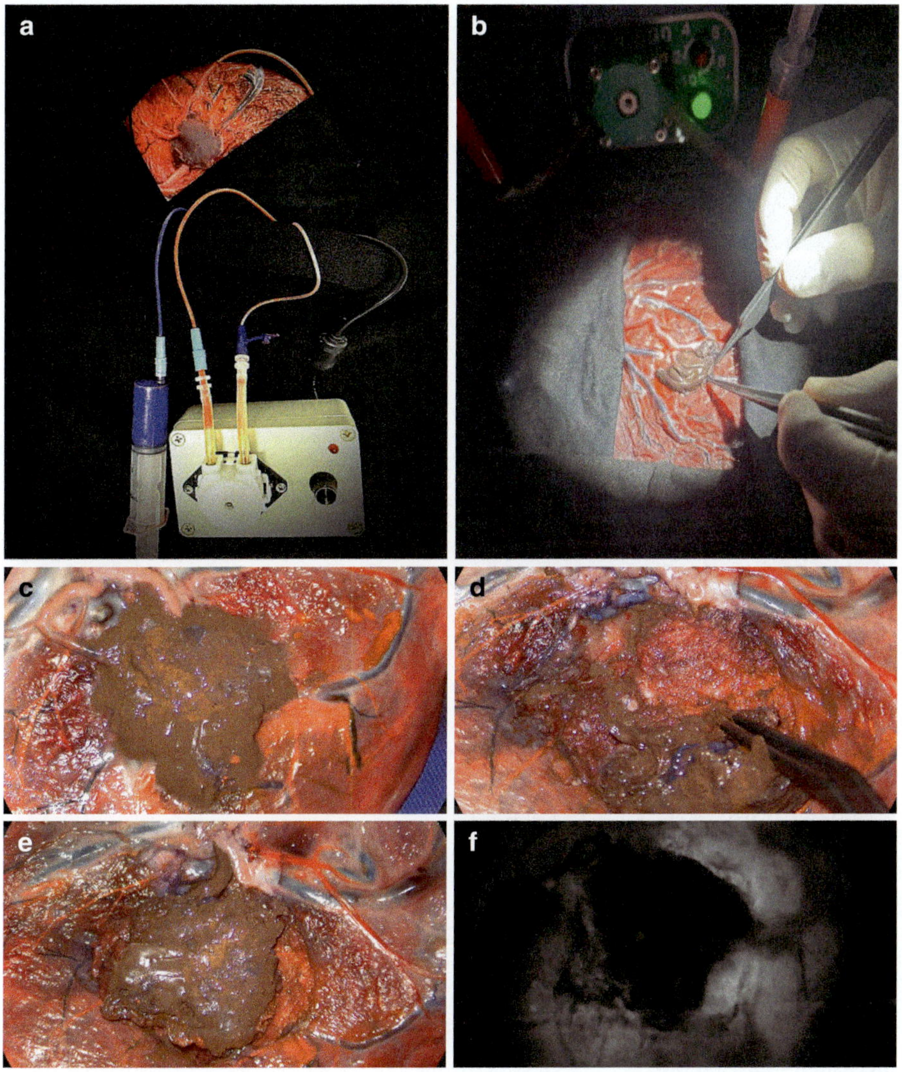

Fig. 3.5 Microsurgical training for the resection of an arteriovenous malformation (model) in human placenta. (**a**) Arteriovenous malformation model created using synthetic materials. Note the connection between the pumping system and the dynamic flow. (**b**) Execution of technical maneuvers during training. (**c**) Initial appearance of the synthetic nidus with evidence of feeding arteries shown in red and draining veins shown in blue. (**d–e**) Deep dissection of the nidus with bipolar and final appearance after circumferential dissection of the model. (**f–i**) Flow verification using indocyanine green (ICG) injection. Note details, such as the execution of temporary clipping and final resection of the nidus. (**j**) Final aspect of the placental bed where the AVM nidus was resected. (**k**) Nidus resected en bloc

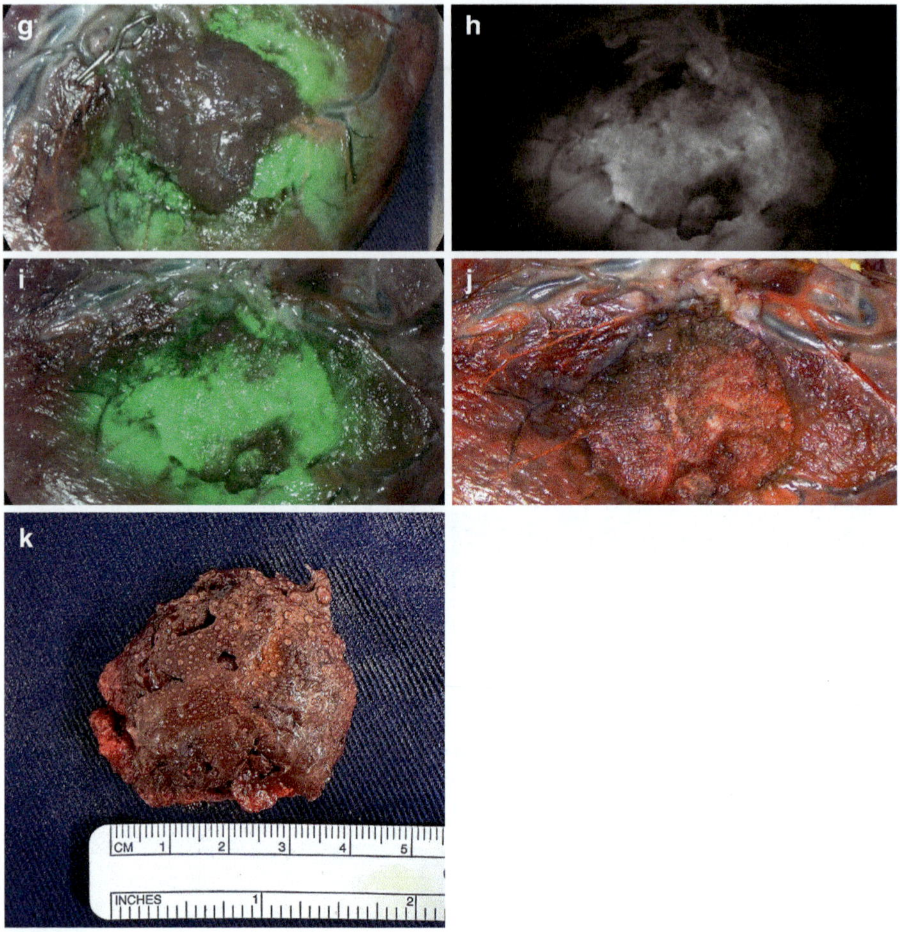

Fig. 3.5 (continued)

Once the brain fixation process for training purposes is completed, other steps are usually carried out.

The initial step involves the meticulous "cleaning" procedure, which entails the removal and dissection of the arachnoid membranes. Although seemingly simple, this step is integral to laboratory training. Under a microscope, the arachnoid membranes are delicately removed using a microscissor and tweezers, marking the beginning of acquiring microsurgical skills. Mastery in microsurgery is a gradual process that demands extensive dedication and practice. The removal of arachnoid membranes with the same caution and care as in real surgical scenarios is crucial for skill advancement.

For anatomical studies of the cerebral sulci, gyri, and ventricles, preserving cleaned specimens in absolute alcohol (70%) suffices (Fig. 3.6). Prior to brain dissection, thorough examination of the surface sulci and gyri and recognizing all

Table 3.1 Comparison of the most common models used in the laboratory, according to their preparation, usefulness, technique, purpose, and flow reproduction

Type	Preparation	Objective	Flow reproduction
Human placenta, chicken wing, and rodents	Capture, washing, and vascular injection with dyes Preservation and durability average: 7–14 days = rodents as models have a usefulness of hours (which vary according to the training objective)	Microsurgical and vascular techniques Membrane dissection, aneurysm clipping, anastomosis or bypass (and its variants), tumor resection, vessel skeletonization, and creation and microsurgical resection of arteriovenous malformations and others	Useful model to reproduce continuous flow during training
Human specimen and encephalon	Collection, washing, injection with resin-silicone, and fixation in alcohol-formaldehyde The reproduction of techniques can be carried out after the injection and completion of the fixation process Average durability and usefulness of the preparation 6 months to 2 years *brains for white fiber dissection techniques must additionally undergo a continuous freezing process averaging 3–4 weeks	Microsurgical techniques, approaches, study of microsurgical anatomy, endoscopic techniques, topographical anatomy, white fibers, and vascular anatomy	Models with poor applicability for continuous flow reproduction during training
Other models may comply with some of the features mentioned during the description but have considerable limitations in order to reproduce most of the features required for training as close as possible to the conditions found in real surgery			

Comparison of the most common models used in the laboratory for training. The process of assessing the preparation aspects, average utility time, objectives, and flow exposure is similar to that of surgery

possible anatomical aspects of the specimen are imperative. Extracting all possible information from the specimen before proceeding with further steps is emphasized.

In our laboratory, the internal encephalic anatomy is examined through a systematic and organized dissection of cuts, following the anatomical points and sections.

The dissection begins by making an axial longitudinal cut at the level of the inferior frontal sulcus (supramarginal gyrus), which exposes the ventricular system as

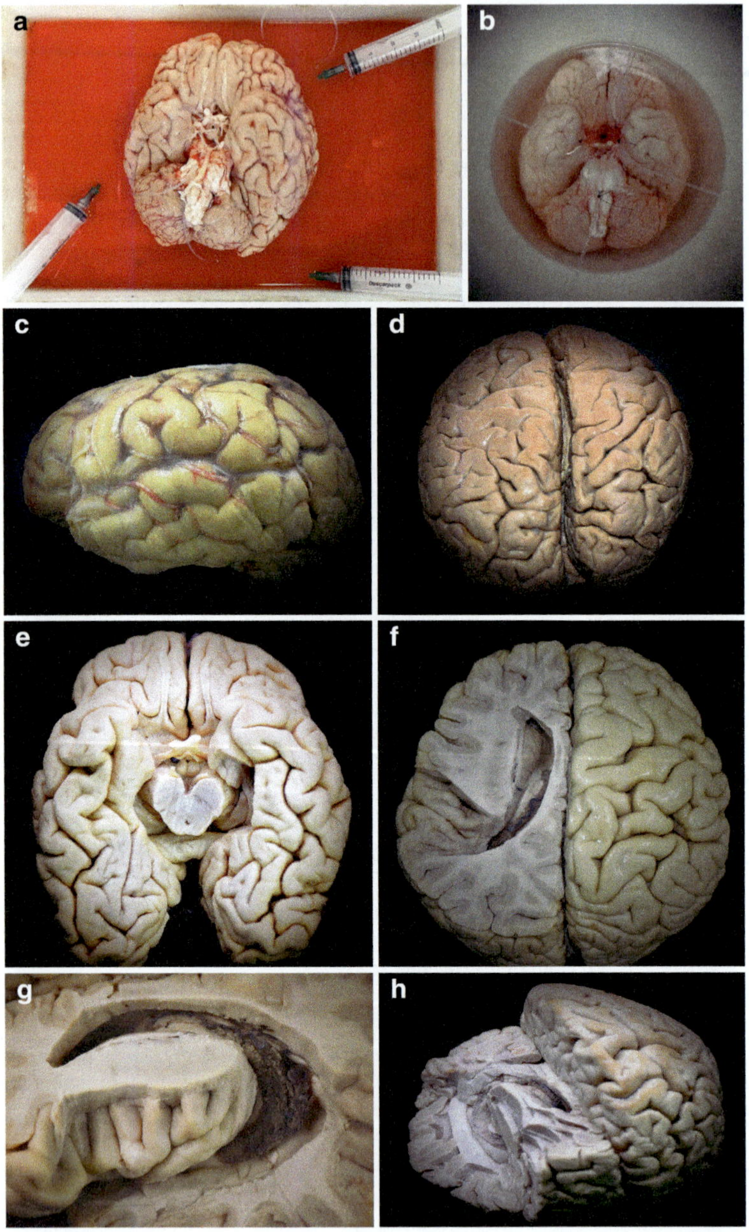

Fig. 3.6 Encephalon for the study of sulci, gyri, and ventricles anatomy. (**a**) Brain preparation after the cranial vault removal. Note the placement of the catheters in the carotid and vertebrobasilar circuits. Intravascular lavage for clot and debris removal (**b**) formalin-fixed brains. Suspension and buoyancy are important for avoiding tissue damage or deformation. (**c**) Lateral view of the brain showing the arachnoid membrane and vascular structures. (**d–e**) Top view and basal side of the brain after membrane removal and fixation. This begins with the study of the external configuration, grooves, turns, and repair points related to deep structures. (**f–h**) Superior, lateral, and anterolateral views of a brain preparation showing exposure of the ventricular system to contiguous structures

the inferior frontal sulcus aligns with the surface projection of the corpus callosum. This incision allows for the identification of the frontal horn and body of the lateral ventricle, as the body of the corpus callosum forms the roof of this part of the lateral ventricle. Subsequently, a cut is made from the supramarginal gyrus toward the ventricular atrium, as the supramarginal gyrus corresponds to the surface projection of the atrium of the lateral ventricle. Additionally, a longitudinal dissection of the temporal lobe is made at the level of the middle temporal gyrus (T2) to expose the temporal horn, followed by a sagittal section at the level of the central core (insula).

If the objective is to examine the white fibers, the brain undergoes cryopreservation using the Klingler method. This involves preserving the brain in a container with water, preferably at a temperature of 0 °C to 4 °C for 21 days.

During this process, the water molecules (under established thermal conditions) expand, facilitating easier dissection of the brain. This method, known as "Cryodissection," is simple yet highly effective (Fig. 3.7).

Subsequently, the water crystals are removed by melting at room temperature, and the gray matter is removed as previously described.

Although the traditional method involves freezing the brain without preservation media or vehicles, we used it with or without liquid media (water) in a protective container. This ensured the nondeformation of the encephalon without substantial changes to the final cryodissection objective.

Table 3.1 outlines the characteristic steps in the technical preparation of the brain according to the purpose of the study.

3.3.3 3D Printing

The 3D printing training models aim to simulate anatomical details and simulate certain lesions or vascular and/or tumor conditions. Although these models may lack the consistency and/or texture of real tissues, they allow technical maneuvers to be executed repeatedly in the same model.

These models can accurately replicate the human anatomy, aiding in the spatial understanding and identification of relevant structures and landmarks.

Using 3D printed models can reduce the costs associated with the consumption of medical supplies and surgical equipment. In addition, they are reusable, allowing repeated training without incurring additional costs. These types of models do not pose significant biological risks, do not require special storage conditions, but cannot simulate anatomical variables of soft tissues.

Some of the conditions or lesions that 3D printing models can reproduce include aneurysms and their variants (saccular, fusiform, and multiple), tumors of the cranial base, vascular anastomosis, drilled bone, membrane dissection, and others (Fig. 3.8).

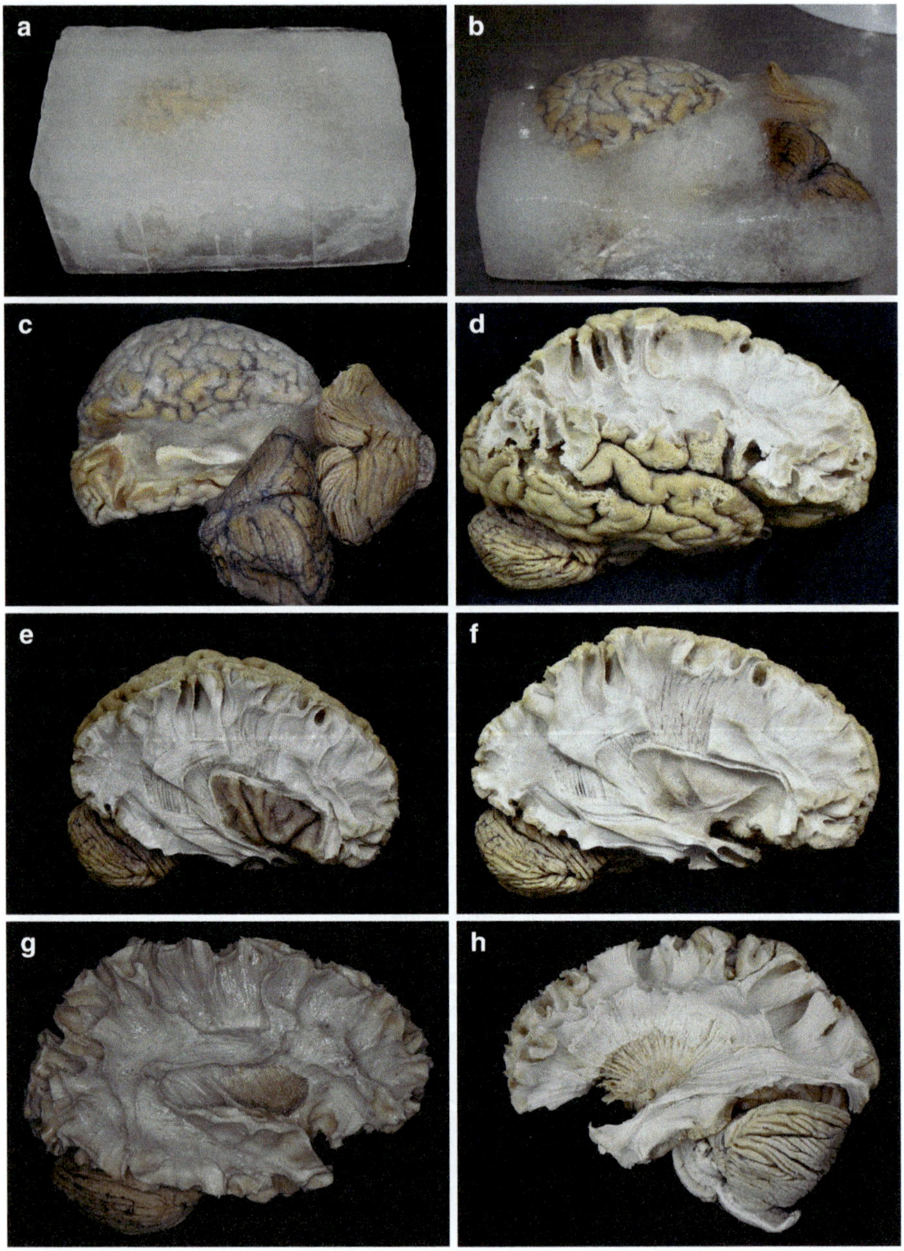

Fig. 3.7 Cryodissection process/Klingler method. (**a–b**) Encephalic preparation subjected to freezing for 4 weeks; note the appearance of the tissue immersed in ice. (**c**) Thawing at room temperature. (**d–h**) Dissection of white fibers in their initial aspect for subsequent exposure of the central nucleus, superior longitudinal fasciculus, and arcuate before removal of the cortex, and U-shaped fibers of the frontal, parietal, and temporal lobes in the lateral aspect. This technique allows for optimal exposure of the white encephalic fibers and anatomical relationships. Organized dissection, starting from the cortex to the depth

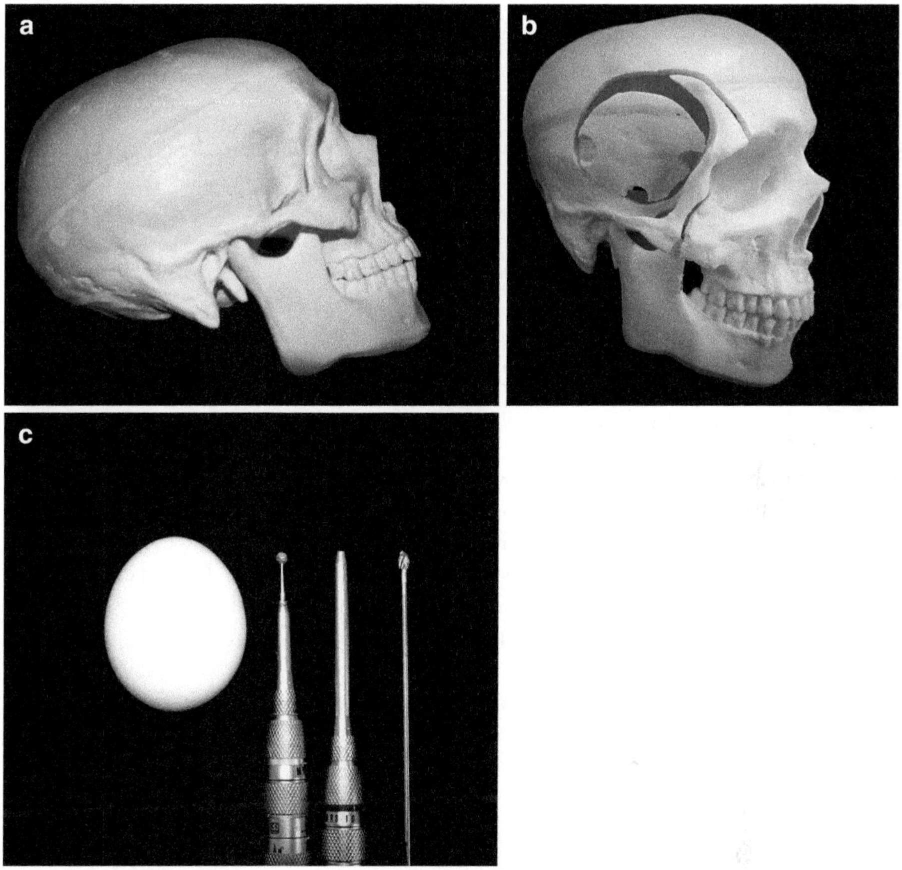

Fig. 3.8 Three-dimensional printing models and others. (**a–b**) Three-dimensional-printed skull with synthetic material with a 1:1 dimension (real size). Note the repair points that can be used and their applicability to craniotomies. (**c**) Egg as training model for fine drilling. Owing to the thinness of the cortex, it has become a very useful model for reducing tremors and improving maneuverability during surgery

3.3.4 Chicken Egg and Wing

Under conditions where access to more advanced biological or synthetic models is limited, simpler models with low or medium structures are highly useful for domestic or laboratory training. Chicken wings are a microsurgical training model with great utility and applicability. The characteristics of its tissue, accessibility, low biological risk, and minimum cost, make them particularly suitable for practicing surgical skills and abilities.

Table 3.2 Comparison of different methods of microsurgery training performed in the laboratory

Type	Biologic	Synthetic	Ethical aspects	Cost
Human placenta	X		Low	Low
Encephalon	X		High	Low
3D printing		X	Without limitations	High
Chicken wing	X		Without limitations	Low
Pig's and/or mutton's head	X		Medium	Medium
Rodents	X		Low	Low
Virtual reality		X	Without limitations	High

Aspects of various models used in the laboratory for training. Assessment of their biological or synthetic origin, the ethical factors that may or may not limit their acquisition, and the comparative costs between them

It is useful for training in various techniques:

Dissection and suturing: Chicken wings can be used to perform dissection and suturing techniques. The process involves identifying and dissecting different tissues, muscles, tendons, vascular structures, and nerves.

Vascular anastomosis: The consistency of chicken wing tissue, the presence of various structures in the vascular plane, and the diameter of the blood vessels, which are relevant and very useful features, make them suitable for practicing vascular anastomosis techniques.

Assessment of dexterity and precision: Chicken wings provide a platform for assessing the dexterity, precision, and the use of magnification, which are essential for the applicability of microsurgical maneuvers.

Although this type of model presents a few limitations in terms of access, low biological risk, and/or ethical considerations, it may not accurately simulate more complex microsurgical maneuvers (Table 3.2).

The chicken egg serves as an easily accessible model with suitable characteristics for training fine and shallow drilling maneuvers. Because of the diameter of the rind, the chicken egg is an ideal model for initial training and mastering drilling techniques (Fig. 3.8).

Various drills, including grooved and diamond drills of various thicknesses (6 mm, 3 mm, 1.4 mm, and others) can be used for this purpose. In addition, linear, circumferential, and diagonal drills can be used for comprehensive training.

3.3.5 Rodents

Rodents, such as rats and mice, share similar anatomical and physiological characteristics with human tissues. This makes them suitable models for practicing microsurgical techniques. Their size requires the precise handling of surgical instruments, providing good training for performing microsurgical maneuvers.

Rodents are readily available as training models at a relatively low cost. This makes them an affordable option compared with other larger or more specialized animal models.

Various measures, such as size; the administration of various anesthetic agents; and analgesia techniques can ensure animal welfare and ethics during surgical procedures or training (Fig. 3.9).

Vascular anastomosis is one of the primary techniques performed during training in rodents, which is considered an excellent model owing to certain characteristics such as tissue consistency, blood flow, and vessel caliber that simulate real surgery.

Figure 3.9 demonstrates the step-by-step preparation of the training model and execution of the vascular anastomosis technique.

3.3.6 Human Specimen

Using human heads as models for microsurgery training offer significant advantages due to their anatomical realism. Human anatomy is complex and unique, and practicing on the human head can provide a more accurate representation of the anatomy and tissue structure that can be used in clinical practice, particularly in cranial approaches.

However, the use of human heads for training has significant legal and ethical limitations. Therefore, access to human heads for microsurgery training is limited and heavily relies on the availability of donated bodies.

Here, we describe the steps for preparing the model for training.

Following the ethical and legal guidelines, we identified the cervical level of the C6 segment and the cervical carotid-jugular vascular bundle.

The ideal time for preparing a cadaver as a model is within 48 h postmortem; however, we considered a maximum limit of 7 days postmortem, considering the cause of death and the quality of the soft and encephalic tissues.

Complete cervical transverse dissection is performed with subsequent bilateral cannulation of six important vessels, including the common carotid artery, internal jugular vein, and vertebral artery. Using feeding catheters tailored to the caliber of each vessel, the head is fixed to the end of the blood vessel with suture threads.

First, the specimen is washed with water or an intravascular physiological solution, either manually or preferably by continuous infusion. Lavage is initiated on one side while keeping the contralateral side open for content and hematological material exit. The washing volume is estimated to be 3–4 liters for the initial lavage, ensuring thorough removal of clots to achieve cleaner vessels and more vibrant colors in the final model. The quality of the specimens varied depending on the preparation steps and the condition of the donor.

The specimen is placed in a container with 70% formalin for 3 weeks, with repeated interdaily washings of the cannulated vascular tree during the first 7 days (two to three times a day).

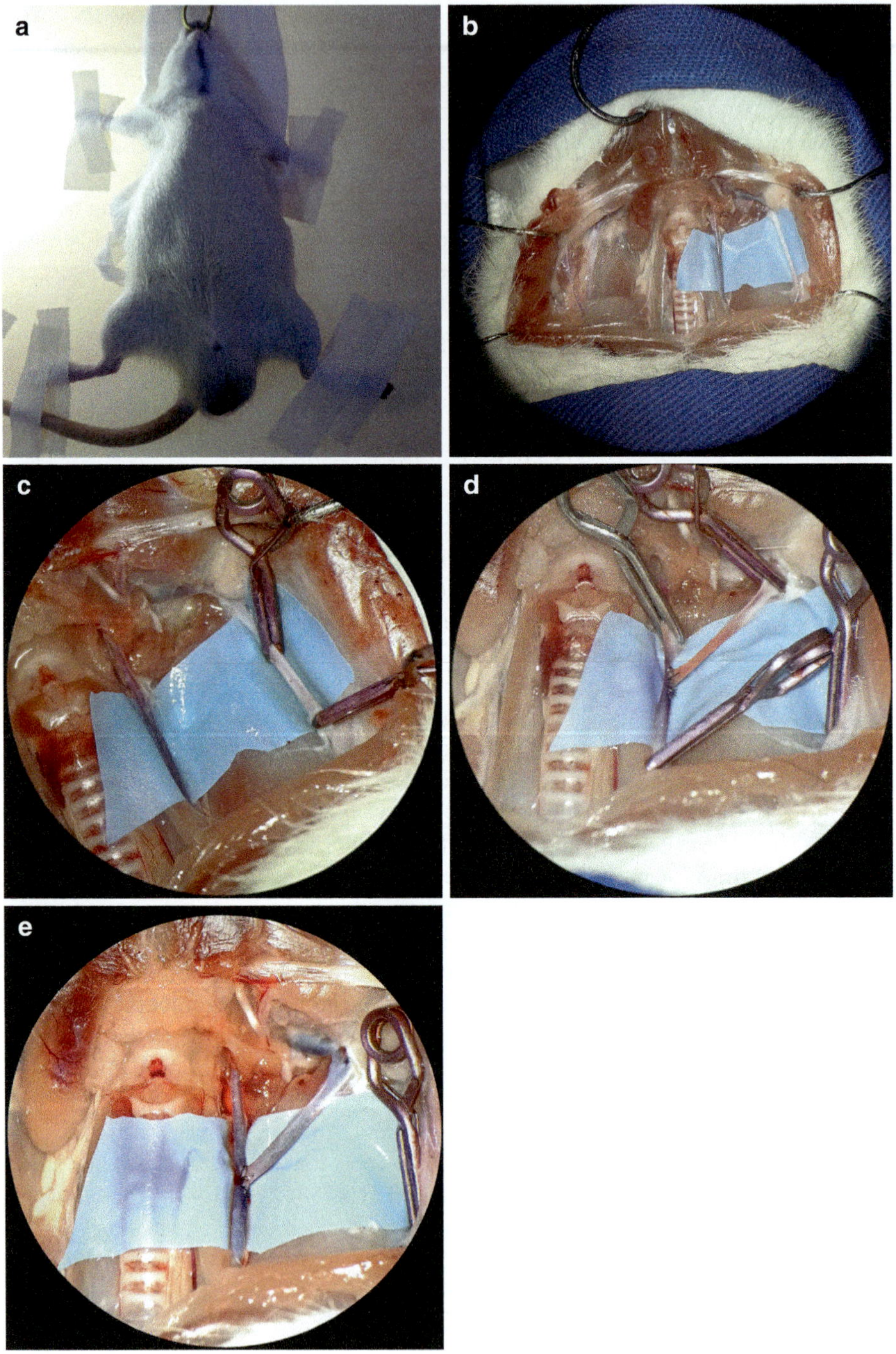

Fig. 3.9 Rodents as training models for vascular microsurgery. (**a**) Positioning and fixation of previously anesthetized rodents at the training station. Fixation at strategic and secure points allows for thoracocervical midline dissection, as shown in (**b**). Additionally, the retraction sites were visualized using surgical hooks. (**c–d**) Dissection, exposure, and temporary clipping of the vessels for the reproduction of the end-to-end and end-to-side vascular anastomoses (bypass). (**e**) Final view of an end-to-side anastomosis

Once the 7-day period had elapsed, vascular injection is performed using colored silicone, with blue silicone indicating veins and red silicone indicating arteries (other materials such as liquid latex or polyester resin can also be used for injection). Table 3.1 lists the detailed steps and materials used in vascular injection.

The average volumes of materials injected intravascularly are 90–100 ml for arteries and 60–80 for veins. The material is injected in the right common carotid artery, thus occluding all other ipsilateral and contralateral arteries. This maneuver is repeated for each cannulated arterial and venous vessel. The injection sequence typically progresses from the anterior or carotid circuit, then to the vertebrobasilar circuit, and finally to the venous system.

During vascular injection, the outflow of the injected material through very small vessels may be observed, indicating vessel occlusion and ensuring adequate injection.

Once the fixation period is complete, the specimen is ready for the execution of different techniques, making it highly advantageous, similar, and applicable to existing training models for anatomy, approaches, and surgical techniques (Fig. 3.10).

3.3.7 *Other Animal Models: Goats, Swine, and Bovines*

Accessing human biological models for training is often restricted by ethical and/or legal regulations in various countries. As a result, animal models become valuable alternatives due to their resemblance to human tissues, such as blood vessels, connective tissue, muscles, bones, and cavity configuration.

Therefore, access to animal specimens such as pigs, goats, and cattle has been deemed highly beneficial. Despite the potential variations in the anatomical configuration compared with humans, these models are instrumental in training fundamental microsurgery concepts, surgical techniques, and even endoscopic approaches.

Table 3.2 outlines the characteristics and advantages of these models compared with other alternatives, along with the key points for preparing and conditioning the model for laboratory training, including the execution of approaches, encephalic dissection, and bone drilling.

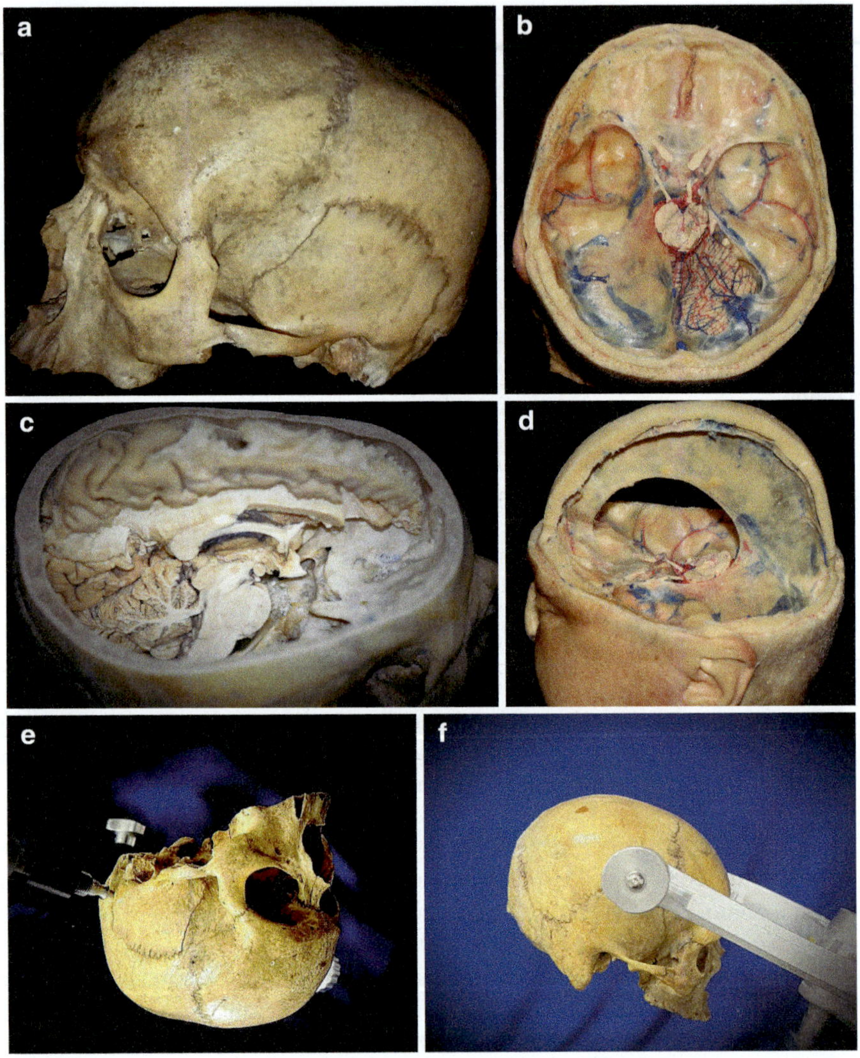

Fig. 3.10 Human skulls and encephalons/biological models for training of surgical techniques and approaches. (**a**) Specimens useful for studying the anatomy, craniometric points, cranial configuration, and references. (**b**) Preparation for studying the skull base anatomy. (**c–d**) Relationship of the brain in the sagittal section with the skull base; a useful tool for planning surgical approaches for the treatment of intracranial lesions. (**e–f**) Procedures requiring fixation with a three-pin head holder: Examples include the posterior cranial fossa and pterional approaches. This is a key tool for consolidating knowledge on the positioning of the patient's head according to the pathology to be treated. (**g**) Position and marking for execution of the right pterional approach in human preparation. (**h–i**) Human preparation during anatomical dissection. Note the relationships between the vascular, bony, cerebral, and neural structures in the lateral and posterior views. (**j–k**) View of a Sylvian fissure (lateral-superficial portion) with evidence of vascular structures, in the right middle cerebral artery and its branches. Additionally, a posterior view of the structures of the posterior cranial fossa, brain stem, vertebral artery, and lower cranial nerves X and XI. Such insights are particularly valuable for complex approaches in regions such as the far lateral approach

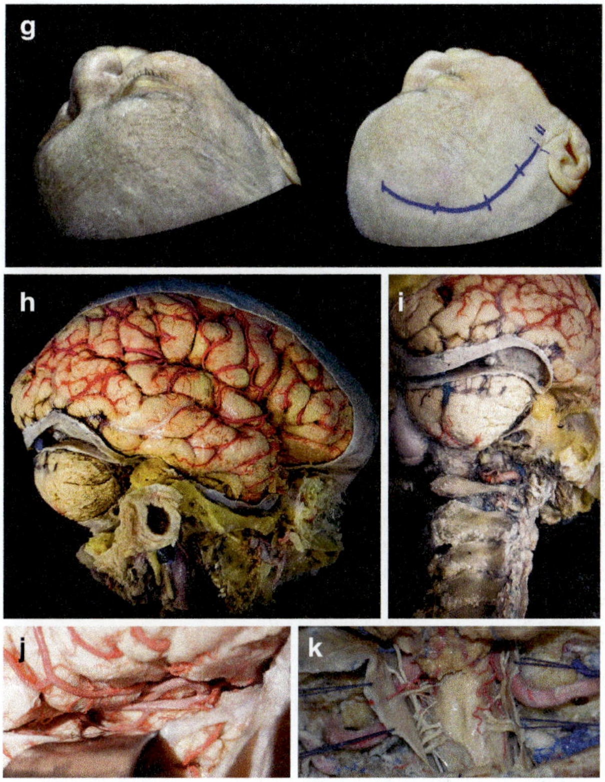

Fig. 3.10 (continued)

Bibliography

1. Goldstein M. Use of fresh human placenta for microsurgical training. J Microsurg. 1979;1(1):70–1.
2. Romero FR, Fernandes ST, Chaddad-Neto F, Ramos JG, Campos JM, Oliveira E. Microsurgical techniques using human placenta. Arq Neuropsiquiatr. 2008;66(4):876–8.
3. Apaza RA, Canache LA, Salvagni F, Biondi LG, Tenelema ED, Vilcahuamán AF, Wuo R, Chaddad-Neto F. Topographical systematization of human placenta model for training in microneurosurgery. World Neurosurg. 2023.
4. Biondi LG, Holanda VM, Veloso G, Biondi AG, Monteiro M, Ahumada JC, Salvagni F, Oliveira ML, Canache LA, Reghin M, Chaddad-Neto F. The technique for transorbital ventricular puncture: an anatomic approach. Oper Neurosurg 2023.
5. Gurses ME, Gungor A, Gökalp E, Hanalioglu S, Karatas Okumus SY, Tatar I, Berker M, Cohen-Gadol AA, Ture U. Three-dimensional modelling and augmented and virtual reality simulations of the white matter anatomy of the cerebrum. Oper Neurosurg (Hagerstown). 2022;23(5):355–66.
6. Oliveira MMR, Ferrarez CE, Ramos TM, et al. Learning brain aneurysm microsurgical skills in a human placenta model: predictive validity. J Neurosurg. 2018;128(3):846–52.

7. Cikla U, Sahin B, Hanalioglu S, Ahmed AS, Niemann D, Baskaya MK. A novel, low-cost, reusable, high-fidelity neurosurgical training simulator for cerebrovascular bypass surgery. J Neurosurg. 2018;11:1–9.
8. Shurey S, Akelina Y, Legagneux J, Malzone G, Jiga L, Ghanem AM. The rat model in microsurgery education: classical exercises and new horizons. Arch Plast Surg. 2014;41(3):201–8.
9. Gélinas-Phaneuf N, Choudhury N, Al-Habib AR, et al. Assessing performance in brain tumor resection using a novel virtual reality simulator. Int J Comput Assist Radiol Sur. 2014;9(1):1–9.
10. Sanan A, Abdel Aziz KM, Janjua RM, van Loveren HR, Keller JT. Colored silicone injection for use in neurosurgical dissections: anatomic technical note. Neurosurgery. 1999;45(5):1267–71.
11. Ahumada-Vizcaino JC, Wuo-Silva R, Hernández MM, Chaddad-Neto F. The art of combining neuroanatomy and microsurgical skills in modern neurosurgery. Front Neurol. 2023;13:1076778.
12. Goiri MA, de Amorim BL, Sarti TM, da Costa MD, Chaddad-Neto F. Building a microneurosurgical laboratory in Latin America: challenges and possibilities. Surg Neurol Int. 2021;12:573.
13. Altunrende ME, Hamamcioglu MK, Hıcdonmez T, Akcakaya MO, Bırgılı B, Cobanoglu S. Microsurgical training model for residents to approach to the orbit and the optic nerve in fresh cadaveric sheep cranium. J Neurosci Rural Pract. 2014;5(2):151–4.
14. Hicdonmez T, Hamamcioglu MK, Tiryaki M, Cukur Z, Cobanoglu S. Microneurosurgical training model in fresh cadaveric cow brain: a laboratory study simulating the approach to the circle of Willis. Surg Neurol. 2006;66(1):100–4.
15. Pojskić M, Čustović O, Erwin KH, Dunn IF, Eisenberg M, Gienapp AJ, Arnautović KI. Microscopic and endoscopic skull base approaches hands-on cadaver course at 30: historical vignette. World Neurosurg. 2020;142:434–40.
16. Alvernia JE, Pradilla G, Mertens P, Lanzino G, Tamargo RJ. Latex injection of cadaver heads: technical note. Neurosurgery. 2010;67(2 Suppl Operative):362–7.
17. Lee WJ, Kim YH, Hong SD, Rho TH, Kim YH, Dho YS, Hong CK, Kong DS. Development of 3-dimensional printed simulation surgical training models for endoscopic. Endonasal and transorbital surgery. Front Oncologia. 2022;12:966051.
18. Olabe J, Olabe J, Sancho V. Human cadaver brain infusion model for neurosurgical training. Surg Neurol. 2009;72(6):700–2.
19. Gurses ME, Gungor A, Rahmanov S, Gökalp E, Hanalioglu S, Berker M, Cohen-Gadol AA, Türe U. Three-dimensional modeling and augmented reality and virtual reality simulation of fiber dissection of the cerebellum and brainstem. Oper Neurosurg (Hagerstown). 2022;23(5):345–54.
20. Uhl JF, Sufianov A, Ruiz C, Iakimov Y, Mogorron HJ, Encarnacion Ramirez M, Prat G, Lorea B, Baldoncini M, Goncharov E, Ramirez I, Céspedes JRC, Nurmukhametov R, Montemurro N. The use of 3D printed models for surgical simulation of Cranioplasty in Craniosynostosis as training and education. Brain Sci. 2023;13(6):894.
21. Jiménez LÁC, Salvagni FP, Biondi-Soares LG, et al. Model of Arteriovenous Malformation Created in Human Placenta for Training in Vascular Microneurosurgery. Oper Neurosurg (Hagerstown). 2025;28(3):418-426.

Chapter 4
Laboratory Documentation: Photographs and Videos

Neurosurgery has evolved exponentially in recent years. The hard work, publications, and accumulated experience from various reference centers have enriched this field, emphasizing the use of relevant tools in the documentation process. The ability to investigate, together with the effort to graphically capture these works, has been a fundamental part of the process. To date, photo-video graphic support is one of the primary factors that garners significant attention and provides valuable information to individuals seeking knowledge through an experience that has already been presented.

The authors also acknowledge the importance of written and graphic documentation, which enables the capture, reproduction, and transmission of knowledge acquired during anatomical and technical training sessions in the laboratory. It is paramount to meticulously capture each of the photographs and videos of the dissections and microsurgical techniques performed during surgery in a neat, didactic, and artistic manner (Fig. 4.1).

In this chapter, we present a simple and precise guide outlining each of the necessary steps to obtain photographs and/or videos of the dissections conducted in the laboratory. Our objective is to facilitate training and refine our techniques and skills. To achieve this, various tools facilitate the acquisition of high-quality two-dimensional (2D) and three-dimensional (3D) photographs, as well as representative videos of various microsurgical procedures.

Before proceeding with the reproduction or capture of photographic materials, it is imperative to ensure three aspects, which will be elaborated in the following sections.

Considering these factors ensures the acquisition of excellent photographic materials, encompassing aspects related to the means of capture (camera and accessories), environment or place of capture (photographic station or video), and the physical characteristics of the specimen or preparation to be showcased (Fig. 4.2).

F. Chaddad-Neto, M. D. S. da Costa, *Microneuroanatomy and Lab*,
https://doi.org/10.1007/978-3-031-91026-5_4

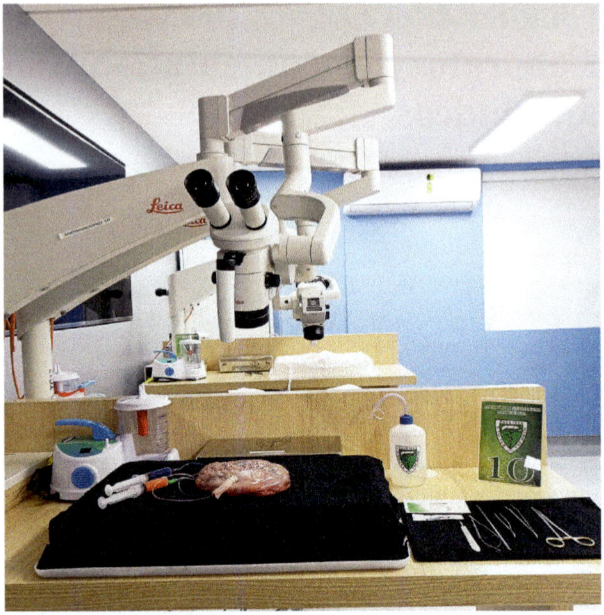

Fig. 4.1 Dissection station in the laboratory, where the preparations or models to be documented are conditioned and where the various technical maneuvers are executed and trained

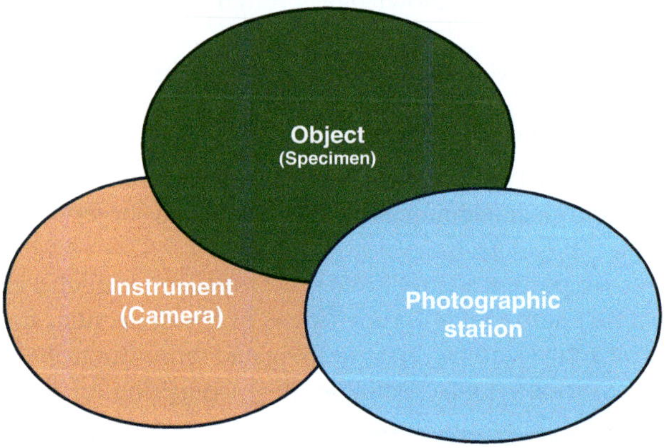

Fig. 4.2 The three factors necessary for the realization of a photograph or video are object (anatomical preparation, training model, dissection material, others); instrument (camera, accessories, magnifying lenses, stand, light ring); photographic station (microenvironment for positioning the lens, with adequate background, lighting, focus, sharpness, and shadow reduction)

In graphic documentation, meticulous cleaning and/or removal of residues, tissues, artifacts, and other contaminants from the specimen are essential, because these distort the intended objective and compromise the aesthetic appeal of images.

Otherwise, sequential capture serves as an invaluable tool. During the dissection process, focusing solely on the dissection itself rather than on photographic capture may lead to overlooking valuable details essential for knowledge acquisition and dissemination.

4.1 Camera and Accessories

We consider a professional camera in the laboratory as a valuable tool. The utility of the professional camera is augmented by its integration with a tripod support, enabling the capture of photographs from various angles, heights, and peripheral areas, and facilitating precise millimetric adjustments. This setup enables the achievement of the highest quality standards in terms of focus, sharpness, and lighting.

A three-point support facilitates precise maneuverability to capture photographs from desired angles, favors a constant distance between the lens and the capture point, and offers versatility for adapting the millimetric ruler in 3D photos, video playback, and other applications (Fig. 4.3).

It is essential to consistently ensure placement on a flat and level surface, maintaining an adequate distance relative to the objective, and in a position that allows unobstructed access to the object to be photographed.

The place of capture should be meticulously prepared to optimize lighting, focus, sharpness, color rendition, and accentuation of key regions, among other factors. We utilize backgrounds with black or blue fabric to direct attention to the target and avoid unwanted light reflections (Fig. 4.4). At times, we moisten the background fabric and the object with water to enhance contrast and to emphasize our focal point in the preparation. The use of water can be particularly advantageous for 2D photography. However, in 3D photography, where image duplication occurs, the indiscriminate use of water on the object may alter the desired 3D appearance.

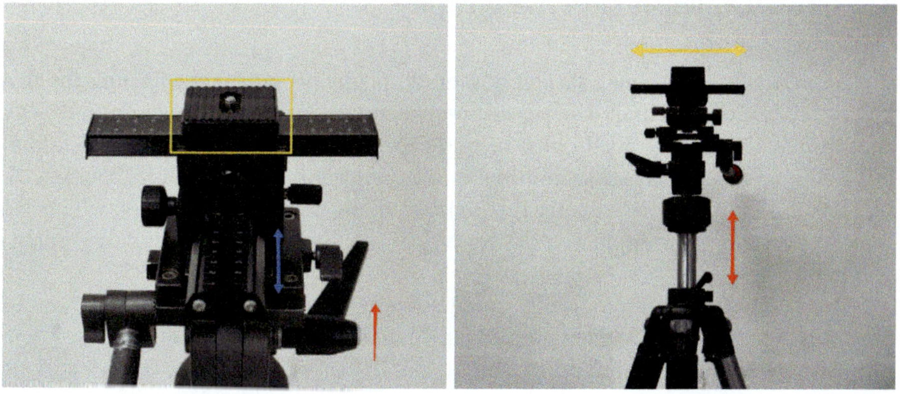

Fig. 4.3 Direction axes of the millimeter ruler. We show the arrangement of the camera attachment point to the millimeter ruler (yellow box) always centered on the horizontal axis, as indicated by the yellow arrows in a level view. On the anteroposterior axis, as shown by the blue arrows, it allows us to move the lens closer to or further away from the objective. Finally, the red arrows indicate the height of the support head in relation to the objective on the lower-upper axis

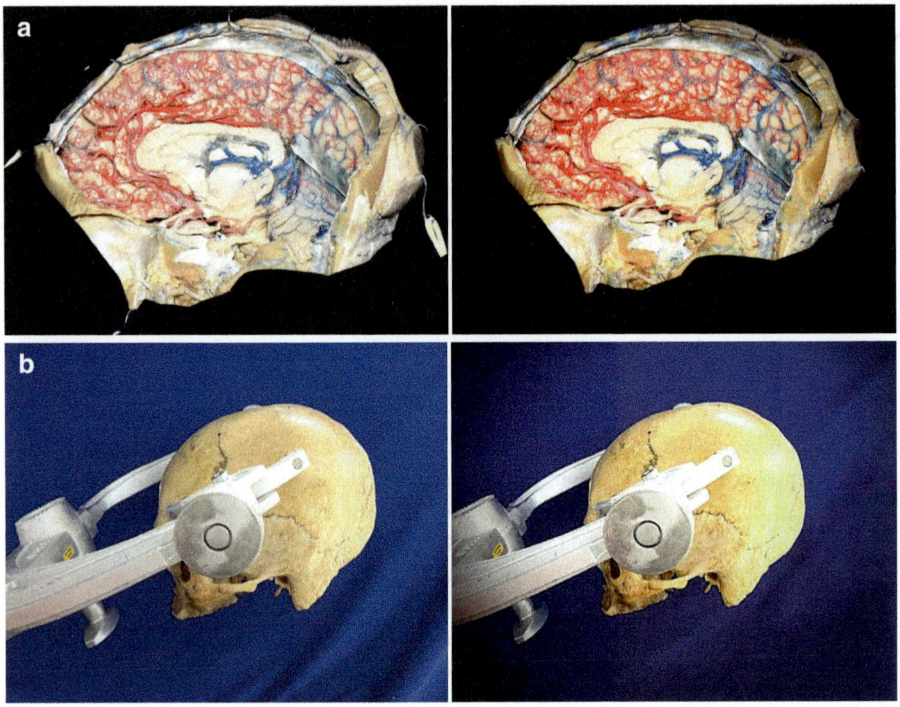

Fig. 4.4 Photographic background: We use black (A) or blue (B) fabric to facilitate light absorption and prevent its reflection on the lens. Additionally, we take care of every detail in terms of sharpness, saturation, light homogeneity, and contrast

4.2 Two-Dimensional Photography

Our approach to capturing a basic photograph is always aimed at fulfilling the following conditions: centered composition, adequate lighting, a background with appropriate contrast (typically blue or preferably black), focus on the desired point to highlight, good sharpness, minimal shadowing, and other essential factors. To achieve this, we explore various methods to adapt to the environment where we want to take the photograph and ensure proper cleaning of the object being photographed (Fig. 4.5).

When considering photography, understanding the advantages and features of the equipment or camera is essential, factors such as camera stability, focus, zoom level according to the central point, height, and distance between the 0 point and the object. In our laboratory, we use an equipment equipped with tripod support.

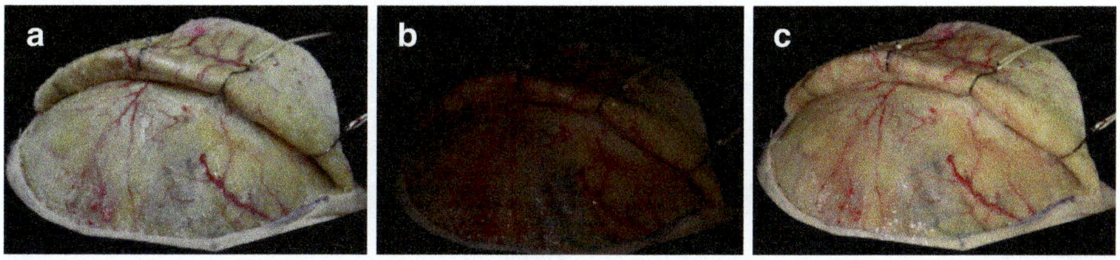

Fig. 4.5 Illumination and contrast. A sequence of photos is observed under different light intensities. Demonstrating the fundamentals of balanced illumination of the target. (**a**) Diffuse light without a light source, (**b**) absence of a light source and shaded regions, and (**c**) standard photograph of the target with adequate illumination and contrast

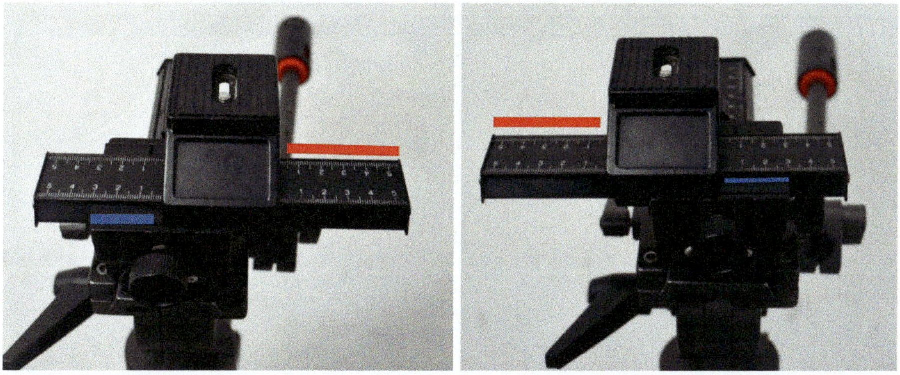

Fig. 4.6 Lateral displacement: We indicate the path of the base or support, as indicated by the blue lines on the left and right for each capture, and its starting point with the end of the red lines. Note that the displacement of the camera on the millimeter ruler ranges between 2.5 and 3 cm in both directions

4.3 Three-Dimensional Photography

When capturing a 3D photograph, additional considerations are necessary to achieve the desired 3D effect. We utilize a ruler fixed to our camera tripod to facilitate this process. This ruler (Fig. X) allows us to capture separate photographs in different dimensions in the X, Y, and Z planes.

To begin, we move our camera to the left to capture the left photo, typically employing a lateral displacement of 2.5–3 cm. After ensuring that our focus is centered on the desired point, we proceed with the capture. Similarly, we repeat this process for the right photo, using the same displacement measure used in capturing the left photo. In daily practice, we prioritize capturing the left photograph, followed by the right photo (Fig. 4.6).

A displacement of precisely 2.5–2.5 or 3–3 cm must be ensured for each photo to achieve the desired effect. After ensuring that our focus is centered on the desired point according to the camera's focus grid, the right photo is captured.

After obtaining both photos, we digitally export them to an exhibition format. Using the PowerPoint application, we orient the screen horizontally and divide it into four equal quadrants (Fig. 4.7).

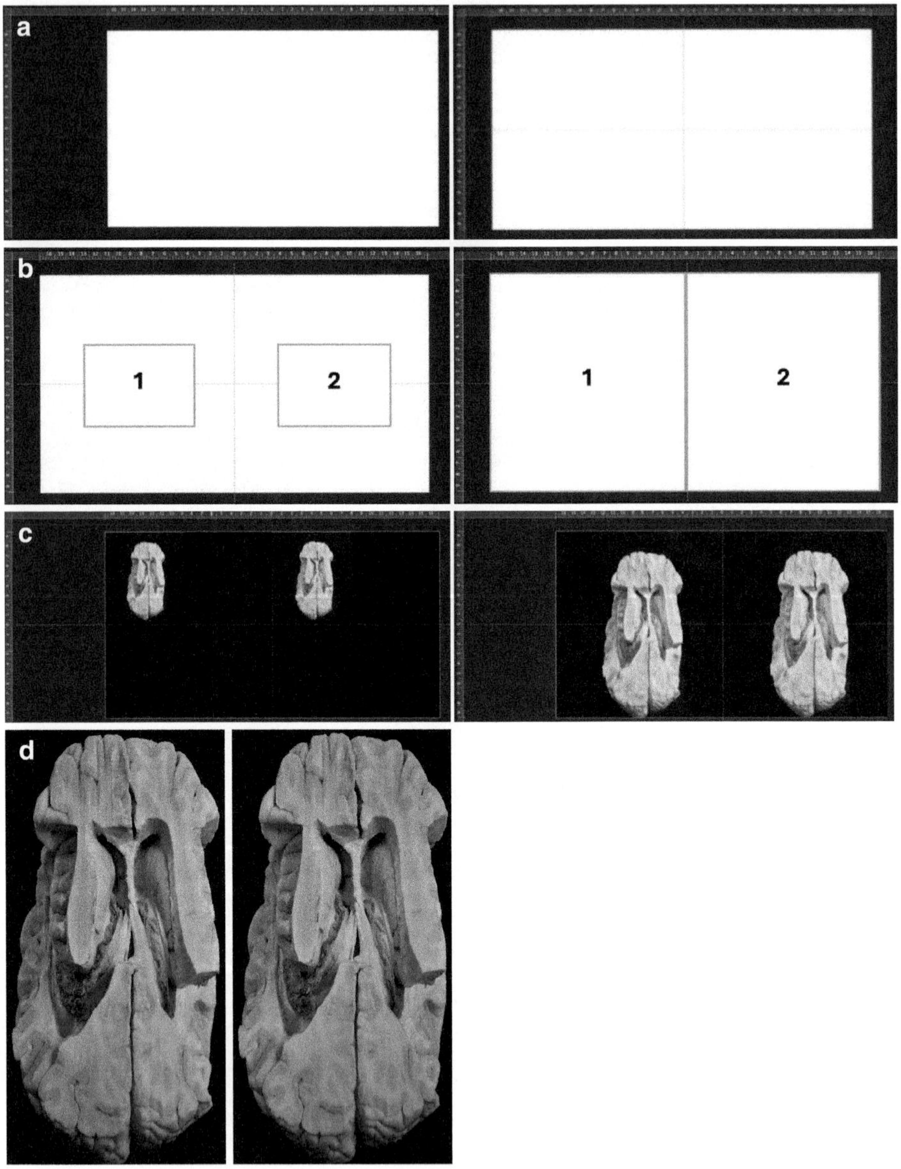

Fig. 4.7 3D assembly. (**a**) Screen layout with power point application, and its identification with linear reference in four quadrants: left top and bottom and right top and bottom. (**b–c**) Layout diagram, centering and enlargement on screen, photo 1 (left), photo 2 (right). (**d**) Photos centered for 3D projection

Segmented in this manner, we place each photograph accordingly, making adjustments in their dimensions to align with the lateral and upper-lower diameters of the screen, as demonstrated.

The arrangement of both photographs facilitates merging, thereby achieving the desired 3D effect.

4.4 Environment and Photographic Station

For photographic and video capture, we ensure adequate space to position and expose the preparation intended for documentation. This includes optimizing the light source, using a contrasting background, centering the subject in the photographic frame, and ensuring flexibility for capturing images from various angles such as front, top, diagonal, and lateral sides.

We emphasize that maintaining optimal conditions for exposure, capture points, and other aspects is crucial for obtaining a high-quality photographic material.

Several key aspects are considered in each photograph and video that we reproduce:

Background: We carefully select an appropriate background (black or dark blue) color to create a contrast with the preparation. In addition to ensuring low brightness, the background should be free of debris, fabrics, or artifacts. Moistening the background with water to achieve a darker tone is a good alternative.

Lighting and shade: Photographs should have sufficient lighting to prevent shadowing of important areas or structures. Additionally, careful consideration of the light source, whether natural or artificial, and the angulation of capture is essential.

Sharpness: This aspect in a photograph is of utmost importance to accurately convey the intended details. Maintaining proper focus in the center of the preparation is essential. Additionally, selecting the appropriate lens according to the space and cavity requirements is important.

Center: When discussing this factor, we refer to positioning the preparation at the center of our capture point. This allows for peripheral captures, gradually approaching maximum magnification. Sequential captures from higher to lower zoom or magnification, with similar angulation, can be performed accordingly (Fig. 4.8).

Schematically, we divide our screen into three zones in relation to the center (Fig. 4.9). The most peripheral area is labeled as Z3, the intermediate area as Z2, and the center area as Z1. Each area represents 1/3 of the total surface and serves as a practical way to consistently maintain a reference pattern.

Examples of artifacts that can be avoided when having a good focus include synthetic materials, instruments, and the presence of the operator's hands. Materials such as retractors, suture thread, and forceps, which aid in capturing the anatomical

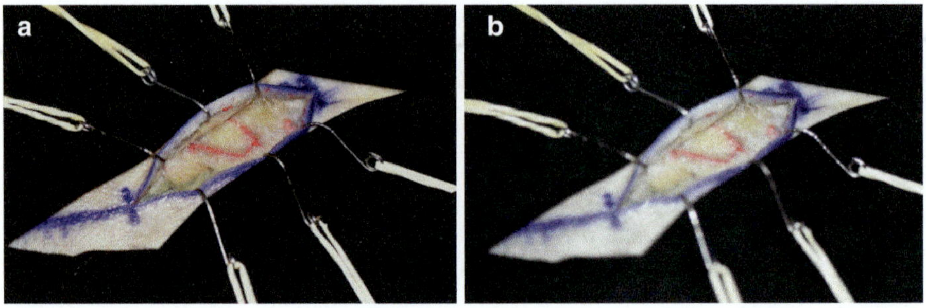

Fig. 4.8 Angulation and center. (**a**) Objective with focused center, adequate contrast, respecting peripheral areas. The objective in this image is to highlight the subcutaneous tissue and exposed vascular structures, while in (**b**), the focus is observed in the upper region, not centered, low contrast and poor lower sharpness. Considering that both captures present the same angulation

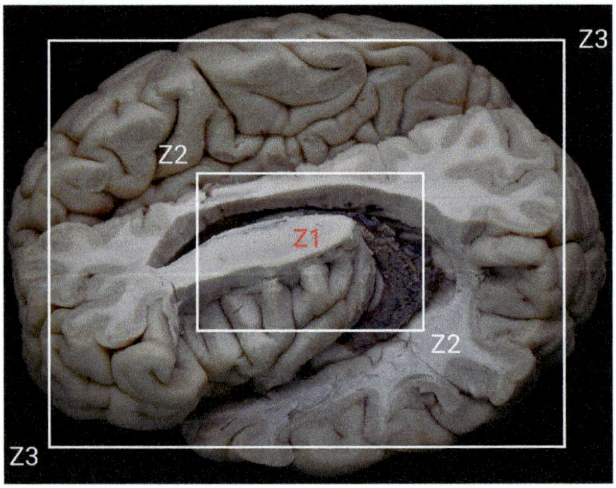

Fig. 4.9 We always try to distribute our rectangular capture screen over the entire length of the lens. Dividing it into three zones: (Z1) main center, (Z2) intermediate zone, and (Z3) peripheral zone. Note that in this way, we obtain an adequate center and avoid unwanted cuts of the lens

structures in depth and their relationship with the surface, are generally not considered artifacts.

When discussing videos, it is essential to maintain focus and prevent the operator's hands from appearing inside the working or dissection field.

What tools or materials do we need to obtain a photograph or video?

In our laboratory, we use various tools to capture photographs and/or videos of dissections and preparations. These tools include a Nikkon camera with lens, tripod support, three-plane ruler, light ring, photographic box, and black tissue.

When creating a video of an anatomical dissection, microsurgical training, or any technical procedure, we have two options for obtaining it: either through direct

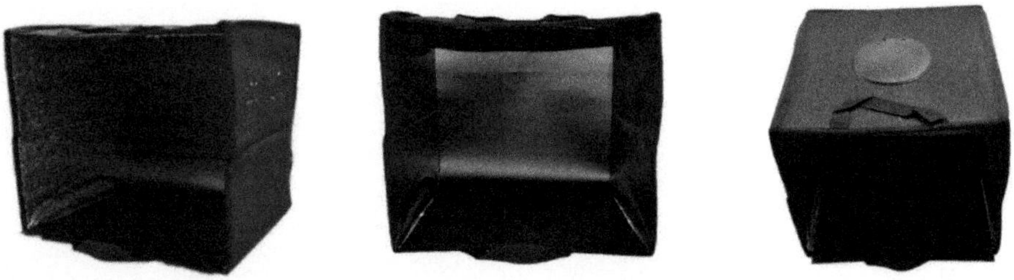

Fig. 4.10 Capture box. Among other tools for proper photographic capture, we use this box, preferably black. If it does not have these characteristics, we cover it with fabric of the same color. In order to avoid reflections and external light entering our objective. Note its three-dimensional characteristics in various projections

macroscopic vision or the use of magnification equipment such as a surgical or laboratory microscope (Fig. 4.10).

In this second scenario, we typically utilize laboratory microscopes, to which we mount a camera for 2D and 3D video capture. We must maintain proper illumination and central and peripheral magnification to ensure optimal visibility of anatomical structures and focus on the central point.

4.5 Photogrammetry

Photogrammetry offers a powerful tool for creating highly detailed, 3D models of anatomical structures. This technology can be particularly valuable in neurosurgery education, allowing students to explore complex neural pathways and brain structures in an interactive way. In contrast with laser scanners for creating models, photogrammetry yields higher-quality images when executed correctly. However, it requires training and expertise to achieve optimal results.

When considering materials and preparation for photogrammetry in neuroanatomy, the small dimensions of the neuroanatomical structures and the requirement for high-resolution and detailed textures pose specific challenges when planning photogrammetry. Low-quality models may be interesting for entertainment purposes, but they lack the detail necessary for comprehensive neuroanatomical study.

A high-resolution digital single-lens reflex or mirrorless camera is ideal. Manual controls for shutter speed, aperture, and ISO are crucial. Alternatively, smartphones with powerful camera capabilities can also be used. However, lower-quality photos may compromise the textures of the 3D model and lead to flaws and errors in the final output. To ensure image stability and consistent framing, a tripod is required.

The lighting is crucial, with every part of the model requiring well-detailed and evenly exposed textures. To achieve this, diffused lighting is essential, which can be achieved using soft boxes or ring lights to avoid harsh shadows. Alternatively, photos can be taken outdoors on sunny and cloudy days with minimal shadows.

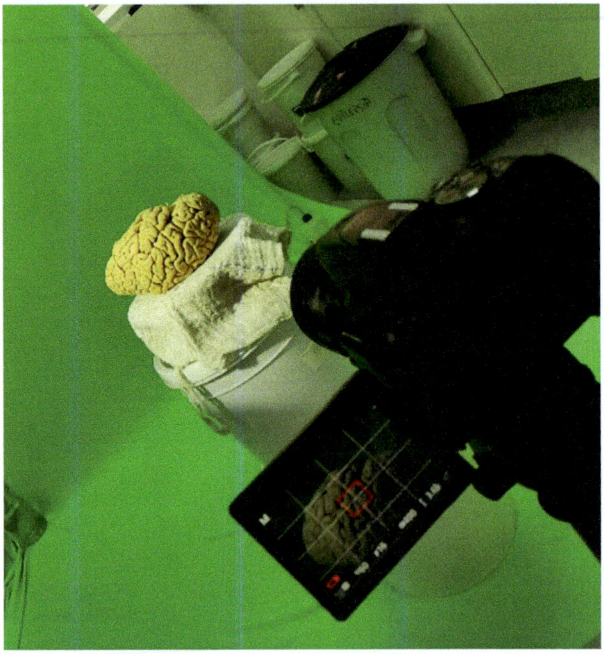

Fig. 4.11 Moment of photographic capture, note the position of the camera, lens, and background fabric

Diffusing the light source minimizes shadows and ensures even illumination across the entire specimen. In camera settings, the manual mode must be activated, with an adequate aperture chosen for sufficient depth of field (f/8 or higher). ISO and shutter speed adjustments are made until a balanced exposure is achieved. White balance should be set to a neutral setting like daylight or flash (Fig. 4.11).

When photographing anatomical pieces, the object colors might be too homogeneous for the photogrammetry software to understand slight differences and correctly create the model. In this case, marking pins with contrasting heads can be pinned into the object to define specific anatomical landmarks, aiding in later 3D model refinement. Additionally, using a printed checkerboard pattern helps the photogrammetry software identify common points between images.

Before beginning the photography process, the anatomical specimen of interest must be prepared. For brain specimens, a stabilizing solution must be used to maintain tissue integrity.

For image capture, after material and environmental preparation, the first step is to include the calibration target in several photos, ensuring it is visible and positioned at different orientations within the frame.

A systematic approach is key to a successful capture. Circle the specimen, taking a series of overlapping photos from various angles, from top to bottom. Aim for a complete circumferential capture, ensuring that the entire structure is documented. Capture additional close-up shots of intricate details. The level of detail in the object determines the number of images needed. Capturing between 100 and 250 images is typically sufficient for small and detailed structures. If moving the camera proves

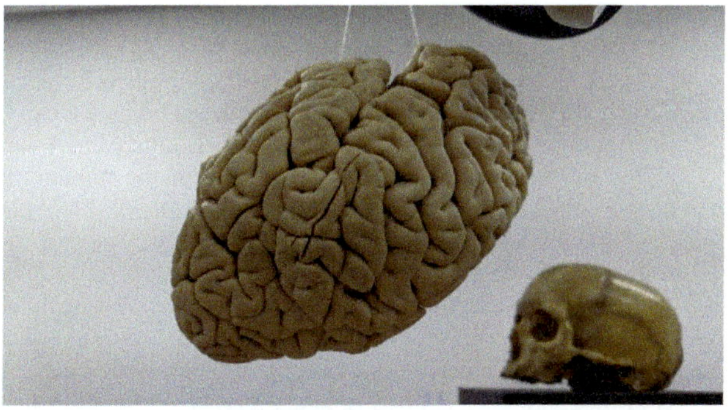

Fig. 4.12 Anatomical preparation (human brain) suspended, when we want to obtain photographs with a remote capturer

challenging, a turntable can be used with the camera in a fixed position while the object rotates. A green screen is necessary to prevent the software from using the background for reference, as it remains consistent in every photo.

Close attention is required to capture the undersurface of the neurological structure. If this area is necessary for the 3D model, the object should be suspended to ensure visibility of all surfaces simultaneously. If suspension is not feasible, the object must be photographed both upright and upside down. However, the latter option requires more challenging post-processing for image fusion into a single model.

When using marking pins to highlight specific landmarks, ensure that they are visible in multiple photos from different angles.

For optimal results, a consistent distance from the specimen throughout the capture process should be maintained. The use of a remote shutter release minimizes camera shake. Tethering the camera to a computer during shooting allows for real-time image review and adjustments. Capturing more photos than initially planned is advisable (Fig. 4.12).

After capturing, transfer the images to a computer. The photogrammetry software will then use them to generate a 3D point cloud and ultimately a textured mesh model. Certain software allow for manual refinement of the 3D model, allowing adjustments to data points and addressing imperfections in the 3D model.

Note that batch processing of high-resolution images requires a computer with robust video and processing specifications.

Following these steps and best practices enables the creation of high-fidelity 3D models for enhanced neurosurgical education.

Bibliography

1. Acosta MA, Loof de Amorim B, Martins TH, Dovanir Silva M, Chaddad-Neto F. Building a microneurosurgical laboratory in Latin América: challenges and possibilities. Surg Neurol Int. 2021;23(12):573. https://doi.org/10.25259/SNI_978_2021.

2. Krause KJ, Mullins DD, Kist MN, Goldman EM. Developing 3D models using photogrammetry for virtual reality training in anatomy. Anat. Sci Educ. 2023;16(6):1033–40. https://doi.org/10.1002/ase.2301. Epub 2023 May 29
3. Krogager ME, Fugleholm K, Mathiesen TI, Spiriev T. Simplified easy-accessible smartphone-based photogrammetry for 3-dimensional anatomy presentation exemplified with a photorealistic cadaver-based model of the intracranial and extracranial course of the facial nerve. Oper Neurosurg (Hagerstown). 2023;25(2):e71–7. https://doi.org/10.1227/ons.0000000000000748. Epub 2023 Jun 15
4. Ahumada JC, Wuo Silva R, Moreno M, Chaddad-Neto F. The art of combining neuroanatomy and microsurgical skills in modern neurosurgery. Front Neurol. 2023;13:1076778. https://doi.org/10.3389/fneur.2022.1076778.
5. Trandzhiev M, Vezirska DI, Maslarski I, Milev MD, Laleva L, Nakov V, Cornelius JF, Spiriev T. Photogrammetry applied to neurosurgery: a literature review. Cureus. 2023;15(9):e46251. https://doi.org/10.7759/cureus.46251. PMID: 37908958; PMCID: PMC10614469
6. Gonzalez-Romo NI, Mignucci-Jiménez G, Hanalioglu S, Gurses ME, Bahadir S, Xu Y, Koskay G, Lawton MT, Preul MC. Virtual neurosurgery anatomy laboratory: a collaborative and remote education experience in the metaverse. Surg Neurol Int. 2023;14:90. https://doi.org/10.25259/SNI_162_2023. PMID: 37025523; PMCID: PMC10070459
7. De Benedictis A, Nocerino E, Menna F, Remondino F, Barbareschi M, Rozzanigo U, Corsini F, Olivetti E, Marras CE, Chioffi F, Avesani P, Sarubbo S. Photogrammetry of the human brain: a novel method for three-dimensional quantitative exploration of the structural connectivity in neurosurgery and neurosciences. World Neurosurg. 2018;115:e279–91. https://doi.org/10.1016/j.wneu.2018.04.036. Epub 2018 Apr 13. PMID: 29660551.
8. Aydin SO, Barut O, Yilmaz MO, Sahin B, Akyoldas G, Akgun MY, Baran O, Tanriover N. Use of 3-dimensional modeling and augmented/virtual reality applications in microsurgical neuroanatomy training. Oper Neurosurg (Hagerstown). 2023;24(3):318–23. https://doi.org/10.1227/ons.0000000000000524. Epub 2022 Nov 28. PMID: 36701556.
9. de Oliveira ASB, Leonel LCPC, LaHood ER, Hallak H, Link MJ, Maleszewski JJ, Pinheiro-Neto CD, Morris JM, Peris-Celda M. Foundations and guidelines for high-quality three-dimensional models using photogrammetry: a technical note on the future of neuroanatomy education. Anat Sci Educ. 2023;16(5):870–83. https://doi.org/10.1002/ase.2274. Epub 2023 Apr 13. PMID: 36934316.
10. Gurses ME, Hanalioglu S, Mignucci-Jiménez G, Gökalp E, Gonzalez-Romo NI, Gungor A, Cohen-Gadol AA, Türe U, Lawton MT, Preul MC. Three-dimensional modeling and extended reality simulations of the cross-sectional anatomy of the cerebrum, cerebellum, and brainstem. Oper Neurosurg (Hagerstown). 2023;25(1):3–10. https://doi.org/10.1227/ons.0000000000000703. Epub 2023 Apr 21. PMID: 37083688
11. Gurses ME, Gonzalez-Romo NI, Xu Y, Mignucci-Jiménez G, Hanalioglu S, Chang JE, Rafka H, Vaughan KA, Ellegala DB, Lawton MT, Preul MC. Interactive microsurgical anatomy education using photogrammetry 3D models and an augmented reality cube. J Neurosurg. 2024;26:1–10. https://doi.org/10.3171/2023.10.JNS23516. Epub ahead of print. PMID: 38277660.
12. Serrato-Avila JL, Paz Archila JA, Silva da Costa MD, et al. Three-Dimensional Quantitative Analysis of the Brainstem Safe Entry Zones Based on Internal Structures. World Neurosurg. 2022;158:e64-e74. https://doi.org/10.1016/j.wneu.2021.10.100

Chapter 5
Dissecting the Brain Surface

5.1 Introduction

We aimed to identify the disparities in the methods employed when examining the cerebral sulci and gyri between the laboratory and operating room settings, emphasizing that the study of anatomy extends beyond mere memorization of the structures. Instead, it involves determining the correlation between these two structures and, most importantly, developing microsurgical skills. Handling specimens in the laboratory can enhance microsurgical ability. In this chapter, we explored the methods for handling specimens in a laboratory based on the anatomical information obtained.

The brain is composed of the brainstem, cerebellum, and cerebrum, with the latter consisting of the telencephalon and diencephalon. The telencephalon comprises the cerebral hemisphere and three telencephalic commissures: the anterior or rostral commissure, fornix commissure, and corpus callosum.

The diencephalon consists of five structures, with the thalamus serving as its core and being surrounded by other structures. This anatomical view of the thalamus as the center of the brain significantly aids in understanding the arrangement of other structures within the diencephalon and telencephalon. The subthalamus, positioned beneath the thalamus, is anatomically continuous with the midbrain, while the hypothalamus, situated beneath the thalamus, does not share this continuity with the midbrain. The epithalamus is situated behind the thalamus and is connected through the epithalamic or posterior commissure, while the metathalamus is located on the sides of the thalamus.

The surface of the brain contains depressions known as sulci, which separate convolutions called gyri. The brain has three anatomical surfaces, lateral, medial, and inferior (or basal), all of which are explored in this section. In this chapter, the connections between the surface structures and deeper structures of the brain, such

F. Chaddad-Neto, M. D. S. da Costa, *Microneuroanatomy and Lab*,
https://doi.org/10.1007/978-3-031-91026-5_5

as the corpus callosum, were explored by examining the lateral surface of the brain and linking them to the cranial structures.

The initial step in dissecting the cerebral surface involves removing the entire arachnoid and vessels from the gyri and sulci, under microscopic guidance. This procedure requires manual dexterity and microsurgical training. Surgeons learn to stabilize their hand on the hypothenar eminence, manipulate toothless delicate forceps, use the microscope at a fixed focal distance, and manipulate straight microscissors. At this stage, neurosurgeons begin to recognize the topography of various surface reliefs while also undergoing microsurgical training in manipulating instruments. They become adept at distinguishing various sulcus arrangements and lobes. In the laboratory, the process of arachnoid removal should not be regarded as a mere repetitive and mechanical task but rather as an opportunity for training.

5.2 Lateral Surface of the Cerebrum

Division

The lateral surface is the largest cerebral surface and is divided into two parts by the lateral sulcus of the cerebrum, also known as the Sylvian fissure: the superolateral and inferolateral parts. Therefore, the initial step in dividing the lateral surface of the cerebrum is to locate the Sylvian fissure, which is the only sulcus that remains entirely continuous on the lateral surface. Recognizing this structure is crucial for understanding the entire cerebral surface, since lobe division relies on its identification. The frontal and parietal lobes lie above the Sylvian fissure, while the temporal lobe lies below it.

During arachnoid removal, this fissure is profoundly deep and exhibits distinctive characteristics, including its division into three branches and the presence of another lobe at its depth, the insular lobe. These aspects will be discussed in detail throughout the chapter. The Sylvian fissure follows an oblique path, running parallel to the lesser wing of the sphenoid bone, with medial to lateral, bottom to top, and anterior to posterior trajectories. It comprises a main trunk that trifurcates into the anterior, ascending, and posterior branches at the anterior Sylvian point.

The adjacent structures bordering the Sylvian fissure are commonly recognized as the operculum, frontal, parietal, and temporal lobes. These structures "hide" the insular lobe, which lies at the depth of the Sylvian valley. The Sylvian fissure houses the middle cerebral artery. Therefore, knowledge of its anatomical trajectory is crucial for proper positioning of the head during the performance of surgical procedures involving the middle cerebral artery, temporal lobe, insula, and opercular region (Fig. 5.1).

A Sylvian fissure is also visible on the cranial surface. The anterior portion of the squamous suture, extending up to its highest part, externally represents the Sylvian fissure. The apex of the squamous suture corresponds to the point at which the central sulcus approaches the Sylvian fissure, also known as the inferior Rolandic point. Additionally, it can be located by palpating the preauricular fold and measuring

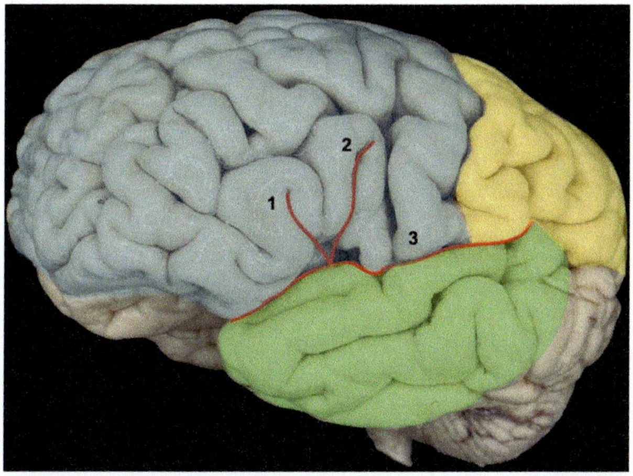

Fig. 5.1 Sylvian fissure. Lateral view of the brain. The Sylvian fissure is highlighted (red line), along with its horizontal (1), ascending (2), and posterior (3) branches. On its surface, the Sylvian fissure clearly marks the boundaries of the frontal lobe (blue) at its supero-anterior border, the postero-superior parietal lobe (yellow), and the temporal lobe (green) at its inferior border

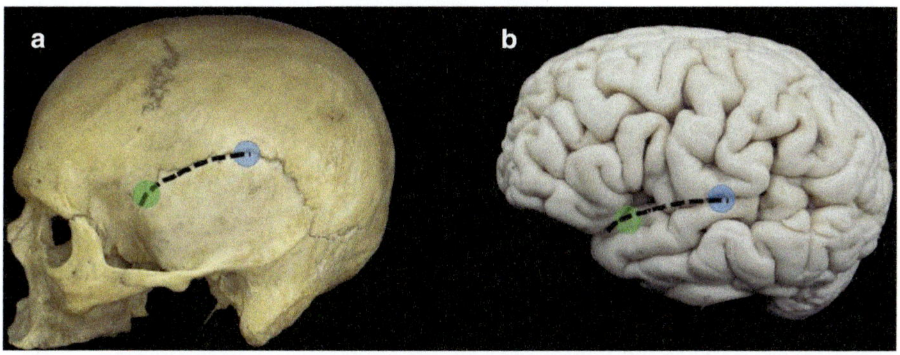

Fig. 5.2 Relationship of points on the cranial surface (A) with the Sylvian fissure (B). The ascending portion of the squamous suture (black dashed line) up to its highest point (blue circle) corresponds to the Sylvian fissure. This point (blue circle) corresponds to the inferior Rolandic point, the region where the central sulcus approaches the Sylvian fissure. The anterior Sylvian point is located at the apex of the triangular area (green circle)

7 cm along a straight line. On the cranial surface, the anterior Sylvian point, where the Sylvian fissure trifurcates, is represented by a region known as the pterion. The pterion is characterized by the convergence of the frontosphenoidal, temporosphenoidal, parietosphenoidal, temporoparietal, and frontoparietal or coronal sutures (Fig. 5.2).

The next step in dividing the lateral surface of the brain involves identifying the central sulcus. A useful method for locating it, which is applicable in anatomical studies, surgical procedures, and imaging examinations, involves searching for a

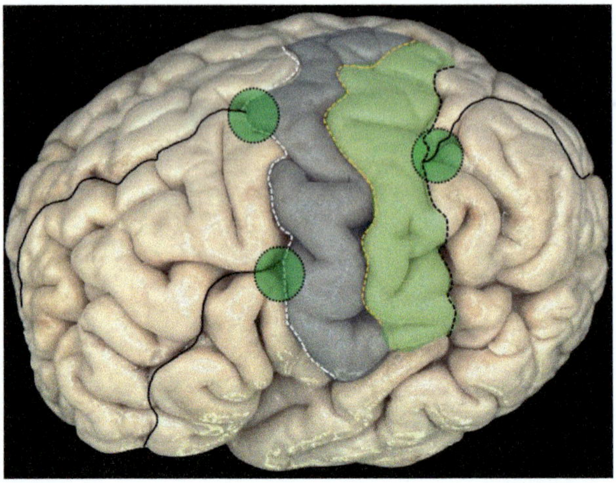

Fig. 5.3 Identification of the vertical sulci. Superolateral view of the brain. Initial identification of the two vertical sulci that connect with the horizontal sulci (green circles): The precentral sulcus (white dashed line) forms the anterior portion, while the postcentral sulcus (black dashed line) forms the posterior portion, with the central sulcus (yellow dashed line) located between these structures

vertical sulcus that connects to a horizontal sulcus to form a termino-lateral connection. This sulcus will necessarily be either the precentral sulcus or the postcentral sulcus. In the anteroposterior direction, the first vertical sulcus connected to the horizontal sulcus is the precentral sulcus, followed by the precentral gyrus, central sulcus, postcentral gyrus, and postcentral sulcus. In the posteroanterior direction, the postcentral sulcus is the vertical sulcus that connects to another horizontal sulcus (Figs. 5.3 and 5.4).

The central sulcus is a crucial anatomical landmark that divides the lateral surface of the brain into frontal, located anteriorly, and parietal, located posteriorly. It exhibits a double S shape with two convexities and is not connected to a horizontal sulcus, which is essential for distinguishing it from the precentral and postcentral sulci. The central sulcus follows an oblique course and has superior to inferior, medial to lateral, and posterior to anterior orientations. Typically, the central sulcus does not extend to the Sylvian fissure and terminates at the frontoparietal operculum, a gyrus-like structure also referred to as the subcentral gyrus or "plea of passage" (Fig. 5.5).

Frontal Lobe

The exploration of the lobes of the lateral surface of the brain begins by examining the frontal lobe. This lobe's lateral surface contains the vertical sulcus and gyrus (precentral sulcus and precentral gyrus), alongside two horizontal sulci (superior and inferior frontal sulci) that determine the three horizontal gyri (superior, middle, and inferior frontal gyri) (Fig. 5.6).

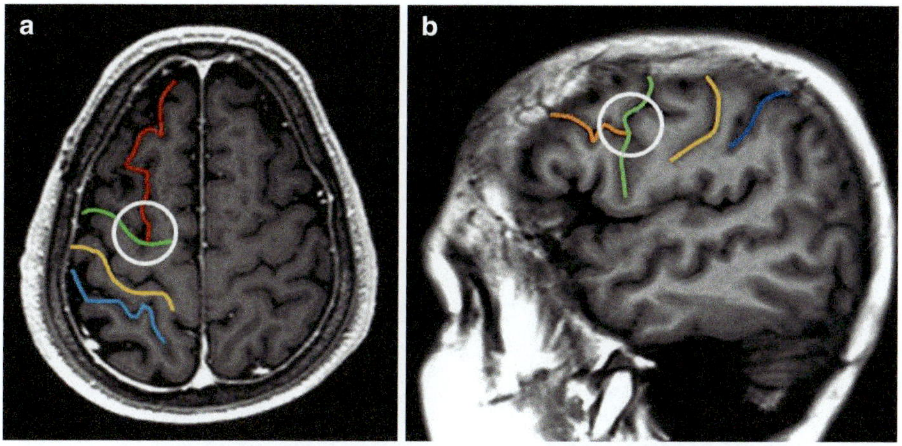

Fig. 5.4 Identification of the vertical sulci on magnetic resonance imaging. (A) Axial T1-weighted magnetic resonance imaging (MRI): Initial identification of a vertical sulcus connecting (white circle) to a horizontal sulcus (superior frontal sulcus, white); as the connection is located anteriorly, this vertical sulcus is identified as the precentral sulcus (green), followed by the central sulcus (yellow) and postcentral sulcus (blue). (B) Sagittal T1-weighted MRI: Initial identification of a vertical sulcus connecting (white circle) to a horizontal sulcus (inferior frontal sulcus, orange); as the connection is anterior, this vertical sulcus is the precentral sulcus (green), followed by the central sulcus (yellow) and postcentral sulcus (blue)

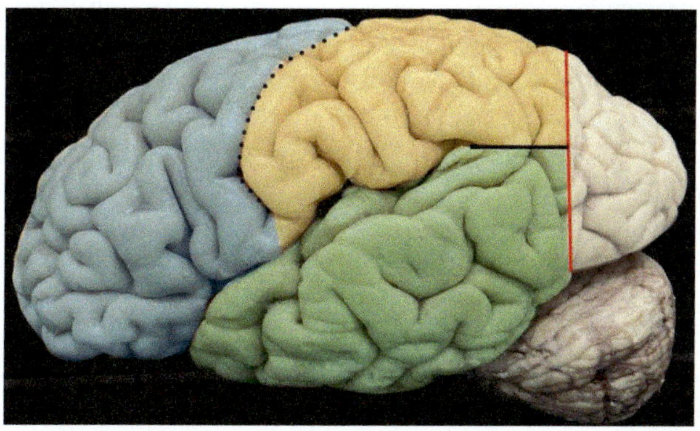

Fig. 5.5 Lateral surface of the brain. Lateral view of the brain divided into cerebral lobes: frontal lobe (blue), parietal lobe (yellow), temporal lobe (green), and occipital lobe (natural). The central sulcus (black dashed line) separates the frontal lobe from the parietal lobe; an imaginary line (black line) extending from the most posterior portion of the Sylvian fissure delineates the parietal and temporal lobes, while a vertical imaginary line (red) extending from the preoccipital incisure further divides the occipital lobe posteriorly

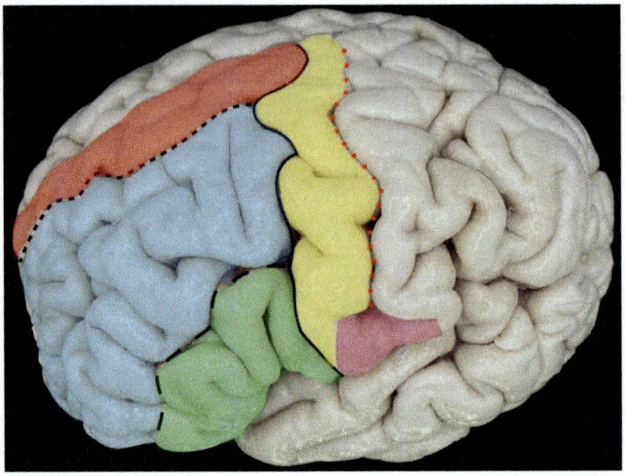

Fig. 5.6 Frontal lobe. Lateral surface of the frontal lobe, illustrating three sulci and four gyri. The superior frontal sulcus (thin black line) and inferior frontal sulcus dashed black line) depict, from superior to inferior, the superior frontal gyrus (red), middle frontal gyrus (blue), and inferior frontal gyrus (green). The anterior verticalized sulcus is the precentral sulcus (black line), posterior to which lies the precentral gyrus (yellow), followed by the central sulcus (red dashed line). The passage pleat (pink) connects the precentral gyrus and the postcentral gyrus, bridging the frontal and parietal lobes

The precentral sulcus, the first vertical sulcus connecting with the horizontal sulci, serves as the anterior boundary of the precentral gyrus and is demarcated posteriorly by the central sulcus. Notably, the precentral sulcus is one of only two sulci found on the lateral surface of the brain that exhibit complete discontinuity, due to interruption by the middle frontal gyrus, which remains connected with the precentral gyrus.

The recognition of the precentral gyrus is of paramount importance, especially during surgical procedures, as it serves as the primary motor area. Hence, comprehending not only its relationship with the adjacent sulci and gyri but also its associations with the cranial surface is crucial. With regard to the cranial boundaries of the precentral gyrus, the superior point of the precentral sulcus is located 3 to 3.5 cm posterior to the bregma, while the superior point of the central sulcus, also known as the superior Rolandic point, is located 5 cm posterior to the Bregma. The previously discussed inferior Rolandic point corresponds to the point where the central sulcus approaches the Sylvian fissure and aligns with the highest point of the squamous suture on the cranial surface (Fig. 5.7).

Another important craniometric point in the identification of lateral surface structures is the Stephanion, which is the junction point of the coronal suture and superior temporal line and internally corresponds to the junction of the inferior frontal sulcus and precentral sulcus (Fig. 5.8).

The superior frontal sulcus was identified by locating the first horizontal sulcus below the interhemispheric fissure; it separates the superior frontal gyrus from the

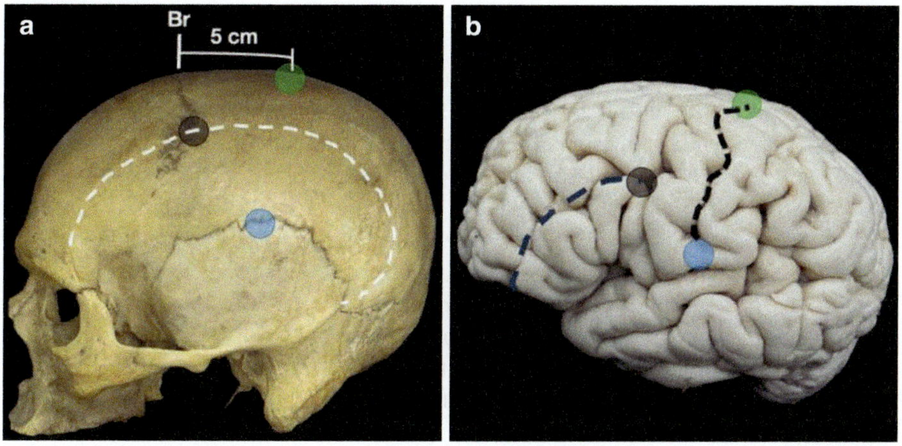

Fig. 5.7 Relationship of points on the cranial surface (A) with the lateral surface of the brain (B). The superior Rolandic point (green circle), located 5 cm posterior to the bregma, corresponds to the superior point of the central sulcus. The inferior Rolandic point (blue circle), found at the highest point of the squamous suture, corresponds to the point where the central sulcus approaches the Sylvian fissure. The stephanion (black circle) is the junction point of the coronal suture and the superior temporal line, corresponding internally to the junction of the inferior frontal sulcus and precentral sulcus. The anterior portion of the superior temporal line (white line) corresponds internally to the inferior frontal sulcus

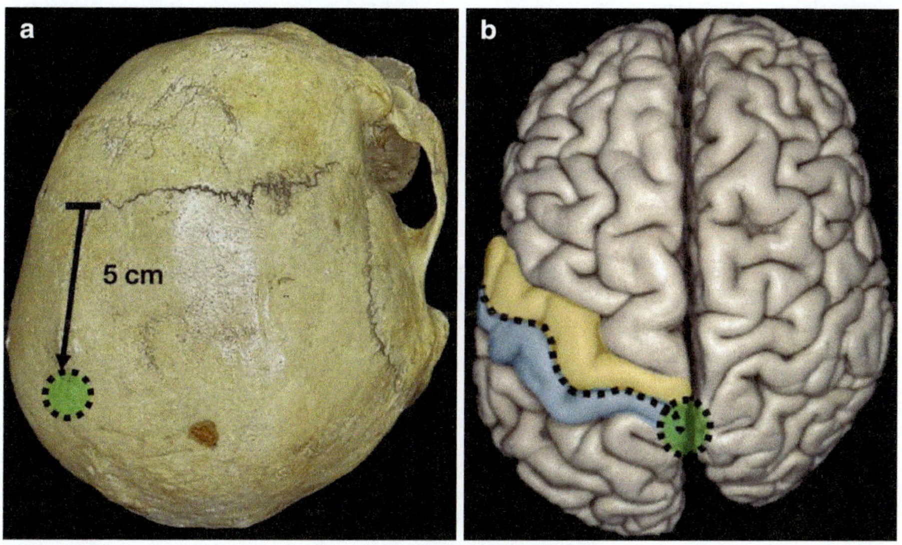

Fig. 5.8 Relationship of points on the cranial surface (**a**) with the brain surface (**b**). The superior Rolandic point (green circle) is located 5 cm posterior to the bregma and corresponds to the superior point of the central sulcus (black dashed line), which separates the precentral gyrus (yellow) from the postcentral gyrus (blue)

middle frontal gyrus. Its connection to the precentral sulcus serves as a crucial anatomical reference and is widely utilized by radiologists for the localization and identification of brain structures in the lateral surface. This connection induces an indentation and determines a convolution in the precentral gyrus known as the "omega" shape, which functionally corresponds to the hand motor area (Fig. 5.9).

The inferior frontal sulcus can be easily recognized as the first horizontal sulcus above the Sylvian fissure, which separates the middle frontal gyrus from the inferior frontal gyrus. On the cranial surface, the inferior frontal gyrus corresponds to the superior temporal line and serves as an important reference point for performing craniotomy. In some individuals, an intermediate frontal sulcus may exist, which divides the middle frontal gyrus into superior and inferior portions. The anterior portion of the middle frontal gyrus forms the base of the frontal pole. Posteriorly, it interrupts the precentral gyrus before seamlessly merging with it (Fig. 5.10).

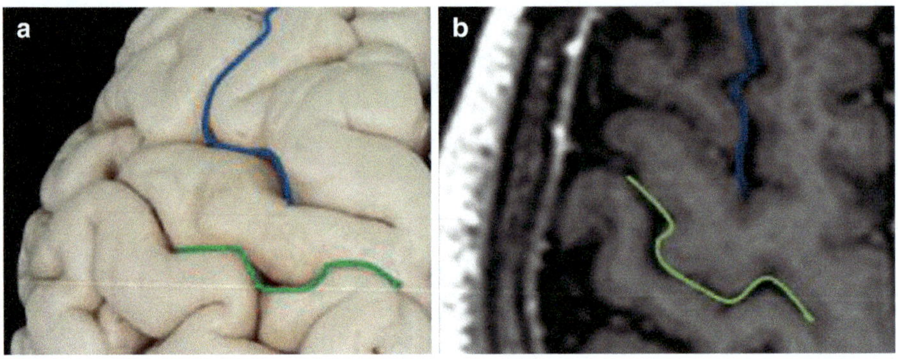

Fig. 5.9 Omega. The superior frontal sulcus (blue line) creates an indentation in the precentral gyrus, determining a convolution called omega, which can be recognized in anatomical specimens (**a**) and imaging studies (**b**)

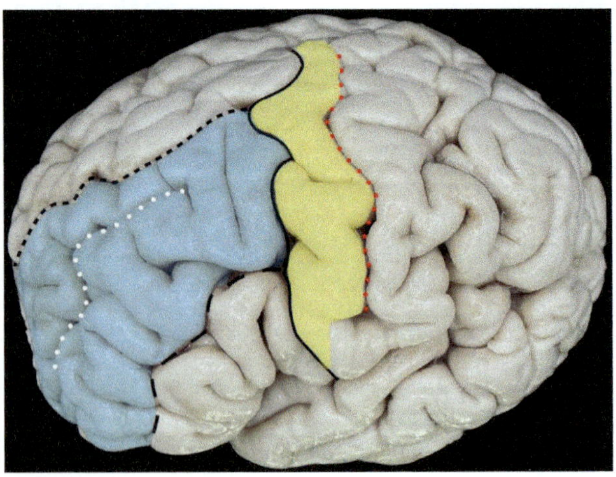

Fig. 5.10 Intermediate frontal sulcus. The middle frontal gyrus divided into superior and inferior portions by a less common sulcus, the intermediate frontal sulcus (white dashed line)

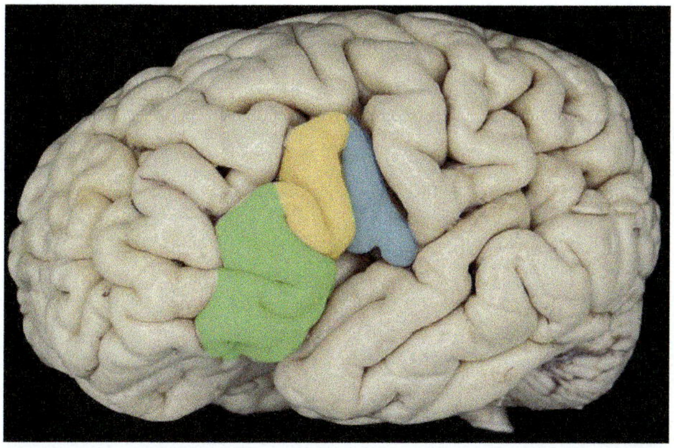

Fig. 5.11 Frontal operculum. Inferior frontal gyrus divided into the orbital part (green), triangular part (yellow), and opercular part (blue). The pars triangularis points toward the anterior Sylvian point, which marks the location of the greatest retraction of the Sylvian fissure

Understanding the three subdivisions of the inferior frontal gyrus, which are delineated by the anterior, ascending, and posterior branches of the Sylvian fissure, is essential (Fig. 5.11).

- **Orbital Part:** This anterior portion is situated below the anterior branch of the Sylvian fissure, resting on the orbital roof.
- **Triangular Part:** This part is located between the anterior and ascending branches of the Sylvian fissure; it has a triangular shape, with its apex pointing toward the limen of the insula. The greatest retraction of the lateral fissure of the brain can be identified at this point.
- **Opercular Part:** This posterior portion of the inferior frontal gyrus is situated between the ascending branch of the Sylvian fissure and the precentral sulcus. It forms a convolution that drapes over the Sylvian fissure; hence, it is referred to as the opercular part.

In the dominant hemisphere, typically the left hemisphere in most individuals, the triangular and opercular parts are responsible for language expression, commonly referred to as the Broca's area.

Temporal Lobe

To understand the lateral surface of the temporal lobe, it is necessary to identify the presence of the two horizontal sulci (superior and inferior temporal sulci) that delineate the three horizontal gyri (superior, middle, and inferior temporal gyri).

Initially, the superior temporal sulcus, which is the first horizontal sulcus situated below the Sylvian fissure, must be recognized. It traverses from the anterior to the posterior regions and terminates in the parietal lobe in a "Y"-shaped pattern, where it splits into the angular and anterior occipital branches, forming the angular gyrus between them. The inferior temporal sulcus is one of the only two sulci on the lateral surface of the brain that are completely discontinuous.

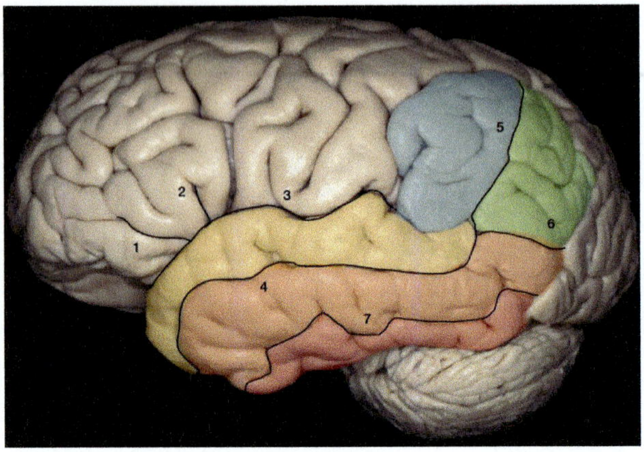

Fig. 5.12 Temporal lobe. Lateral surface of the temporal lobe. The temporal lobe is located inferiorly to the Sylvian fissure, with its uppermost portion comprising the superior temporal gyrus (yellow). The Sylvian fissure divides into the horizontal ramus (1), ascending ramus (2), and posterior ramus (3). The superior temporal sulcus (4) terminates in a Y-shaped pattern, branching into the angular ramus (5) and the anterior occipital ramus (6). The inferior temporal sulcus (7) serves as the lower boundary of the middle temporal gyrus (orange) and the upper boundary of the inferior temporal gyrus (red). The gyri are the superior temporal gyrus, which posteriorly becomes the supramarginal gyrus (blue); the middle temporal gyrus (orange), which later becomes the angular gyrus (green); and the inferior temporal gyrus (red)

The superior temporal gyrus continues posteriorly as the supramarginal gyrus, also known as the temporoparietal operculum, which covers the posterior limit of the Sylvian fissure. The anterior portion of the middle temporal gyrus forms the base of the temporal pole and has an important anatomical relationship with the greater wing of the sphenoid bone. Additionally, the inferior temporal gyrus connects the lateral and basal brain surfaces (Fig. 5.12).

Parietal Lobe

The lateral surface of the parietal lobe exhibits a vertical sulcus and gyrus (postcentral sulcus and postcentral gyrus) as well as a horizontal sulcus (intraparietal sulcus) that divides the lobe into superior and inferior parietal lobules (Fig. 5.13).

To anatomically delimitate the parietal lobe, we utilized the method previously described and identified the second vertical sulcus in the anteroposterior direction that connects with a horizontal sulcus (intraparietal sulcus). This sulcus is referred to as the postcentral sulcus, which is the posterior boundary of the postcentral gyrus and is bounded anteriorly by the central sulcus. The postcentral gyrus is a functional primary somatosensory area.

The next step involves the identification of the intraparietal sulcus, achievable by discerning a horizontal sulcus connected to the postcentral sulcus. This sulcus is the intraparietal sulcus, dividing the parietal lobe into the superior parietal lobule and the inferior parietal lobule. These lobules are formed by the supramarginal gyrus and the angular gyrus, both separated by the angular branch of the superior temporal sulcus (Fig. 5.14).

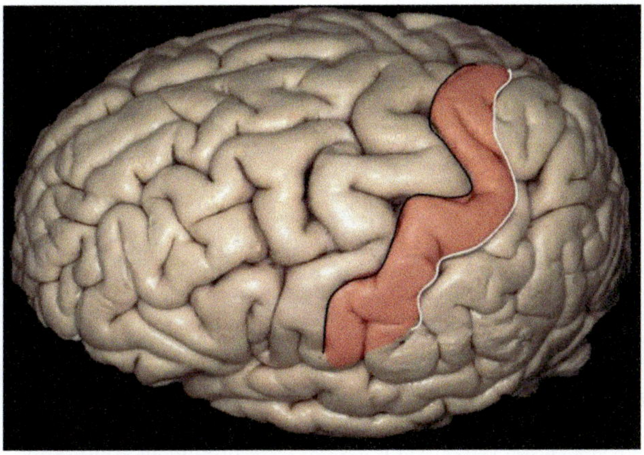

Fig. 5.13 Postcentral gyrus. Anatomical boundaries of the postcentral gyrus (red), central sulcus (black line), and postcentral sulcus (white line)

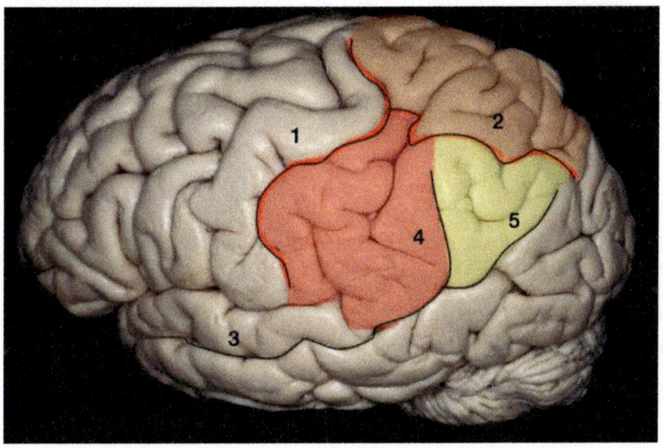

Fig. 5.14 Parietal lobe. Parietal lobe and its divisions. Postcentral sulcus (1). The presence of a horizontal sulcus (2) dividing the parietal lobe into the superior parietal lobule (orange) and the inferior parietal lobule, which is subdivided into the supramarginal gyrus (red) and the angular gyrus (yellow), separated by branches of the superior temporal sulcus (3) and its terminal branches, the angular branch (4) and the anterior occipital branch (5)

The supramarginal gyrus is a continuation of the superior temporal gyrus and surrounds the posterior ascending limb of the Sylvian fissure. Its anterior, superior, inferior, and posterior boundaries are delineated by the postcentral sulcus, intraparietal sulcus, superior temporal sulcus, and angular branch of the superior temporal sulcus, respectively.

In the dominant hemisphere, the supramarginal gyrus, also known as the Wernicke's area, is associated with language comprehension. On the cranial surface, the supramarginal gyrus may be related to the euryon (Fig. 5.15). This

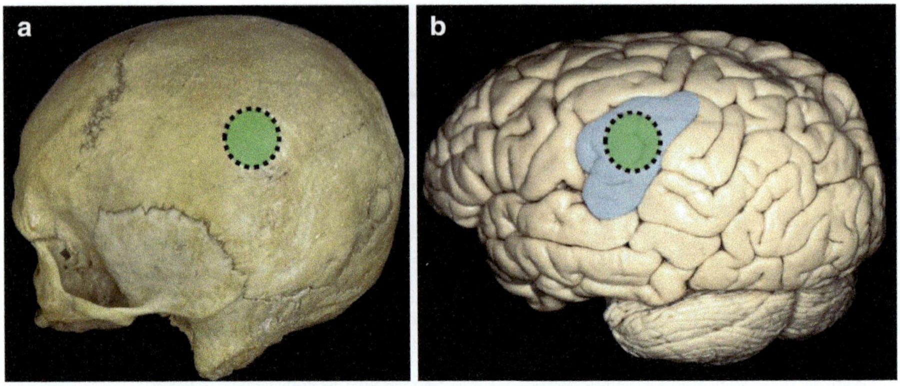

Fig. 5.15 Eurion. The eurion (green circle) is the most prominent point of the parietal boss and corresponds to the supramarginal gyrus (blue)

craniometric point corresponds to the center of the parietal tuberosity and is easily palpated as it is the most prominent cranial area of the parietal region.

5.3 Medial Surface of the Brain

Corpus Callosum
The primary structure for examining the medial surface of the brain is the corpus callosum, which consists of a telencephalic commissure composed of four parts: the rostrum, genu, body, and splenium. The two primary sulci on the medial surface of the brain are situated around the corpus callosum (Fig. 5.16).

Frontal and Parietal Lobes
We will study the frontal and parietal lobes on the medial surface of the brain because the two main horizontal sulci present on this surface (the callosal sulcus and calcarine sulcus) traverse both lobes.

The callosal sulcus surrounds the corpus callosum and is one of the two continuous sulci on the medial surface of the brain. Originating below the rostrum, it acts as a boundary between the corpus callosum and the cingulate gyrus. The cingulate sulcus is parallel to the callosal sulcus and superiorly delimits the cingulate gyrus. During anatomical dissection, it is important to identify that the pericallosal artery is located in the callosal sulcus, while the marginal callosal artery is located in the cingulate sulcus (Fig. 5.17).

The cingulate gyrus wraps around the corpus callosum, bordered by the callosal and cingulate sulci. In the posterior portion of the cingulate gyrus, the gyrus narrows into an isthmus, demarcated anteriorly by the splenium of the corpus callosum and pericallosal artery, inferiorly by the anterior portion of the calcarine sulcus and posterior cerebral artery, and posteriorly by the parieto-occipital sulcus. This

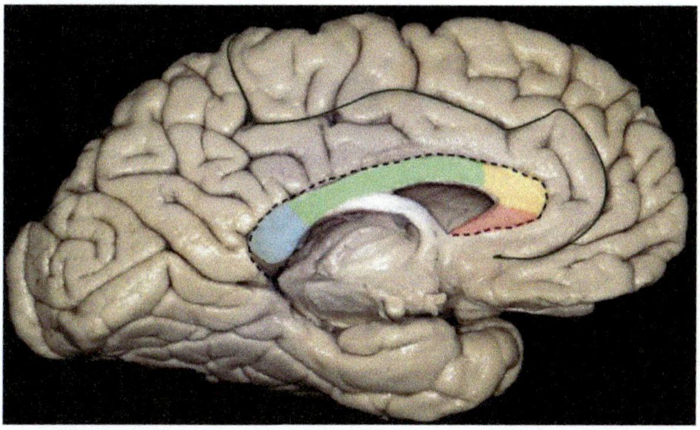

Fig. 5.16 Corpus callosum. Corpus callosum and its portions: rostrum (red), genu (yellow), body (green), and splenium (blue). Callosal sulcus (black dashed line) and cingulate sulcus (black line)

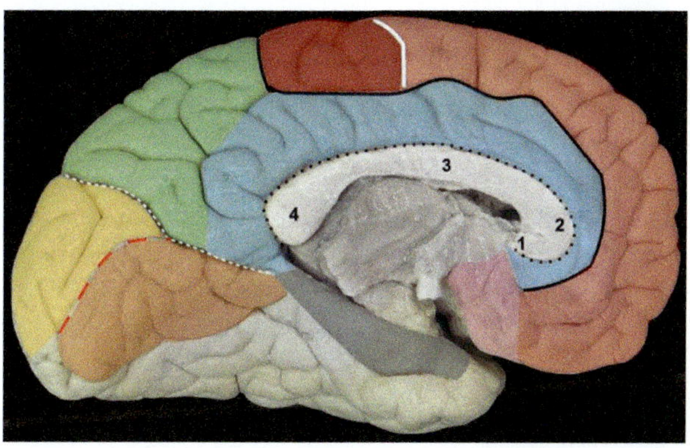

Fig. 5.17 Medial surface of the brain. Corpus callosum (white) and its portions: rostrum (1), genu (2), body (3), and splenium (4). Callosal sulcus (black dashed line), cingulate sulcus, and its marginal branch (black) in an ascending direction. Parieto-occipital sulcus (white dashed line), crossed with the calcarine sulcus (red dashes) in its anterior portion. The gyri on the medial aspect include the medial frontal gyrus (red), paracentral lobule (brown), cingulate gyrus (blue), precuneus or quadrangular lobule (green), cuneus (yellow), lingula of the occipital lobe (orange), parahippocampal gyrus (gray), and parolfactory area (pink)

isthmus marks the medial boundary of the lateral ventricular atrium and is considered a non-eloquent area potentially used for surgical access to the ventricular atrium.

In the posterior portion, the cingulate sulcus is divided into the marginal branch and the subparietal sulcus. The marginal branch, oriented superiorly, aids in anatomically localizing the structures on the medial brain surface by creating an indentation in the postcentral gyrus. Using this reference, we identified the central sulcus, precentral gyrus, central sulcus, and medial aspect of the superior frontal gyrus.

The precentral and postcentral gyri on the medial surface of the brain form the paracentral lobule. This lobule is anteriorly bounded by the paracentral sulcus, posteriorly by the marginal branch of the cingulate sulcus, and inferiorly by the cingulate sulcus.

Posterior to the paracentral lobule lies the quadrangular or precuneus lobe, bounded anteriorly by the marginal branch of the cingulate sulcus, inferiorly by the subparietal sulcus, and posteriorly by the parieto-occipital sulcus, which marks the posterior limit of the parietal lobe.

The parieto-occipital sulcus is a deep sulcus, a significant landmark during laboratory dissection. It is the second continuous sulcus on the medial surface of the brain, extending uninterrupted to the calcarine sulcus. This sulcus separates the parietal lobe from the occipital lobe on the medial surface of the brain, serving as the posterior boundary of the precuneus and the anterior boundary of the cuneus.

Occipital Lobe
The medial surface of the occipital lobe has two important sulci: the parieto-occipital sulcus, which constitutes the anterior limit of the occipital lobe, and the calcarine sulcus.

The calcarine sulcus originates beneath the splenium of the corpus callosum and extends toward the occipital pole. Along its course, the parieto-occipital sulcus divides it into two parts: an anterior portion, non-eloquent part, and a posterior portion, which is integral to the primary visual area. The trajectory of the calcarine sulcus can be used during surgery as a guide during the performance of procedures to access the quadrigeminal lamina cistern and the posterior part of the brainstem.

Situated between the parieto-occipital and calcarine sulci is the cuneiform lobe or cuneus. The lingual gyrus of the occipital lobe lies below the calcarine sulcus.

Temporal Lobe
On the medial surface, the temporal lobe presents a parahippocampal gyrus that is continuous with the isthmus of the cingulate gyrus. It is bound superiorly by the hippocampal sulcus and inferiorly by the collateral sulcus.

The anterior bend of the parahippocampal gyrus is called the uncus, which has a pyramidal shape and is divided into the anterior, apex, and posterior parts, each with important anatomical relationships:

Anterior part of the uncus: covering the amygdaloid body.
Apex of the uncus: medially oriented, related to the oculomotor nerve.
Posterior part of the uncus: covering the head of the hippocampus (Fig. 5.18).

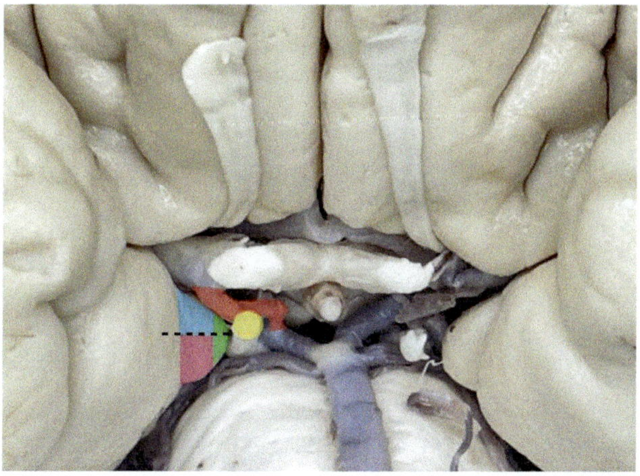

Fig. 5.18 Uncu. The uncus exhibiting a pyramidal shape. The anterior portion (blue) is closely related to the posterior communicating artery (red), while the apex (green) and posterior portion (pink) are closely related to the oculomotor nerve (yellow). The division between the anterior and posterior portions is marked by an imaginary line (black dashed) originating at the apex

5.4 Basal Surface of the Brain

Frontal Lobe

To divide the basal surface of the frontal lobe, the olfactory sulcus, located superior to the olfactory bulb and tract, should initially be identified. The olfactory sulcus lies medially in the straight gyrus and laterally in the orbital gyri. The straight gyrus derives its name from its linear appearance and is positioned atop the cribriform plate of the ethmoid bone, while the orbital gyri appear concave in shape and rest on the roof of the orbit.

The olfactory nerve is a telencephalic projection that extends anteriorly to posteriorly along the olfactory bulb and tract. The olfactory tract bifurcates into the medial and lateral olfactory striae. The olfactory sulcus is covered by the olfactory bulb and tract (Fig. 5.19).

The straight gyrus is continuous with the superior frontal gyrus and connects the basal and medial surfaces of the brain. The orbital gyri are divided into four segments (lateral, medial, anterior, and posterior orbital gyri) by the orbital sulcus, which has an "H"-shaped appearance. The medial orbital gyrus is separated from the straight gyrus by an olfactory sulcus. The lateral orbital gyrus continues along the lateral surface of the brain as an orbital part of the inferior frontal gyrus.

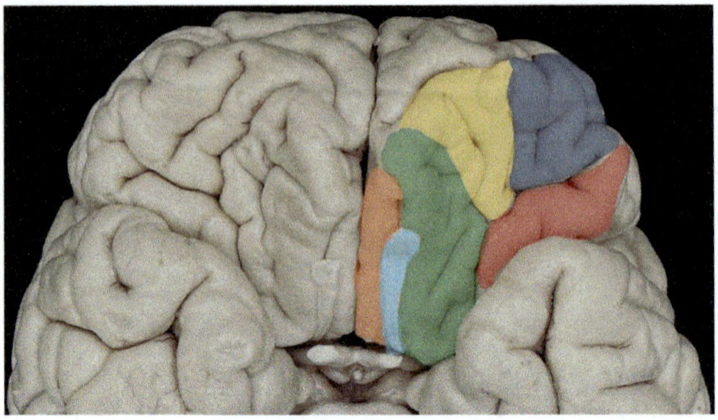

Fig. 5.19 Basal surface of the frontal lobe. Inferior view of the frontal lobe. Straight gyrus (orange); olfactory nerve (light blue); and anterior (yellow), lateral (blue), posterior (red), and medial (green) orbital gyri

Temporal Lobe

The basal surface of the temporal lobe presents two longitudinal sulci (the temporo-occipital sulcus and collateral sulcus), delineating three gyri (the lateral temporo-occipital gyrus, medial temporo-occipital gyrus (fusiform gyrus), and parahippocampal gyrus).

The collateral sulcus is the most medial sulcus on the basal surface of the temporal lobe, continuing posteriorly as the rhinal gyrus and is the only continuous sulcus on the basal surface of the brain. This represents the lateral boundary of the parahippocampal gyrus.

The parahippocampal gyrus occupies the transitional area between the basal and medial surfaces of the temporal lobe. The anterior bend of the parahippocampal gyrus is termed the uncus and is divided into the anterior, apex, and posterior portions. The rhinal incisure separates the anterior border of the uncus, located laterally and medially from the temporal pole (Fig. 5.20).

The temporo-occipital sulcus is located lateral to the collateral sulcus and separates the medial temporo-occipital gyrus from the lateral temporo-occipital gyrus. When the collateral sulcus meets the temporo-occipital sulcus, the gyrus formed between them, instead of being called the medial temporal gyrus, is termed the fusiform gyrus owing to its spindle shape. The lateral occipitotemporal gyrus continues laterally with the inferior temporal sulcus, facilitating communication between the basal and lateral brain surfaces.

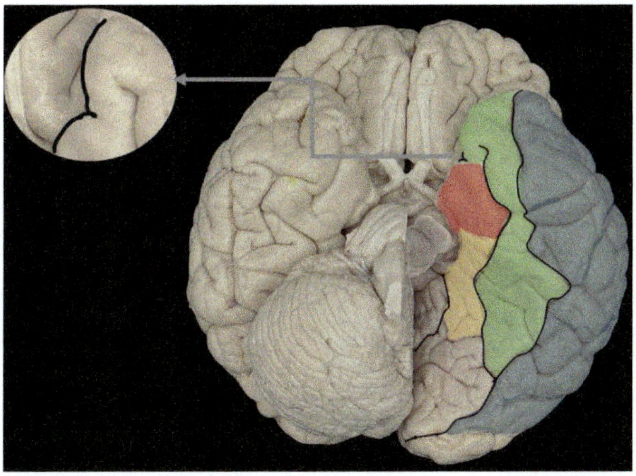

Fig. 5.20 Basal surface of temporal lobe. From the lateral to the medial direction, we observed the inferior temporal gyrus, which on the basal surface is referred to as the lateral occipitotemporal gyrus (yellow), occipitotemporal sulcus (black), medial occipitotemporal or fusiform gyrus (green), collateral sulcus (red), parahippocampal gyrus (blue), calcarine sulcus (orange), and uncus (pink)

Bibliography

1. Chaddad-Neto F, da Costa MDS. Microneuroanatomy and surgery—a practical anatomical guide. 1st ed. Cham: Springer; 2022.
2. Alves RV, Ribas GC, Parraga RG, et al. The occipital lobe convexity sulci and gyri. J Neurosurg. 2012;116(5):1014–23.
3. Ono M, Kubik S, Aberbathey C. Atlas of the cerebral sulci. Stuttgart: Thieme; 1989.
4. Ribas GC. The cerebral sulci and gyri. Neurosurg Focus. 2010;28(2):E2.
5. Ribas GC, Yasuda A, Ribas EC, et al. Surgical anatomy of microneurosurgical sulcal key points. Neurosurgery. 2006;59(4):ONS177–210.
6. Rodrigues TP, Rodrigues MA, Paz Dde A, Costa MD, Centeno RS, Chaddad Neto FE, Cavalheiro S. Orbitofrontal sulcal and gyrus pattern in human: an anatomical study. Arq Neuropsiquiatria. 2015b;73(5):431–5.
7. Rodrigues T, Rodrigues M, Paz D, Costa MD, Santos B, Braga V, Paiva Neto M, Centeno R, Cavalheiro S, Chaddad-Neto F. Is the omega sign a reliable landmark for the neurosurgical team? An anatomical study about the central sulcus region. Arq Neuropsiquiatr. 2015a;73(11):934–8.
8. Ten Donkelaar HJ, Tzourio-Mazoyer N, Mai JK. Toward a common terminology for the gyri and sulci of the human cerebral cortex. Front Neuroanat. 2018;12:93.
9. Effgen EA, Teyssandier M, Giovannini SJM, et al. Anatomical aspects, technical nuances, and a case series of the resection of the inferior temporal gyrus as a strategy to access the basal surface of the temporal lobe and the lateral incisural space. Surg Neurol Int. 2025;16:59. Published 2025 Feb 21. https://doi.org/10.25259/SNI_1016_2024

Chapter 6
Brain Surface White Fibers

6.1 White Matter Anatomy and Principles of High-Definition Fiber Tractography

The myelinated fiber tracts representing the white matter of the brain are classified as association, projection, and commissural fibers.

Short or long association fibers interconnect cortical regions in the same hemisphere. The arcuate bundles, or "U" fibers, are short association fascicles located immediately below the cerebral cortex. The prominent long associative bundles are the cingulum, uncinate fasciculus, occipitofrontal fascicle, and superior, middle, and inferior longitudinal fasciculi.

Projection fibers link the cerebral cortex with the brainstem and spinal cord, shaping the corona radiata and internal capsule.

The commissural fibers traverse the midline and connect the two hemispheres. These fibers consist of the corpus callosum, anterior commissure, and hippocampal commissure.

The use of a combination of dissection techniques and advanced imaging strategies promotes an integrated analysis of the location, design, and trajectory of white matter fibers, even detecting potential functional roles.

Magnetic resonance imaging (MRI) with diffusion tensor imaging (DTI) is a revolutionary imaging technique for various neurological and neurosurgical pathologies.

Originally proposed by Basser in 1994, DTI exploits the diffusion tensor to obtain in vivo brain white matter reconstructions. This technique visually reproduces language, optic, and corticospinal tracts. DTI measures the translational movements of water molecules. The pattern of water propagation in the central nervous system depends on the structural organization of the tissue, which differs significantly between neurons and white matter fibers. Diffusion is defined as isotropic, without a privileged direction, in uniform tissues such as the neuronal

F. Chaddad-Neto, M. D. S. da Costa, *Microneuroanatomy and Lab*,
https://doi.org/10.1007/978-3-031-91026-5_6

bodies. In the white matter, the axons serve as barriers to the diffusion of water molecules, resulting in an anisotropic diffusion in multiple directions, with the maximum coefficient equal to the principal orientation.

The water movement along the main axis was faster than the perpendicular movement, and the DTI analysis was based on the difference between these two movements.

DTI scans are acquired in multiple directions, via tensor decomposition, and extract diffusivities parallel and perpendicular to the fibers (also called main diffusivities, $\lambda//$ and λ). The anisotropic pattern is measured using the apparent diffusion coefficient (the mean of diffusivity) and fractional anisotropy (FA, the normalized standard deviation of diffusivity). The FA was numerically set between 0 and 1 and reflected the degree of anisotropy in the tissue. FA is higher in the white matter, reflecting the quick diffusivity along the fibers, while FA is close to 0 in the gray matter, since the diffusivity is similar in all directions (Fig. 6.1).

DTI data can be employed to create three-dimensional fields, where each vector describes a fiber's orientation. These three-dimensional 3D white matter reconstructions utilize an advanced imaging method known as *tractography*.

Tractography is a three-dimensional modeling technique that visually represents fiber bundles. The structural information provided was unsuitable for grayscale representation; therefore, specific color-coded maps were introduced in 1999. The red-green-blue map assigns color to each orientation of the fibers: Red denotes the left-to-right direction, green denotes the antero-posterior direction, and blue denotes fibers that run in the bottom-up direction. This color-coded scheme displays the fibers in a 3D coordinate system, called "anisotropic map" (Fig. 6.2).

Despite its success in outlining the anatomy and architecture of the white matter, tractography presents significant limitations in spatial resolution. In 2009, the University of Pittsburgh Learning Research and Development Center launched the Pittsburgh Brain Competition to encourage research groups to propose imaging strategies aimed at identifying the components of the visual pathway. The winner, a scholar from Taiwan, represented the Meyer loop using sophisticated mathematical algorithms. The University of Pittsburgh further refined this technique to create

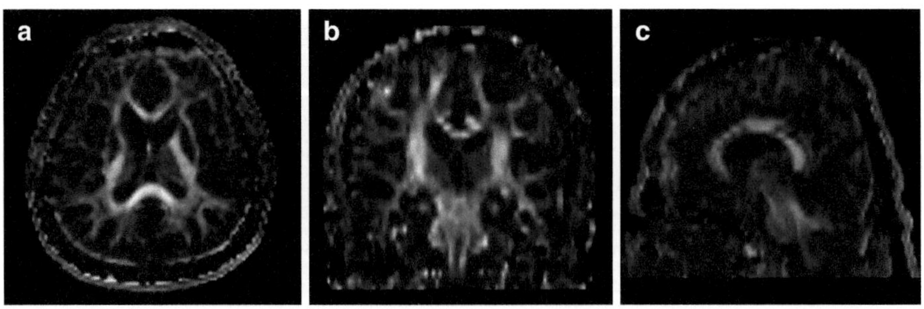

Fig. 6.1 Fractional anisotropy maps based on RMN-diffusion tensor imaging data obtained in the axial (**a**), coronal (**b**), and sagittal (**c**) planes, showing the contrast between the white matter, gray matter, and liquor

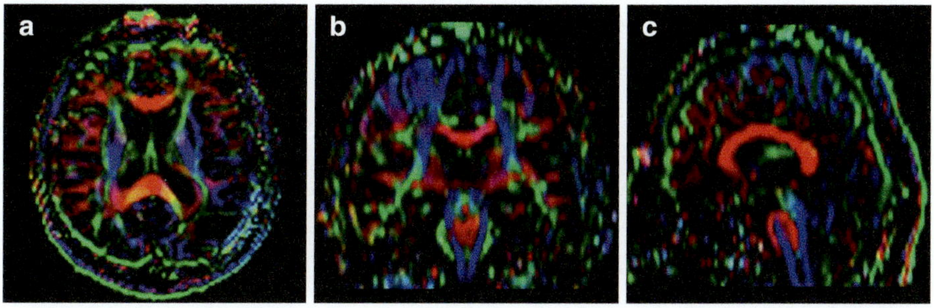

Fig. 6.2 Fractional anisotropy maps based on RMN-DTI data with color coding in the axial (**a**), coronal (**b**), and sagittal (**c**) planes

an innovative high-definition strategy, known as the high-definition fiber tractography (HDFT). HDFT combines DTI data and reconstruction methods developed using computer algorithms and can reproduce fibers with millimeter-level resolution and high definition. This technique overcomes the limitations of a standard DTI by employing indices based on density rather than diffusivity. In addition, HDFT relies on a generalized Q-sampling imaging algorithm, which is a high-resolution angular system that effectively reconstructs multiple orientations of intravoxel fibers.

The HDFT provides an accurate reconstruction of the geometric configuration of the white matter fibers, following the most recent neuroanatomical studies, and allows the distinction of areas of tumor, gliosis, or cerebral edema.

In the context of high-grade glioma surgery, HDFT is helpful for diagnosis, surgical planning, intraoperative strategy, and postoperative evaluation of residual structural connectivity.

6.2 White Matter Anatomy of the Lateral Surface of the Brain

The fiber dissection technique is an invaluable tool for neuroanatomical studies and permits the accurate observation of white matter topography and spatial organization. In 1935, Joseph Klingler promoted a new dissection method, which is still widely used in the present day, advocating for the freezing of specimens beforehand. He relied on the assumption that ice crystals would precipitate between the white matter fasciculi, causing them to expand and separate. This phenomenon facilitates the natural and anatomical splitting of fibers.

The primary dissection instruments include microsurgical tweezers, delicate probes, scalpels, and handmade wooden spatulas of varying tip sizes. Wooden spatulas are extremely useful for peeling away fasciculi and ensuring the safe separation of fibers. Soft wooden spatulas with small, rounded tips permit the precise splitting of extremely thin fibers along the anatomic planes with utmost precision (Fig. 6.3).

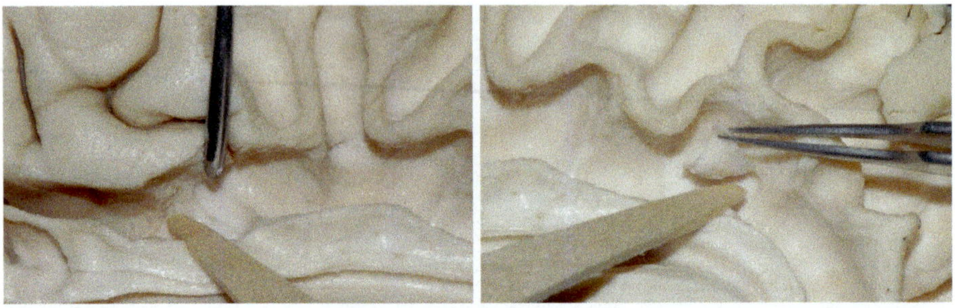

Fig. 6.3 Images of fiber dissection using a soft handmade wooden spatula

Fig. 6.4 Exposure of "U" fibers on the cerebral lateral surface, preserving the central and precentral gyrus

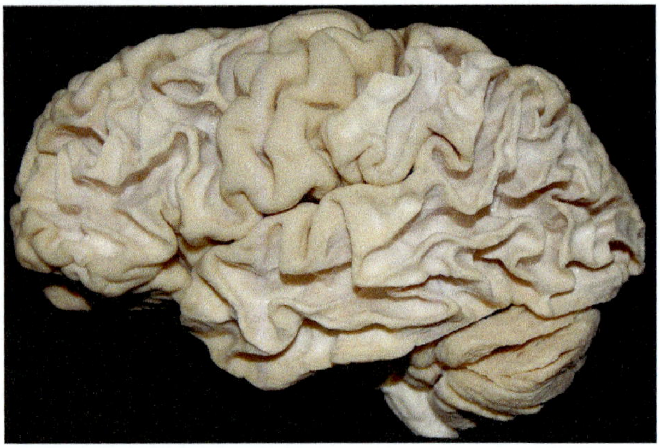

These delicate tools facilitate successful dissection, prevent damage, and reveal the 3D spatial organization of the white matter fasciculi.

The first step of dissection on the cerebral lateral surface involves the removal of the cortical layer to identify short association fibers (Fig. 6.4).

6.3 Longitudinal Association System

The dissection of the "U" fibers, carried out from the middle frontal gyrus and extended to the entire frontal, parietal, and temporal lateral surface, permits the exposition of the *superior longitudinal* fasciculus *(SLF) or arcuate fasciculus.*

The SLF appears as a "C-shaped" bundle, extending around the Sylvian fissure and the insula, and consisting of long fibers connecting between the frontal, parietal, and temporal lobes. This fasciculus is divided into three distinct sections: a

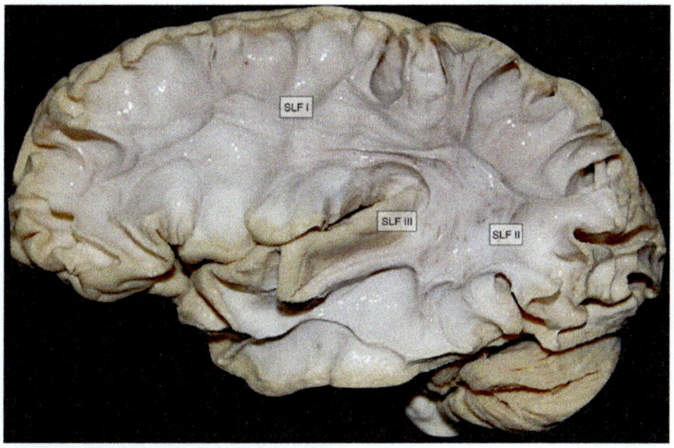

Fig. 6.5 Superior longitudinal fasciculus. Frontoparietal segment (SLF I), temporoparietal segment (SLF II), and frontotemporal/arcuate segment (SLF III)

horizontal or frontoparietal segment (SLF I), which connects the superior and middle frontal lobes to the inferior parietal lobe; a vertical segment; and an arcuate segment. The vertical, or temporoparietal (SLF II), consists of a well-defined group of vertically oriented fibers running between the inferior parietal region and the superior and middle temporal gyri.

In the deeper regions of the temporoparietal area, a cluster of fibers arranged around the posterior peri-insular sulcus can be distinguished, forming connections between the posterior temporal region and the prefrontal area. These fibers collectively constitute the frontotemporal or arcuate segments (SLF III).

The SLF is functionally related to motor control, awareness, and visuospatial attention. In the dominant hemisphere, the arcuate fasciculus connects Broca's area to Wernicke's area, facilitating various functions related to language, motor, and praxis (Fig. 6.5).

The subcortical region of the superior temporal gyrus, the *middle longitudinal* fasciculus *(MLF)*, was observed. The MLF consists of fibers running from the temporal lobe to the inferior parietal lobe, mainly the angular gyrus. The MLF encloses the anterior and posterior components, which can be distinguished at the posteromedial aspect of the anterior transverse temporal gyrus (Heschl). The MLF plays a role in speech, attention, auditory reception, and sound memory.

Removal of the "U" fibers of the inferior temporal lobe exposes a group of fibers lying beneath the SLF II. These fibers extend posteriorly from the temporal pole to the occipital lobe and constitute the superficial and dorsal portion of the temporo-occipital bundle or *inferior longitudinal* fasciculus (*dILF*). The dILF connects the superior, middle, and inferior occipital gyri to the anterior and temporal poles. Considering the ILF cortical endpoints of the occipital and temporal visual associative areas, this fasciculus is functionally associated with visual memory, facial recognition, visual perception, and language (Fig. 6.6).

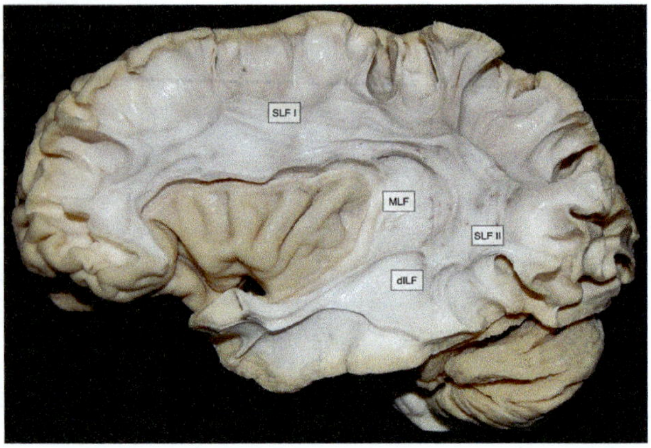

Fig. 6.6 Superior (SLF), middle (MLF), and dorsal inferior (dILF) longitudinal fasciculi

6.4 Insula

The complete removal of the opercular area reveals an insular surface. The triangular-shaped insular lobe is divided by a central sulcus into an anterior surface, comprising the short gyri, and a posterior surface, consisting of the long gyri. The short turns converge at the insular pole on the anteroinferior edge, while the long turns merge with the limen insulae. The limen insulae are located at the sphenoidal and operculoinsular junctions of the Sylvian fissure and extend from the temporal pole to the orbital surface of the frontal lobe (Fig. 6.7).

The dissection of the insular cortex exposes the *extreme capsule*, a white matter bundle of the associative fibers. The extreme capsule is divided into two distinct areas: the posterosuperior-dorsal and anteroinferior-ventral regions. The dorsal part is formed by a thin layer of fibers connecting the insula to the frontal, parietal, and temporal opercula. The removal of these fibers reveals the gray matter of the dorsal claustrum.

The ventral portion of the extreme capsule is formed by two layers: a superficial layer, composed of short fibers that link the insula to the frontal and temporal opercula, and a deeper layer. The latter is the most external component of the *uncinate fasciculus* (*UF*) and *inferior frontal-occipital fasciculus* (iFOF), which crosses the ventral component of the claustrum (Fig. 6.8).

The removal of the dorsal extreme capsule uncovers the *posterosuperior external capsule* and the dorsal claustrum at the level of the insular apex. Instead, the progressive dissection of the extreme ventral fibers highlights the ventral claustrum, iFOF, and UF of the limen [6].

The gray matter of the claustrum is a network of cortical and subcortical circuits involved in multiple functions related to the sphere of conscious sensation.

The external capsule is described as a layer of fibers located between the claustrum and putamen with associative functions. The dissection of the external capsule

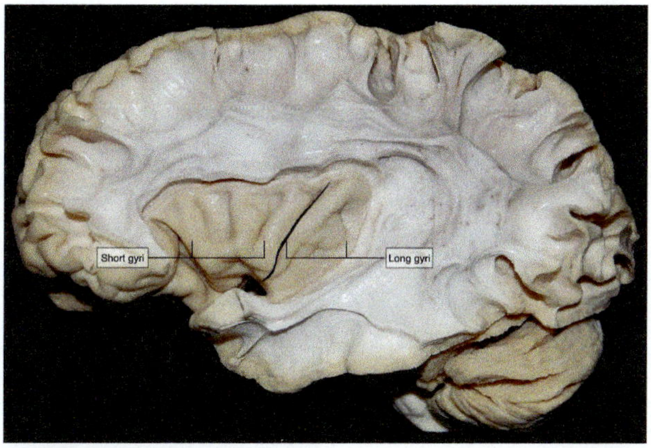

Fig. 6.7 Lateral surface of the insula

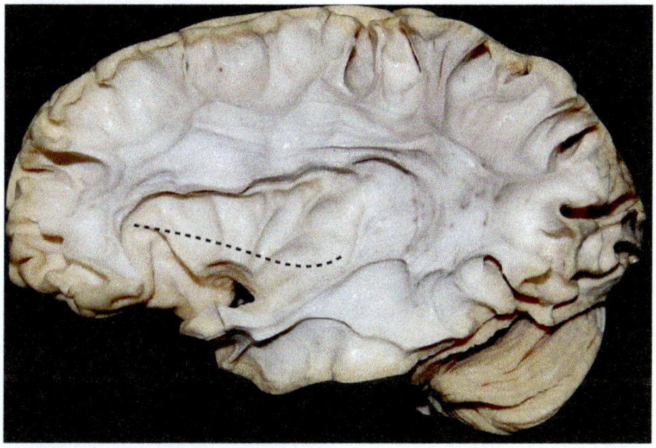

Fig. 6.8 Extreme capsule. The dotted line separates the posterior/dorsal region from the anteroinferior/ventral one

from the periphery in the centripetal direction shows that most of the capsule converged and merged with the dorsal claustrum. In the ventral claustrum, the extreme and external capsules overlap with the UF and iFOF. In the limen, these are integral components of the external capsule (Fig. 6.9).

The UF is an associative fiber involved in emotional processes and language functions. It traverses the insular limen and connects the fronto-orbital cortex to the temporal pole and the anterior portions of the superior and middle temporal gyri.

The iFOF is a long bundle of associative fibers that link the orbitofrontal cortex and occipital lobe from the basal portion of the insula above the FU. The occipital lobe runs parallel to the ILF above the optic radiation. In the temporal lobe, it merges with the FU and the external capsule, forming a double fan corresponding to the limen insulae. The iFOF contributes to various cognitive processes including reading, semantic aspects of language, attention, and visual elaboration.

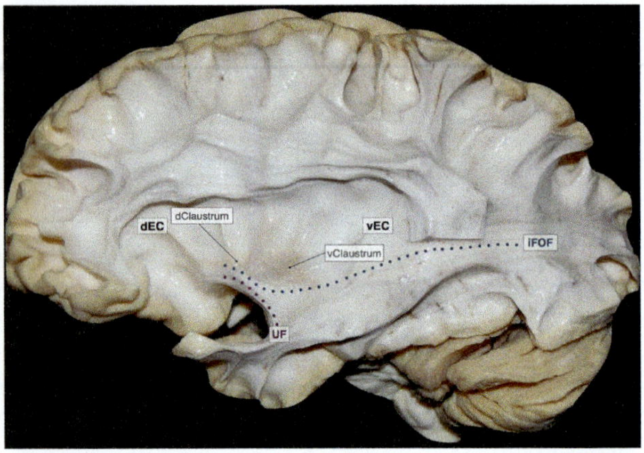

Fig. 6.9 External capsule. *D* dorsal, *EC* external capsule, *iFOF* inferior frontal-occipital fasciculus (blue dotted line), *UF* uncinate fasciculus (purple dotted line), *v* ventral

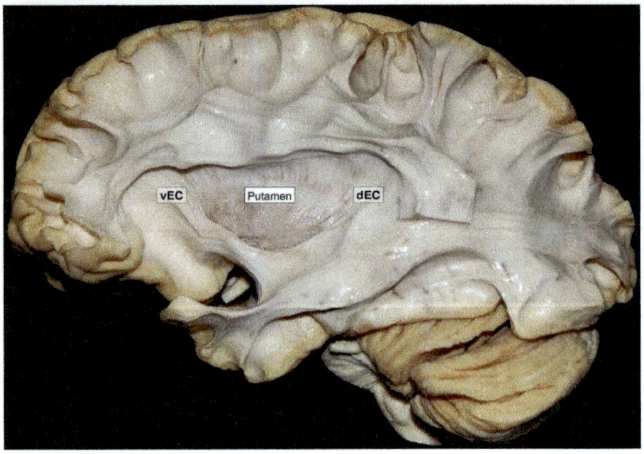

Fig. 6.10 Putamen. *d*,dorsal, *EC* external capsule, *v* ventral

6.5 Basal Ganglia

The lateral surface of the putamen was exposed by dissecting the claustrum and external capsule (Fig. 6.10).

The spongy surface of the putamen was removed, and the globus pallidus was discernible. A thin layer of white substance is located between these two nuclei, which is the external medullary lamina.

After finalizing the dissection of the SLF, the *internal capsule* was continuously exposed along with the *corona radiata*.

The resection of the putamen completely exposes the *internal capsule*. This part consists of white projecting fibers ascending from the thalamus to the cerebral cortex and descending from the frontoparietal cortex to the nuclei of the base and brainstem. At the upper edge of the putamen, along the superior limiting sulcus of the insula, the internal capsule joins the external capsule and forms the *corona radiata*.

The corona radiata projects these fibers to the frontal and parietal lobes, where they merge with the callous fibers to form the central semiovale.

The internal capsule consists of an anterior limb located between the lenticular nucleus and head of the caudate, the genu at the apex of the lenticular nucleus, a posterior limb between the lenticular nucleus and thalamus, and the retrolenticular and sublenticular portions located behind and below the lenticular nucleus.

From a functional point of view, the anterior limb is composed of the frontopontine and thalamic frontal fibers (anterior thalamic radiation). The latter connects the thalamus with the prefrontal cortex and cingulate gyrus, following an oblique orientation and anteroposterior direction. The fibers of the anterior limb are associated with cognitive functions, emotional processing, and decision-making.

In the anterior half of the posterior limb, the corticospinal, corticorubral, and corticopontine fibers can be found. The corticospinal tract originates from the primary motor cortex and premotor areas and constitutes the motor pathway [45]. The corticopontine fibers originate from all areas of the cerebral cortex, ascend to the cerebellum, and terminate in the pontine nuclei, coordinating voluntary motor functions. The corticorubral fibers arise from the primary motor and sensory areas and terminate in the red core.

The posterior third of the posterior limb contains the primary somatosensory connections from the thalamus to the primary sensory area of the postcentral gyrus.

The anterior and posterior limbs converge at right angles, forming the genu. The genu includes the thalamic precentral fibers (superior thalamic radiation) and corticobulbars. These connections link the precentral cortex to the motor nuclei of cranial nerves. Notably, the corticobulbar tract controls the cranial nerves, the movement of facial muscles, chewing, and swallowing.

The retrolenticular portion of the internal capsule is composed of the parietal, temporal, and occipital-pontine fibers, facilitating connections between the pulvinar of the thalamus, parieto-occipital cortex, and optic radiation fibers, which link the lateral geniculate nucleus to the calcarine fissure (posterior thalamic radiation).

The sublenticular part contains the Meyer loop fibers and auditory radiation. These fibers originate from the medial geniculate body of the thalamus and terminate in the transverse temporal gyrus of Heschl (Fig. 6.11).

Tractography enables the identification of different portions of the internal capsule, represented by different color codes (Fig. 6.12).

The anterior commissure was exposed by extending the dissection through the UF and iFOF removal. The *anterior commissure*, located in the Gratiolet's canal, was found below the globus pallidus and medial to the UF (Fig. 6.13).

The anterior commissure is formed by the anterior crus, which connects the olfactory systems of the two hemispheres, forming the olfactory commissure, and the posterior crus. The latter is further subdivided into the temporal tract, which merges with the uncinate fasciculus to the temporal pole, and the occipital tract, which is directed posteriorly toward the *sagittal stratum*.

The anterior commissure is a critical interhemispherical connection between the medial temporal lobes, and its occipital extension is involved in the transmission of olfactory, auditory, and visual information [20].

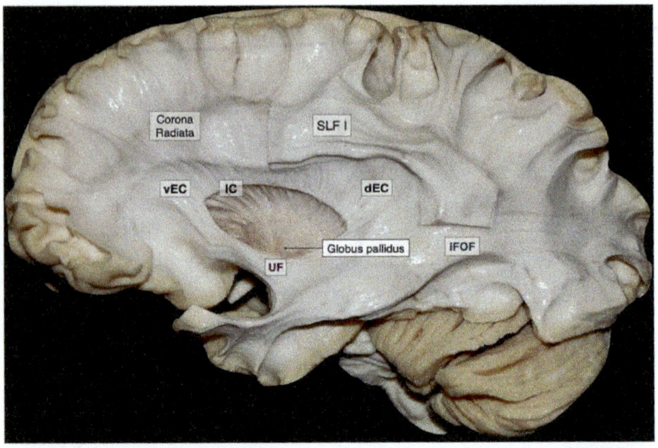

Fig. 6.11 Internal capsule. *d* dorsal, *EC* external capsule, *iFOF* inferior frontal-occipital fasciculus (blue dotted line), *IC* internal capsule, *SLF* superior longitudinal fasciculus, *UF* uncinate fasciculus (purple dotted line), *v* ventral

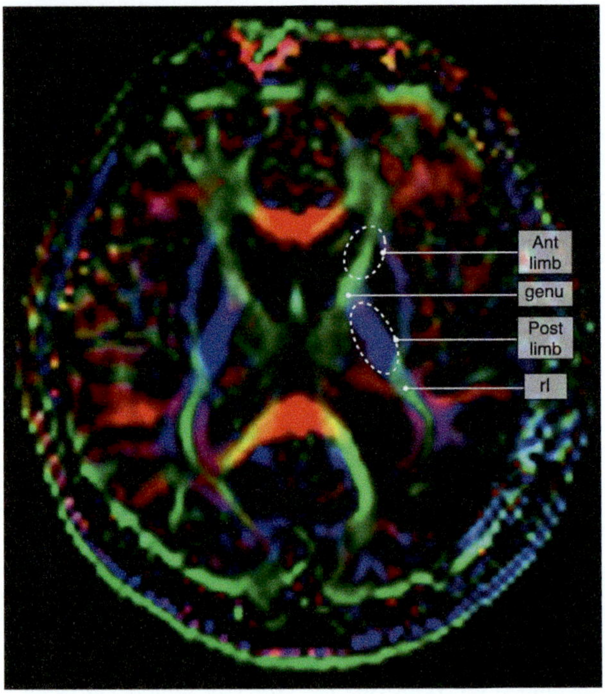

Fig. 6.12 Color-coded diffusion tensor imaging map in the axial plane, showing the components of the internal capsule. Ant, anterior; post, posterior; rt., retrolenticular part

The removal of the internal capsule exposes the thalamus and caudate nucleus. The caudate nucleus wraps around the thalamus and is divided into the head, body, and tail. The head of the caudate nucleus is located on the lateral wall of the frontal horn of the lateral ventricle, the lateral wall of the body of the lateral ventricle, and the tail of the roof of the temporal horn. The anterior part of the thalamus is located on the floor of the body of the lateral ventricle, while the posterior part is located on the anterior wall of the atrium and superomedial side of the temporal horn.

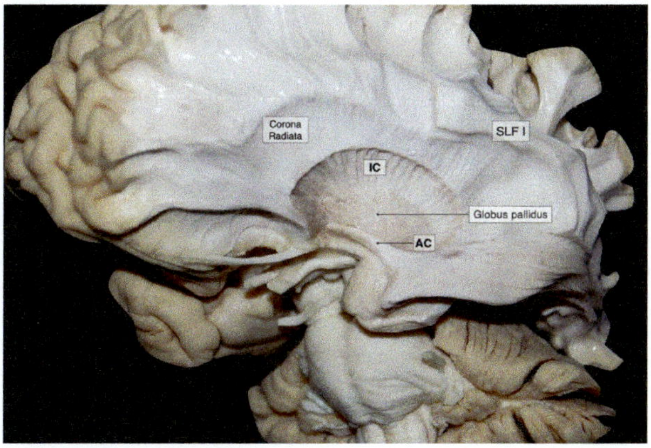

Fig. 6.13 Anterior commissure. *AC* anterior commissure, *IC* internal capsule, *SLF* superior longitudinal fasciculus

6.6 Sagittal Stratum and Visual System

The *sagittal stratum*, which is formed by white matter fibers, is composed of three layers. The superficial layer consists of the MLF and ILF, the middle layer is entirely made up of the iFOF, and the deeper layer consists of optic radiation, part of the ILF, the retrolenticular component of the internal capsule, and the fibers of the anterior commissure.

The *optic tract* consists of contralateral nasal and homolateral temporal fibers. A vast majority of the fibers in the optic tract reach the lateral geniculate body, while only a small portion is directed toward the pulvinar, pretectal nucleus, and upper colliculus. The *optic radiation* arises from the lateral geniculate body and reaches the visual cortex at the upper and lower lips of the calcarine fissures. The optic radiation comprises fibers that carry visual information from the ipsilateral nasal and contralateral temporal retinal halves. Conventionally, the optic radiation is divided into three portions. The anterior component is known as the Meyer loop. It follows an anterolateral trajectory along the roof of the temporal horn, lateral to the amygdala. Anterior to the temporal horn, the fibers form a loop lateral to the temporal horn and traverse through the sublenticular portion of the external capsule, ultimately terminating along the lower lip of the calcarine fissure.

The central part of the optic radiation initially follows the lateral direction through the upper roof of the temporal horn. It then assumed a posterior trend, passing above and through the ILF and ending at the occipital pole. The posterior bundle of the lateral geniculate body crosses the retrolenticular portion of the internal capsule and reaches the sagittal stratum. These fibers form the lateral wall of the atrium and the occipital horn of the lateral ventricle, terminating along the upper lip of the calcarine fissure.

The dissection of the sagittal stratum exposes the tapetum. These vertical corpus callosum fibers cover the superior and lateral walls of the atrium and temporal horn and separate the optic radiation from the ependyma of the lateral ventricle (Fig. 6.14).

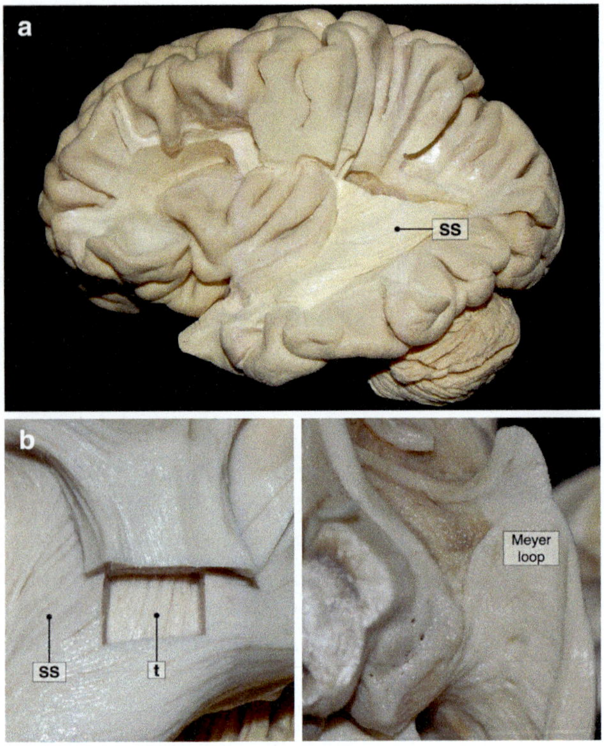

Fig. 6.14 (**a**) Sagittal stratum. (**b**) Section showing the horizontal fibers of the sagittal stratum and the tapetum running vertically. *SS* sagittal stratum, *t* tapetum

6.7 Corticospinal Tract and Medial Lemniscus

Fasciculi extending from the cerebral peduncle to the brainstem were identified on the lateral brain surface. The cerebral peduncles and ventral portions of the midbrain include fibers that connect the cerebral cortex to the nuclei of the pons, cerebellum, and spinal cord. Among these structures are the frontopontine fasciculi, which originate from the frontal lobe and traverse into the anterior limb of the internal capsule to the pons nuclei, temporopontine fibers, and pyramidal system. The pyramidal system consists of a corticobulbar tract, directed to the nuclei of the brainstem, and the corticospinal tract.

The *corticospinal tract* originates from the primary and supplementary motor areas; traverses through the corona radiata, the posterior half of the posterior limb of the internal capsule, and the cerebral peduncles up to the brainstem; and descends into the spinal cord through the pyramidal decussation [49] (Fig. 6.15).

The HDFT enables the delineation of the ascending dorsal fibers posterior to the corticospinal tract, which transmits information related to tactile, proprioceptive, and thermal-dolorific sensitivity. The *primary somatosensory ascending tracts*

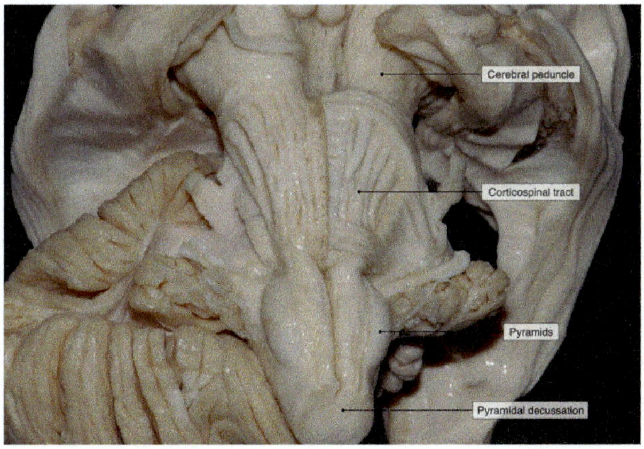

Fig. 6.15 Corticospinal tract

originate in the dorsal columns of the spinal cord and extend through the brainstem to the medial and lateral ventral-posterior thalamic nuclei, forming the *medial lemniscus*. Subsequently, they traverse through the anterior portion of the posterior limb of the internal capsule and terminate in the somatosensory cortex of the postcentral gyrus.

6.8 Thalamic Radiations

The HDFT technique enables the precise identification of thalamic radiation fibers. Thalamic radiations are thalamic-cortical projection tracts consisting of both afferent and efferent fibers. They originate in the thalamus, traverse the internal capsule and the corona radiata, and terminate in specific cortical areas.

The anterior thalamic radiation connects the dorsomedial, dorsolateral, and anterior nuclei to the prefrontal cortex through the anterior limb of the internal capsule. This pathway is implicated in praxis and motor planning.

The superior thalamic radiation connects the ventral thalamic nuclei to the motor and somatosensory cortices through the upper thalamic peduncle, posterior limb, genu of the internal capsule, and corona radiata.

Meanwhile, the inferior radiation connects the thalamus to the temporal lobe, insula, and ventral portion of the frontal lobe through the inferior thalamic peduncle and sublenticular part of the internal capsule. Finally, the posterior thalamic radiation connects the caudal nuclei of the thalamus to the parietal and occipital lobes via the posterior thalamic peduncle. Notably, this pathway includes fibers from the posterior part of the optic radiation.

6.9 From the Bench to the Bedside: Role of HDFT in Planning, Intraoperative Strategy, and Follow-Up

A detailed anatomical description derived following a white matter dissection serves as the foundational step for adapting and validating the use of HDFT in surgery.

In neurosurgical practice, HDFT is useful for diagnosis, surgical planning, intraoperative strategy, and postoperative evaluation of residual structural connectivity. This technique allows the early analysis of fiber integrity and its relationship with the lesion, allowing the identification of eloquent regions, the corticospinal tract, the optic radiation, and the language area. Immediate access to connectivity information streamlines the planning process, simplifies the selection of the surgical trajectory, and minimizes the risk of damage to adjacent fibers.

Beyond structural analysis of the surgical target, tractography permits qualitative and quantitative studies of the surrounding white matter. The growth pattern and intrinsic heterogeneity of brain lesions induce significant perilesional changes. Extra-axial tumors and vascular lesions cause dislocation of adjacent fibers, while malignant and intra-axial tumors alter nearby structures depending on the histopathological grade [60, 61]. High-grade gliomas, which are associated with extensive areas of necrosis and edema, can cause displacement, disruption, or destruction of adjacent white matter.

In 2004, Lu et al. introduced the tumor infiltration index, which distinguishes the neoplastic area from perilesional edema. This index measures the FA variation in the transition areas from neoplastic cells to edema, facilitating the delineation of tumor architecture and its relationships with adjacent structures before surgery.

Therefore, tractography is an important intraoperative technique. HDFT data applied in vivo during surgery maximize the extent of resection, improve patient life expectancy, and limit damage to adjacent fibers. Preoperative reconstructions can also be integrated with the neuronavigation workstation, ensuring continuous and updated navigation to provide real and three-dimensional visualization of white matter fasciculi and their relationships with anatomical structures. Tractography can be integrated with multiple sources of real data, such as microscopy, endoscopy, in vivo fluorescent dyes, cortical/subcortical stimulation, and mapping techniques. The integration of these advanced intraoperative tools facilitates lesion resection and improves functional outcomes.

During follow-up, the HDFT proved to be particularly helpful for the postoperative evaluation of residual structural connectivity. Quantitative parameters, such as FA, are useful for identifying the nature of the damage and formulating prognostic hypotheses related to the reversibility of associated neurological deficits.

Accordingly, the pre-, intra-, and postoperative identification of white matter fibers and awareness of their spatial orientation are pivotal to refining and tailoring the surgical technique, while also adjusting the approach to each patient's unique anatomy to ensure optimal therapeutic outcomes.

In recent years, augmented reality has transitioned from a futuristic concept to an integrated tool in clinical practice. DTI has been applied to various neurological pathologies including developmental disorders, congenital abnormalities, psychiatric pathologies, schizophrenia, demyelinating and neurodegenerative diseases, multiple sclerosis, amyotrophic lateral sclerosis, and stroke.

The literature demonstrates the tremendous value of tractography in quantifying the physiopathological changes in the central nervous system.

In the future, advancements in neuroimaging techniques and the adoption of probabilistic tracking algorithms will facilitate more precise microscopic mapping of cellular architecture and fiber tracts. These advances will allow DTI to be fully included in surgical practice as a tool for diagnosis and an avant-garde therapeutic strategy.

Bibliography

1. Türe U, Yaşargil MG, Friedman AH, Al-Mefty O. Fiber dissection technique: lateral aspect of the brain. Neurosurgery. 2000;47:417–26.; discussion 426–417,. https://doi.org/10.1097/00006123-200008000-00028.
2. Basser PJ, Pajevic S, Pierpaoli C, Duda J, Aldroubi A. In vivo fiber tractography using DT-MRI data. Magn Reson Med. 2000;44:625–32. https://doi.org/10.1002/1522-2594(200010)44:4<625::aid-mrm17>3.0.co;2-o.
3. Mori S. Two and Three-dimensional Analyses of Brain White Matter Architecture Using Diffusion Imaging. CNS Spectrums. 2002;7:529–34. https://doi.org/10.1017/S1092852900018083.
4. Basser PJ, Mattiello J, LeBihan D. Estimation of the effective self-diffusion tensor from the NMR spin echo. J Magn Reson B. 1994;103:247–54. https://doi.org/10.1006/jmrb.1994.1037.
5. Basser PJ, Mattiello J, LeBihan D. MR diffusion tensor spectroscopy and imaging. Biophys J. 1994;66:259–67. https://doi.org/10.1016/s0006-3495(94)80775-1.
6. Catani M, Howard RJ, Pajevic S, Jones DK. Virtual in vivo interactive dissection of white matter fasciculi in the human brain. Neuroimage. 2002;17:77–94. https://doi.org/10.1006/nimg.2002.1136.
7. Catani M, Jones DK, ffytche, D.H. Perisylvian language networks of the human brain. Ann Neurol. 2005;57:8–16. https://doi.org/10.1002/ana.20319.
8. Mori S, van Zijl PC. Fiber tracking: principles and strategies – a technical review. NMR Biomed. 2002;15:468–80. https://doi.org/10.1002/nbm.781.
9. Pierpaoli C, Jezzard P, Basser PJ, Barnett A, Di Chiro G. Diffusion tensor MR imaging of the human brain. Radiology. 1996;201:637–48. https://doi.org/10.1148/radiology.201.3.8939209.
10. Lope-Piedrafita S. Diffusion Tensor Imaging (DTI). Methods Mol Biol. 2018;1718:103–16. https://doi.org/10.1007/978-1-4939-7531-0_7.
11. Alexander AL, Lee JE, Lazar M, Field AS. Diffusion tensor imaging of the brain. Neurotherapeutics. 2007;4:316–29. https://doi.org/10.1016/j.nurt.2007.05.011.
12. Catani M, de Schotten MT. Atlas of Human Brain Connections. Oxford: OUP; 2012.
13. Filler A. The history, development and impact of computed imaging in neurological diagnosis and neurosurgery: CT, MRI, and DTI. Internet J Neurosurg. 2010;7:1–85. https://doi.org/10.1038/npre.2009.3267.5.
14. Pajevic S, Pierpaoli C. Color schemes to represent the orientation of anisotropic tissues from diffusion tensor data: application to white matter fiber tract mapping in the human brain. Magn Reson Med. 1999;42:526–40.

15. Fernandez-Miranda JC, Pathak S, Engh J, Jarbo K, Verstynen T, Yeh FC, Wang Y, Mintz A, Boada F, Schneider W, et al. High-definition fiber tractography of the human brain: neuroanatomical validation and neurosurgical applications. Neurosurgery. 2012;71:430–53. https://doi.org/10.1227/NEU.0b013e3182592faa.
16. Wedeen VJ, Wang RP, Schmahmann JD, Benner T, Tseng WY, Dai G, Pandya DN, Hagmann P, D'Arceuil H, de Crespigny AJ. Diffusion spectrum magnetic resonance imaging (DSI) tractography of crossing fibers. Neuroimage. 2008;41:1267–77. https://doi.org/10.1016/j.neuroimage.2008.03.036.
17. Yeh FC, Wedeen VJ, Tseng WY. Generalized q-sampling imaging. IEEE Trans Med Imaging. 2010;29:1626–35. https://doi.org/10.1109/tmi.2010.2045126.
18. Yeh FC, Wedeen VJ, Tseng WY. Estimation of fiber orientation and spin density distribution by diffusion deconvolution. Neuroimage. 2011;55:1054–62. https://doi.org/10.1016/j.neuroimage.2010.11.087.
19. Verstynen T, Jarbo K, Pathak S, Schneider W. In vivo mapping of microstructural somatotopies in the human corticospinal pathways. J Neurophysiol. 2011;105:336–46. https://doi.org/10.1152/jn.00698.2010.
20. Fernández-Miranda JC, Rhoton AL Jr, Alvarez-Linera J, Kakizawa Y, Choi C, de Oliveira EP. Three-dimensional microsurgical and tractographic anatomy of the white matter of the human brain. Neurosurgery. 2008;62:989–1026.; discussion 1026–1028,. https://doi.org/10.1227/01.neu.0000333767.05328.49.
21. Nimsky C, Ganslandt O, Hastreiter P, Wang R, Benner T, Sorensen AG, Fahlbusch R. Preoperative and intraoperative diffusion tensor imaging-based fiber tracking in glioma surgery. Neurosurgery. 2005;56:130–7.; discussion 138. https://doi.org/10.1227/01.neu.0000144842.18771.30.
22. Nimsky C, Ganslandt O, Fahlbusch R. Implementation of fiber tract navigation. Neurosurgery. 2007;61:306–17.; discussion 317–308. https://doi.org/10.1227/01.neu.0000279224.83998.7d.
23. Abdullah KG, Lubelski D, Nucifora PG, Brem S. Use of diffusion tensor imaging in glioma resection. Neurosurg Focus. 2013;34:E1. https://doi.org/10.3171/2013.1.Focus12412.
24. Brunberg JA, Chenevert TL, McKeever PE, Ross DA, Junck LR, Muraszko KM, Dauser R, Pipe JG, Betley AT. In vivo MR determination of water diffusion coefficients and diffusion anisotropy: correlation with structural alteration in gliomas of the cerebral hemispheres. AJNR Am J Neuroradiol. 1995;16:361–71.
25. Henderson F, Abdullah KG, Verma R, Brem S. Tractography and the connectome in neurosurgical treatment of gliomas: the premise, the progress, and the potential. Neurosurg Focus. 2020;48:E6. https://doi.org/10.3171/2019.11.Focus19785.
26. Luzzi S, Giotta Lucifero A, Martinelli A, Maestro MD, Savioli G, Simoncelli A, Lafe E, Preda L, Galzio R. Supratentorial high-grade gliomas: maximal safe anatomical resection guided by augmented reality high-definition fiber tractography and fluorescein. Neurosurg Focus. 2021;51:E5. https://doi.org/10.3171/2021.5.Focus21185.
27. Klingler J. Erleichterung der makroskopischen Präparation des Gehirns durch den Gefrierprozess. Schweiz Arch Neurol Psychiatr. 1935;36:247–56.
28. Klingler J, Gloor P. The connections of the amygdala and of the anterior temporal cortex in the human brain. J Comp Neurol. 1960;115:333–69. https://doi.org/10.1002/cne.901150305.
29. Ludwig, E. Klingler, J. Atlas cerebri humani.
30. Koutsarnakis C, Liakos F, Kalyvas AV, Sakas DE, Stranjalis G. A laboratory manual for stepwise cerebral white matter fiber dissection. World Neurosurg. 2015;84:483–93. https://doi.org/10.1016/j.wneu.2015.04.018.
31. Peris-Celda M, Martinez-Soriano F, Rhoton AL. Rhoton's Atlas of head, neck, and brain: 2D and 3D images. Thieme; 2017.
32. Makris N, Kennedy DN, McInerney S, Sorensen AG, Wang R, Caviness VS Jr, Pandya DN. Segmentation of subcomponents within the superior longitudinal fascicle in humans: a quantitative, in vivo, DT-MRI study. Cereb Cortex. 2005;15:854–69. https://doi.org/10.1093/cercor/bhh186.

33. Schmahmann J, Pandya D. Fiber pathways of the brain, vol. xviii; 2006.
34. Glasser MF, Rilling JK. DTI tractography of the human brain's language pathways. Cereb Cortex. 2008;18:2471–82. https://doi.org/10.1093/cercor/bhn011.
35. Makris N, Papadimitriou GM, Kaiser JR, Sorg S, Kennedy DN, Pandya DN. Delineation of the middle longitudinal fascicle in humans: a quantitative, in vivo, DT-MRI study. Cereb Cortex. 2009;19:777–85. https://doi.org/10.1093/cercor/bhn124.
36. De Witt Hamer PC, Moritz-Gasser S, Gatignol P, Duffau H. Is the human left middle longitudinal fascicle essential for language? A brain electrostimulation study. Hum Brain Mapp. 2011;32:962–73. https://doi.org/10.1002/hbm.21082.
37. Catani M, Jones DK, Donato R, Ffytche DH. Occipito-temporal connections in the human brain. Brain. 2003;126:2093–107. https://doi.org/10.1093/brain/awg203.
38. Catani M, Thiebaut de Schotten M. A diffusion tensor imaging tractography atlas for virtual in vivo dissections. Cortex. 2008;44:1105–32. https://doi.org/10.1016/j.cortex.2008.05.004.
39. Türe U, Yaşargil DC, Al-Mefty O, Yaşargil MG. Topographic anatomy of the insular region. J Neurosurg. 1999;90:720–33. https://doi.org/10.3171/jns.1999.90.4.0720.
40. Catani M, Mesulam M. The arcuate fasciculus and the disconnection theme in language and aphasia: history and current state. Cortex. 2008;44:953–61. https://doi.org/10.1016/j.cortex.2008.04.002.
41. Doricchi F, Thiebaut de Schotten M, Tomaiuolo F, Bartolomeo P. White matter (dis)connections and gray matter (dys)functions in visual neglect: gaining insights into the brain networks of spatial awareness. Cortex. 2008;44:983–95. https://doi.org/10.1016/j.cortex.2008.03.006.
42. Costa M, Braga VL, Yağmurlu K, Centeno RS, Cavalheiro S, Chaddad-Neto F. A Technical Guide for Fiber Tract Dissection of the Internal Capsule. Turk Neurosurg. 2018;28:934–9. https://doi.org/10.5137/1019-5149.Jtn.20884-17.1.
43. Emos MC, Khan Suheb MZ, Agarwal SN. Internal Capsule. In: StatPearls. Treasure Island (FL): StatPearls Publishing. Copyright © 2023, StatPearls Publishing LLC; 2023.
44. Safadi Z, Grisot G, Jbabdi S, Behrens TE, Heilbronner SR, McLaughlin NCR, Mandeville J, Versace A, Phillips ML, Lehman JF, et al. Functional Segmentation of the Anterior Limb of the Internal Capsule: Linking White Matter Abnormalities to Specific Connections. J Neurosci. 2018;38:2106–17. https://doi.org/10.1523/jneurosci.2335-17.2017.
45. Qian C, Tan F. Internal capsule: The homunculus distribution in the posterior limb. Brain Behav. 2017;7:e00629. https://doi.org/10.1002/brb3.629.
46. Tredici G, Barajon I, Pizzini G, Sanguineti I. The organization of corticopontine fibres in man. Acta Anat (Basel). 1990;137:320–3. https://doi.org/10.1159/000146902.
47. Younes K, Hasan KM, Kamali A, McGough CE, Keser Z, Hasan O, Melicher T, Kramer LA, Schulz PE. Diffusion Tensor Imaging of the Superior Thalamic Radiation and Cerebrospinal Fluid Distribution in Idiopathic Normal Pressure Hydrocephalus. J Neuroimaging. 2019;29:242–51. https://doi.org/10.1111/jon.12581.
48. Natali AL, Reddy V, Bordoni B. Neuroanatomy, corticospinal cord tract. In: StatPearls. Treasure Island (FL): StatPearls Publishing. Copyright © 2023, StatPearls Publishing LLC; 2023.
49. Radwan AM, Sunaert S, Schilling K, Descoteaux M, Landman BA, Vandenbulcke M, Theys T, Dupont P, Emsell L. An atlas of white matter anatomy, its variability, and reproducibility based on constrained spherical deconvolution of diffusion MRI. Neuroimage. 2022;254:119029. https://doi.org/10.1016/j.neuroimage.2022.119029.
50. Serra C, Türe U, Krayenbühl N, Şengül G, Yaşargil DC, Yaşargil MG. Topographic classification of the thalamus surfaces related to microneurosurgery: a white matter fiber microdissection study. World Neurosurg. 2017;97:438–52. https://doi.org/10.1016/j.wneu.2016.09.101.
51. George K, Das JM. Neuroanatomy, Thalamocortical Radiations. In: StatPearls. Treasure Island (FL): StatPearls Publishing. Copyright © 2023, StatPearls Publishing LLC; 2023.
52. Niida R, Yamagata B, Niida A, Uechi A, Matsuda H, Mimura M. Aberrant anterior thalamic radiation structure in bipolar disorder: a diffusion tensor tractography study. Frontiers in Psychiatry. 2018;9 https://doi.org/10.3389/fpsyt.2018.00522.

53. Castellano A, Bello L, Michelozzi C, Gallucci M, Fava E, Iadanza A, Riva M, Casaceli G, Falini A. Role of diffusion tensor magnetic resonance tractography in predicting the extent of resection in glioma surgery. Neuro Oncol. 2012;14:192–202. https://doi.org/10.1093/neuonc/nor188.
54. Nimsky C, Ganslandt O, Merhof D, Sorensen AG, Fahlbusch R. Intraoperative visualization of the pyramidal tract by diffusion-tensor-imaging-based fiber tracking. Neuroimage. 2006;30:1219–29. https://doi.org/10.1016/j.neuroimage.2005.11.001.
55. Berman JI, Berger MS, Mukherjee P, Henry RG. Diffusion-tensor imaging-guided tracking of fibers of the pyramidal tract combined with intraoperative cortical stimulation mapping in patients with gliomas. J Neurosurg. 2004;101:66–72. https://doi.org/10.3171/jns.2004.101.1.0066.
56. Kamada K, Todo T, Morita A, Masutani Y, Aoki S, Ino K, Kawai K, Kirino T. Functional monitoring for visual pathway using real-time visual evoked potentials and optic-radiation tractography. Neurosurgery. 2005;57:121–7.; discussion 121–127. https://doi.org/10.1227/01.neu.0000163526.60240.b6.
57. Kamada K, Todo T, Masutani Y, Aoki S, Ino K, Morita A, Saito N. Visualization of the frontotemporal language fibers by tractography combined with functional magnetic resonance imaging and magnetoencephalography. J Neurosurg. 2007;106:90–8. https://doi.org/10.3171/jns.2007.106.1.90.
58. Henry RG, Berman JI, Nagarajan SS, Mukherjee P, Berger MS. Subcortical pathways serving cortical language sites: initial experience with diffusion tensor imaging fiber tracking combined with intraoperative language mapping. Neuroimage. 2004;21:616–22. https://doi.org/10.1016/j.neuroimage.2003.09.047.
59. Witwer BP, Moftakhar R, Hasan KM, Deshmukh P, Haughton V, Field A, Arfanakis K, Noyes J, Moritz CH, Meyerand ME, et al. Diffusion-tensor imaging of white matter tracts in patients with cerebral neoplasm. J Neurosurg. 2002;97:568–75. https://doi.org/10.3171/jns.2002.97.3.0568.
60. Wei CW, Guo G, Mikulis DJ. Tumor effects on cerebral white matter as characterized by diffusion tensor tractography. Can J Neurol Sci. 2007;34:62–8. https://doi.org/10.1017/s0317167100005801.
61. Faraji AH, Abhinav K, Jarbo K, Yeh FC, Shin SS, Pathak S, Hirsch BE, Schneider W, Fernandez-Miranda JC, Friedlander RM. Longitudinal evaluation of corticospinal tract in patients with resected brainstem cavernous malformations using high-definition fiber tractography and diffusion connectometry analysis: preliminary experience. J Neurosurg. 2015;123:1133–44. https://doi.org/10.3171/2014.12.Jns142169.
62. Nimsky C, Ganslandt O, Fahlbusch R. Implementation of fiber tract navigation. Neurosurgery. 2006;58:ONS-292-303.; discussion ONS-303-294,. https://doi.org/10.1227/01.Neu.0000204726.00088.6d.

Chapter 7
Dissecting the Lateral and Third Ventricles

7.1 Introduction

After we have studied the cortical surfaces of the brain, we intend to study the deep cavities and their surrounding structures. These cavities are called ventricles; the brain ventricles are divided into four large chambers with six communicating pathways connecting them to the subarachnoid space.

The four large chambers are the left and right lateral ventricles, the third ventricle, and the fourth ventricle. Each lateral ventricle connects with the roof of the third ventricle through the intraventricular foramen, more commonly known as Monro's foramen. The third ventricle communicates with the fourth ventricle through the mesencephalic aqueduct (aqueduct of Sylvius). The fourth ventricle communicates with the subarachnoid space through the medial and lateral openings, also known as the foramen of Magendie and the foramen of Luschka, respectively. The foramen of Magendie lies on the most caudal part of the roof of the fourth ventricle, is the largest aperture, and communicates directly with the Magna cistern, the peribulbar cistern of the subarachnoid space. The foramen of Luschka are smaller openings located on the most lateral aspect on each side of the fourth ventricle in communication with the cerebellopontine cistern.

Before dissecting, we need to understand the importance of the thalamus in studying the lateral ventricles. The thalamus is used as a central anatomic landmark to identify each part of the lateral ventricle. Anterior to the thalamus is the frontal horn of the lateral ventricle, above the thalamus is the body, posterior to the thalamus is the atrium and occipital horn, and inferior to the thalamus is the temporal horn, between the thalamus we have the third ventricle.

The importance of studying the brain ventricles very well in the laboratory is to practice and develop a three-dimensional anatomic understanding of the ventricular and periventricular diseases; to understand the pathogenesis and therapeutic strategies of a very common neurosurgical disease, hydrocephalus; and to learn through

F. Chaddad-Neto, M. D. S. da Costa, *Microneuroanatomy and Lab*,
https://doi.org/10.1007/978-3-031-91026-5_7

practical dissections the best and safe pathways to access each part of the ventricular system. In this chapter, we will describe a step-by-step guide to dissecting a fixed brain specimen to study the lateral ventricles.

7.2 In the Laboratory

Necessary items:

- A formaldehyde-fixed and cleaned brain specimen.
- A long, sharp Chef knife with a non-serrated blade edge.
- A laboratory balcony.
- A number 11 blade.
- Two small Adson forceps with and without teeth.
- A simple set of neurosurgical microdissectors.
- A laboratory microscope.

Tips before you start:

- We suggest cutting one hemisphere first and leaving the contralateral side intact for referral purposes.
- As we advance in the process, we improve our technique, and it gives us a chance to do even better cuts on the contralateral side.
- Be sure the knife's blade is sharp enough to avoid a serrating movement.
- The cuts must be executed in one slow movement to avoid an irregular surface.
- We intend to do cuts in multiple levels to not transpose our purpose or waste the specimen.
- Use wet instruments to cut the specimen and avoid damage due to friction.
- Take photos from each step you have done.
- Don't be in a hurry and enjoy each step of the process.

Step by step:

1. The first cut is axial and above the level of the corpus callosum. As we know, the most cephalic parts of the lateral ventricles are the body and the frontal horn of the lateral ventricles, and their roof is constituted by horizontal fibers of the corpus callosum. Therefore, we can use the corpus callosum as the superior landmark on the mesial surface. In the lateral surface, we use two points as landmarks to initiate, level, and direct the blade of the Chef knife movement in this first cut. These landmarks are a point 2 cm above the most posterior point of the lateral fissure and another point on the inferior frontal gyrus at the level where the pars triangularis' base is located (Figs. 7.1, 7.2, and 7.3). This cut must be aimed at the superior limit of the corpus callosum in the midline to preserve the lateral ventricle roof to be opened later, which can be difficult in some hemispheres. If that is the case, this step should be done with more than one movement, with multiple axial cuts, until it reaches the corpus callosum by the midline.

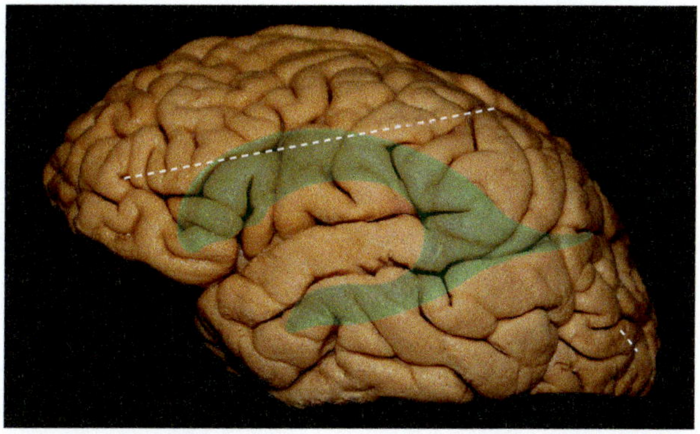

Fig. 7.1 The angle of the axial cut based on the landmarks: the middle point of the base of the pars triangularis in the inferior frontal sulci and a point 2-cm superior to the most posterior end of the Sylvian fissure

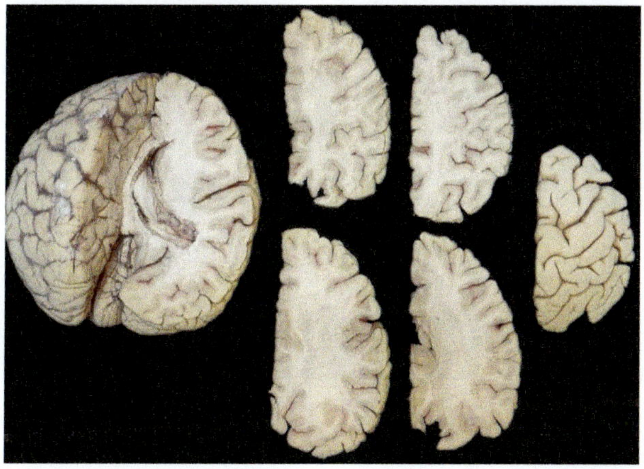

Fig. 7.2 Example of sequential axial cuts to expose the lateral ventricle

2. We remove the remaining roof (corpus callosum fibers and ependyma) of the lateral ventricle preferentially under microscopic view with Adson forceps and a number 11 blade. Try to smoothly bevel the edges uniformly (Figs. 7.4 and 7.5). For this step, you can use a dissector underneath the edges to protect the underlying structures and stabilize the cut movement. At the end of this step, you can identify the anatomic structures of the body and the anterior horns of the lateral ventricle. Take some time to study and take pictures of the specimen. This anatomy is very important for neuroendoscopic procedures and callosotomy procedures.
3. As follows, we aim to expose the atrium and the posterior part of the temporal horn of the lateral ventricle. The first cut is in the coronal plane right dorsal to the pulvinar part of the thalamus. The second cut is oblique and tangential to the mesial wall of the atrium. And the third cut is axial and at the level of the atrium's floor. So we can expose the temporal lobe from the Sylvian fissure, and we can additionally make a sagittal cut at the level of the superior limiting sulcus of the insula.

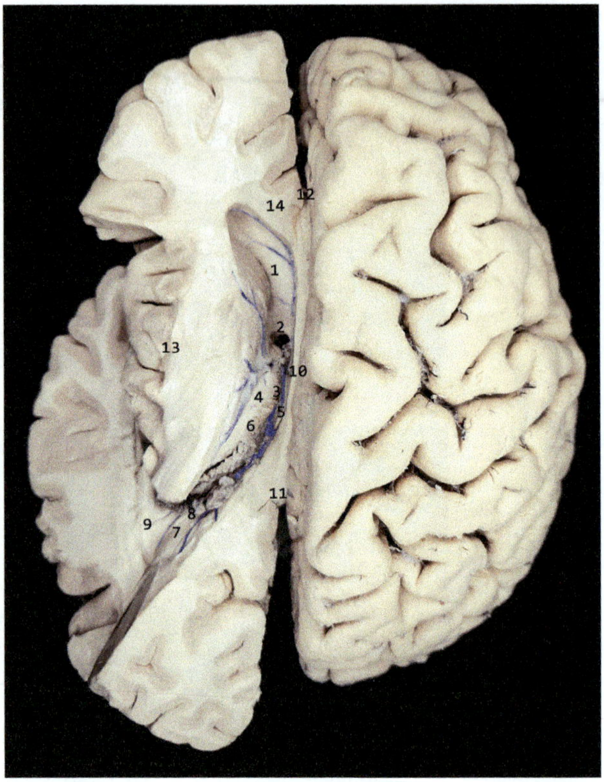

Fig. 7.3 Anatomical structures numbered as exposed: (1) frontal horn of the lateral ventricle, (2) Monroe foramen, (3) choroid fissure harboring the choroid plexus, (4) thalamus, (5) body of the fornix, (6) body of the lateral ventricle, (7) atrium of the lateral ventricle, (8) crura of the fornix, (9) collateral trigone, (10) body of the corpus callosum (roof of the lateral ventricles), (11) splenium of the corpus callosum, (12) knee of the corpus callosum, (13) circular sulci of the insula, (14) forceps minor of the corpus callosum

Fig. 7.4 Sequential cuts, from left to right, to expose the atrium of the lateral ventricle

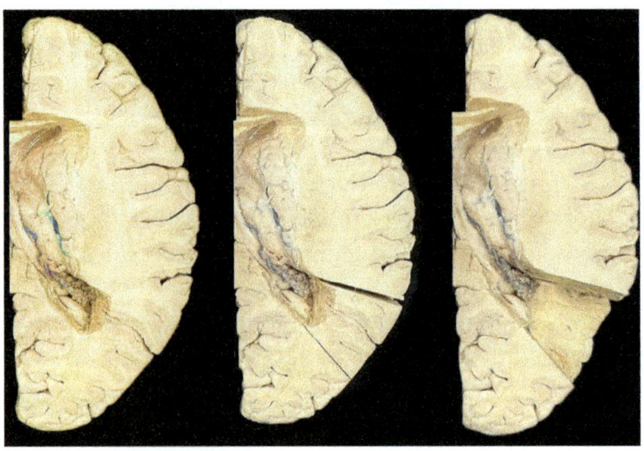

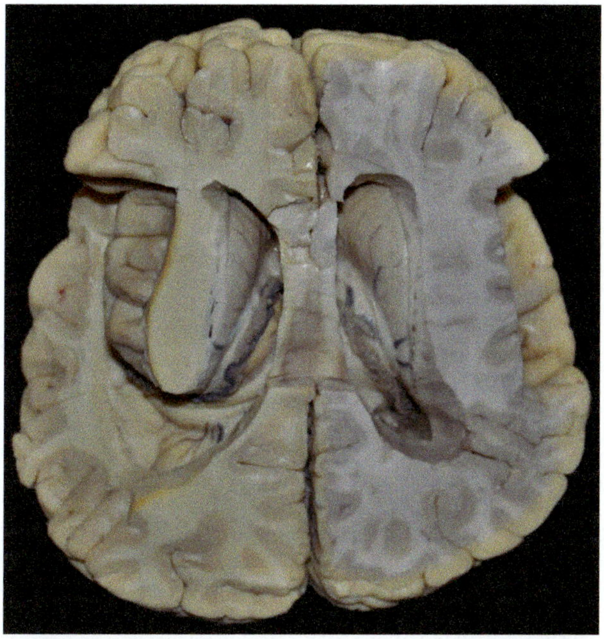

Fig. 7.5 To further study the temporal horn and the close relationship with the insula, we illustrate the subcortical cut necessary to remove the frontoparietal operculum of the Sylvian fissure. The right side the frontoparietal operculum was removed to give the view of the insula in the left side

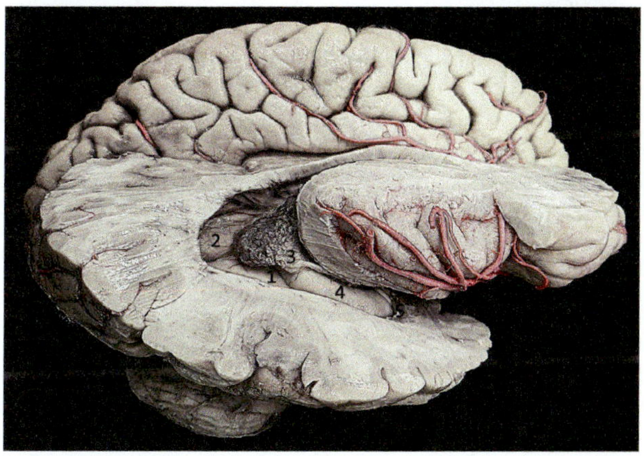

Fig. 7.6 Dissection of the temporal horn Temporal horn: dissection: (1) Collateral trigone; (2) Calcar avis; (3) Choiroid plexus; (4) Hippocampus; (5) Uncal recess

4. To understand the lateral surgical corridors to the lateral ventricle, we need to understand its relationship with the insula. Therefore, the next step is to remove the frontoparietal operculum above the Sylvian fissure. For this step, we use the anterior ascending ramus of the lateral fissure (right behind the pars triangular) and cut first the cortical part of the frontoparietal operculum.
5. To expose the temporal horn of the lateral ventricle (Fig. 7.6) further, we make another sagittal cut at the level of the inferior limiting sulcus of the insula and a

second cut axial at the level of the floor of the temporal horn. The temporal horn is very narrow; therefore, it's best to do this under a microscopic view to reduce the chance of damaging the hippocampus.

6. Notice that the temporal horn and the perimesencephalic cisterns (crural and ambient) are at the same level as the middle temporal gyrus.

Bibliography

1. Mattos JP, Santos MJ, Zullo JF, Joaquim AF, Chaddad-Neto F, Oliveira E, editors. Dissection technique for the study of the cerebral sulci, gyri and ventricles. Arq Neuropsiquiatr. 2008;66(2A):282–7. https://doi.org/10.1590/s0004-282x2008000200034.
2. Rhoton A. Rhoton cranial anatomy and surgical approaches. Oxford University Press Inc; 2019.
3. Chaddad-Neto F, Silva D, da Costa M, Bozkurt B, Leonardo Doria-Netto H, de Araujo Paz D, da Silva Centeno R, et al. Contralateral anterior interhemispheric-transcallosal-transrostral approach to the subcallosal region: a novel surgical technique. J Neurosurg. 2018;129(2):508–14. https://doi.org/10.3171/2017.4.jns16951.
4. Da Costa MDS, Santos BFO, de Almeida B, Guardini F, Chaddad-Neto F. Microsurgical treatment for arteriovenous malformation of the corpus callosum and choroidal fissure. Neurosurg Focus. 2017;43(VideoSuppl1):V12. https://doi.org/10.3171/2017.7.FocusVid.1733.
5. Chaddad-Neto F, Silva MD. Microneuroanatomy and surgery. A practical anatomical guide: Springer; 2022.

Chapter 8
Dissecting the Central Core

8.1 Introduction

The human brain has a complex anatomy, which is better understood when divided topographically into regions. The central core within each cerebral hemisphere is a distinct anatomical region with significant clinical and surgical implications.

8.2 Central Core

The central core stands as a block "on top of the brainstem," at the morphological center of the supratentorial compartment. From lateral to medial, this solid block includes the insular surface, extreme capsule, claustrum, external capsule, putamen, globus pallidus, internal capsule, caudate nucleus, stria terminalis, septal region, and thalamus (Figs. 8.1, 8.2 and 8.3).

The insula acts as a "shield" of the central core, covering it externally and defining its boundaries through its limiting sulci, as illustrated in Fig. 8.3.

The central core also includes the medial part of the anterior commissure and structures located above and posterior to the anterior perforated substance (i.e., the nucleus accumbens, which corresponds to the ventral striatum; the Meynert nucleus; the ventral amygdalofugal pathways; and the substantia innominata, which corresponds to the ventral globus pallidus). It is also connected to the rest of the brain by the cerebral isthmus and inferiorly by fibers projecting from and toward the brainstem (Fig. 8.4).

The boundaries of the central core were initially divided into three planes, each drawn from one of the limiting sulci of the insula toward the lateral ventricle, marking the anterior, superior, and posteroinferior boundaries. Each of these planes

F. Chaddad-Neto, M. D. S. da Costa, *Microneuroanatomy and Lab*,
https://doi.org/10.1007/978-3-031-91026-5_8

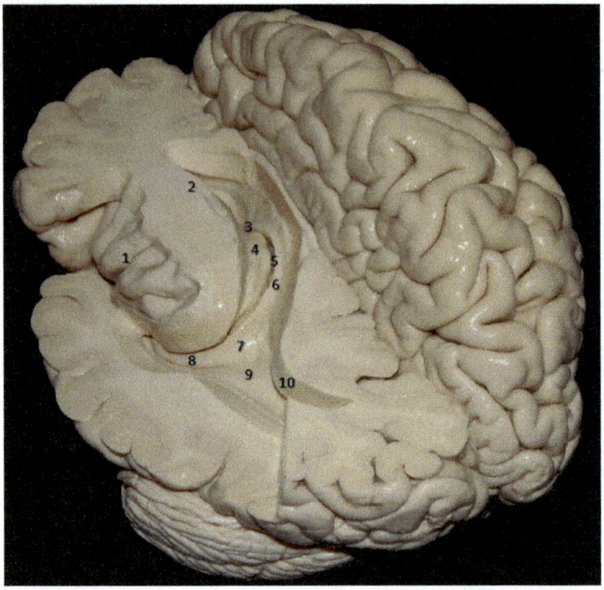

Fig. 8.1 Superolateral view of the structures of the central core (1). Insular lobe, (2) head of the caudate nucleus, (3) foramen of Monro, (4) thalamus, (5) choroidal fissure, (6) crura fornix, (7) tail of the hippocampus, (8) hippocampal body, (9) collateral trigone, and (10) calcar avis

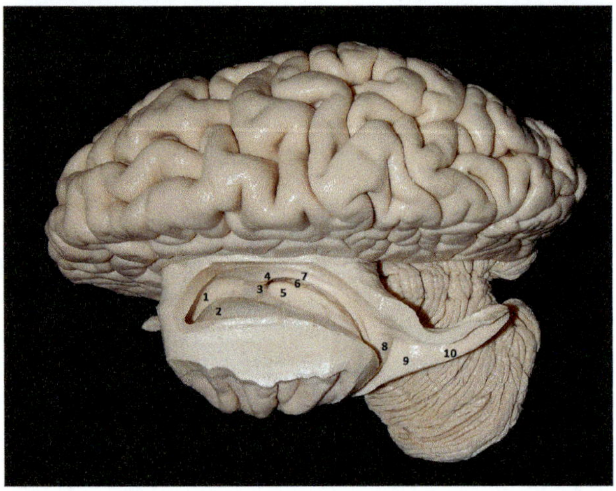

Fig. 8.2 Superior view of the structures of the central core in the axial section (1). Frontal horn of the lateral ventricle, (2) head of the caudate nucleus, (3) fornix column, (4) Monro foramen, (5) thalamus, (6) choroidal fissure, (7) body of the fornix, (8) tail of the hippocampus, (9) atrium of the lateral ventricle, and (10) posterior horn of the lateral ventricle

passes through the cerebral isthmus, transecting connections that link the central core to the other cerebral lobes.

The anterior plane is directed medially and connects the anterior limiting sulcus (Fig. 8.5) to the anterior horn of the lateral ventricle. This plane marks the anterior limit of the central core, leaving the genu of the corpus callosum excluded anteriorly and the entire caudate nucleus included posteriorly. The septal region, which is included as part of the central core, is composed of three small gyri: the anterior paraolfactory gyri, posterior paraolfactory gyri, and paraterminal gyrus (separated by the anterior and posterior paraolfactory sulci).

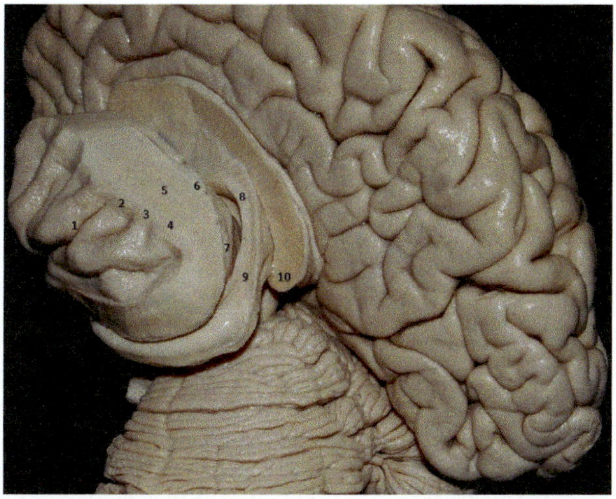

Fig. 8.3 Posterolateral view of the structures of the central core (1). Insular lobe, (2) extreme capsule, (3) claustrum, (4) external capsule, (5) lentiform nucleus, (6) internal capsule, (7) thalamus, (8) body of the fornix, (9) crura fornix, and (10) splenium of the corpus callosum

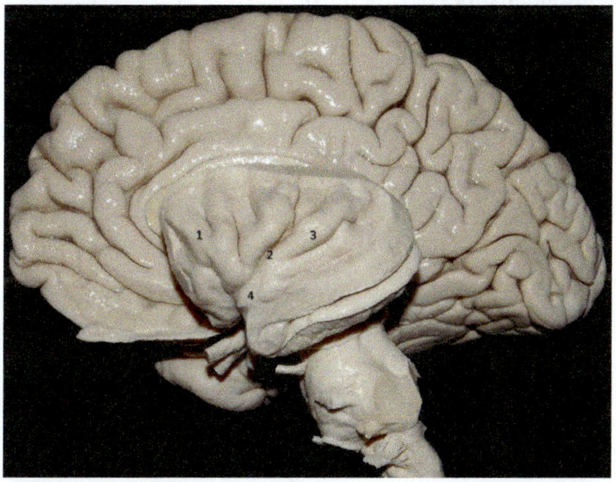

Fig. 8.4 The insula covers the central core like a protective shield (1). Short gyri of the insula, (2) central sulcus of the insula, (3) long gyri of the insula, and (4) apex of the insula

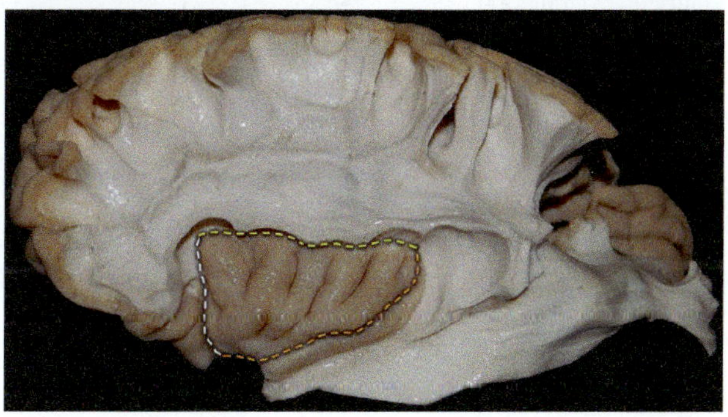

Fig. 8.5 Boundaries of the insular lobe: The dashed lines represent the three limiting sulci of the insula. White dashed line, anterior limiting sulcus; yellow dashed line, superior limiting sulcus; and orange dashed line, inferior limiting sulcus

The superior plane is also directed medially and connects the superior limiting sulcus (Fig. 8.5) to the body and superior aspect of the atrium of the lateral ventricle, which lies superior to the body of the caudate nucleus.

The inferior plane is directed medially at its posterior part and inferiorly at its inferior part, connecting the inferior limiting sulcus (Fig. 8.5) to the atrium and inferior horn of the lateral ventricle, respectively.

When these three planes reach the lateral ventricle, they are connected to the choroidal fissure (Fig. 8.2). The caudate nucleus and stria terminalis (running in the groove between the thalamus and caudate nucleus) are included in the central core. As a result, cuts made at the anterior, superior, and inferior planes detach the central core from the frontal, parietal, and F.

These boundaries depict the central core encircled outside by the lateral ventricles and important structures of the limbic system (fornix and parahippocampal gyrus). Together, these structures form a C-shaped morphology that embraces the superior, posterior, and lateroinferior borders. The third ventricle, hypothalamus, and epithalamus are grouped at the midline between the central cores of the left and right hemispheres (Fig. 8.6).

The hypothalamic sulcus represents the medial-inferior limit of the central core. Meanwhile, the groove between the thalamus and epithalamus, which consists of the pineal body, right and left habenular nuclei, and habenular and posterior commissures, represents the medio-posterior limit of the central core (Fig. 8.7).

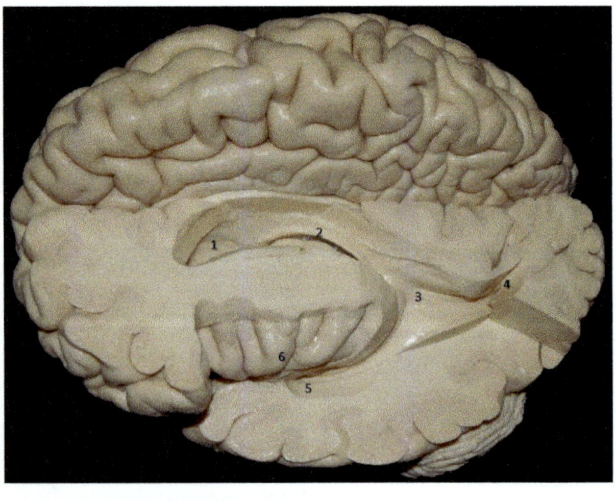

Fig. 8.6 The insula makes up the lateral part of the central core (1). Frontal horn of the lateral ventricle, (2) body of the lateral ventricle, (3) atrium of the lateral ventricle, (4) posterior horn of the lateral ventricle, (5) temporal horn of the lateral ventricle, and (6) insular lobe

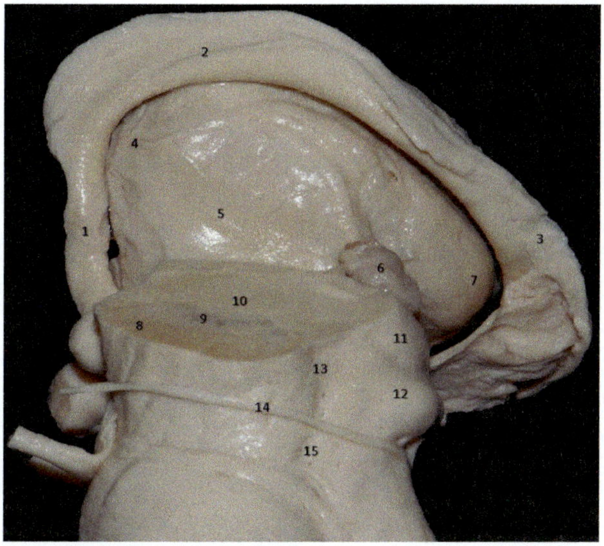

Fig. 8.7 Structures related to the thalamus and central core. (1) Fornix column, (2) body of the fornix, (3) fornix crura, (4) anterior tubercle of the thalamus, (5) hypothalamic sulcus, (6) pineal gland, (7) pulvinar of the thalamus, (8) base of the cerebral peduncle, (9) substantia nigra, (10) mesencephalic tegmentum, (11) superior colliculus, (12) inferior colliculus, (13) mesencephalic lateral sulcus, (14) cranial nerve IV (trochlear nerve), and (15) interpeduncular sulcus

8.3 Insula

The insular lobe is covered by opercular portions of the frontal, parietal, and temporal lobes. To access it, the Sylvian fissure must be opened, or the opercular portions of these lobes must be removed. As mentioned previously, it is a triangular structure that forms the lateral part of the central core, covering it like a protective shield (Figs. 8.3 and 8.4).

The insula begins at the anterior Sylvian point, a retracted point in the subarachnoid space indicated by the apex of the pars triangularis of the inferior frontal gyrus (Fig. 8.4). This point marks the presence of the limen of the insula, where the Sylvian vallecula is located and where the direction of the middle cerebral artery changes from medial to lateral (segment M1) to anterior to posterior (segment M2). The insular lobe ends at the posterior Sylvian point, which is represented by the Heschl's gyrus or the long anterior transverse gyrus.

The insula has a central sulcus, known as the central sulcus of the insula, which is juxtaposed to the central sulcus of the brain. The central sulcus of the insula separates the short insular gyri anteriorly from the long insular gyri posteriorly. The short insular gyri converge at the anteroinferior end of the triangle, which is the apex of the insula (Fig. 8.4).

The insula also has an important relationship with the Sylvian fissure as its presence indicates the region where the fissure can be most easily separated, known as the polar plane of the Sylvian fissure (before the Heschl's gyrus). Beyond the Heschl's gyrus, that is, after the end of the insula, the temporal plane of the Sylvian fissure can be found, where opening the fissure becomes more challenging.

8.4 White Matter

To understand the distribution of structures within the central core, it is essential to understand the white fibers arranged in this region (Figs. 8.8, 8.9 and 8.10).

Extreme Capsule: A set of fibers located distal to the lentiform nucleus. It is composed of "U" fibers that connect the insular gyri to the frontoparietal and temporal opercula (Fig. 8.11).

External Capsule: The external capsule is a bundle of fibers located lateral to the lentiform nucleus. It is primarily formed by the uncinate fascicle, inferior fronto-occipital fascicle, and claustrocortical fibers (Figs. 8.12, 8.13, and 8.14).

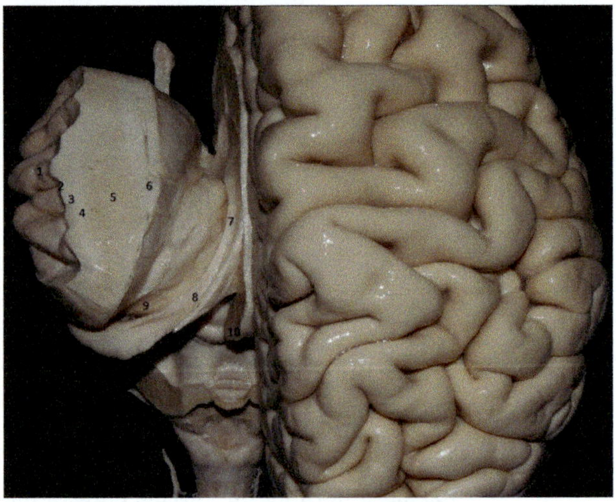

Fig. 8.8 Superior view of the central core in the axial section (1). Insular lobe, (2) extreme capsule, (3) claustrum, (4) external capsule, (5) lentiform nucleus, (6) internal capsule, (7) body of the fornix, (8) crura fornix, (9) pulvinar of the thalamus, and (10) splenium of the corpus callosum

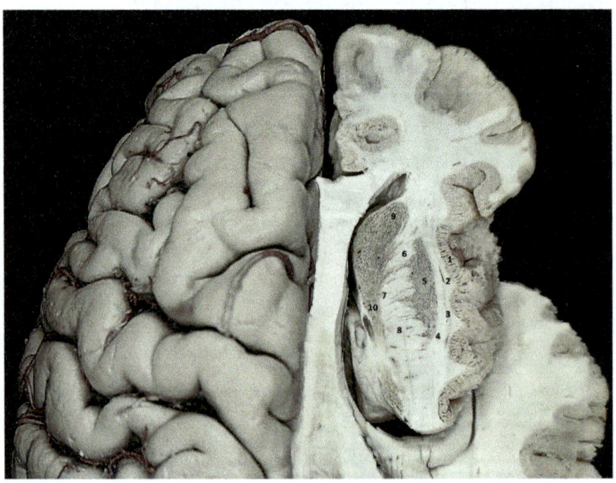

Fig. 8.9 Structures of the central core viewed from the axial region at the level of the inferior frontal gyrus. Superior view (1). Insular cortex, (2) extreme capsule, (3) claustrum, (4) external capsule, (5) lentiform nucleus, (6) anterior limb of the internal capsule, (7) genu of the internal capsule, (8) posterior limb of the internal capsule, (9) head of the caudate nucleus, and (10) body of the caudate nucleus

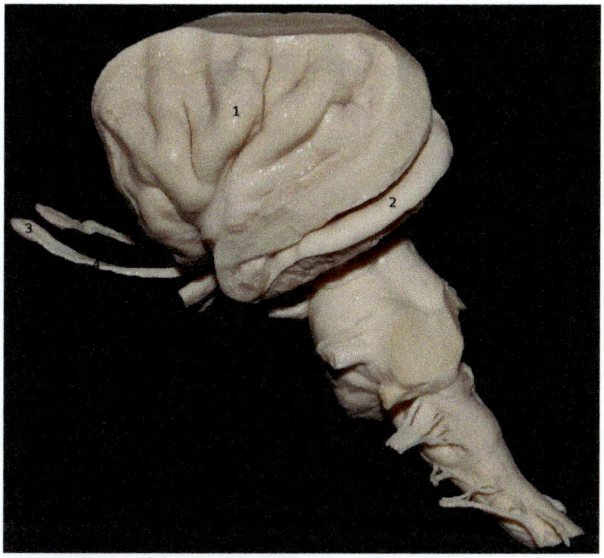

Fig. 8.10 Dissection of white matter related to the central core from lateral to medial (1). Insular lobe, (2) crura fonix, (3) olfactory bulb, and (4) olfactory tract

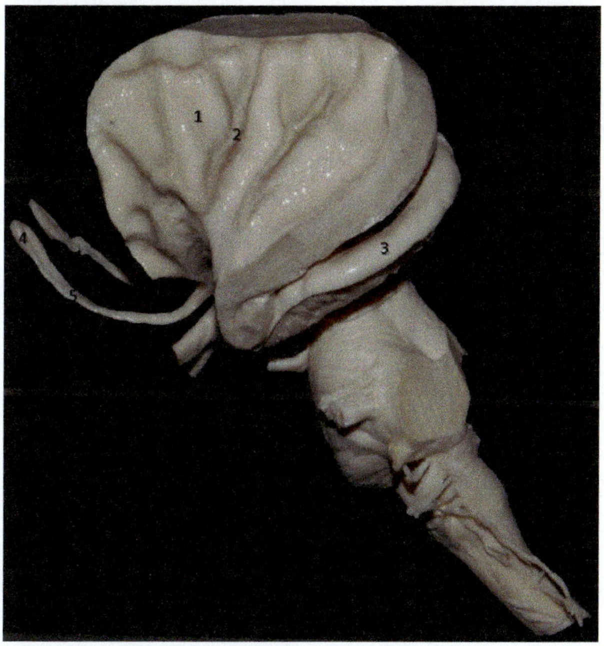

Fig. 8.11 Dissection of white matter related to the central core from lateral to medial (1). Extreme capsule, (2) "U-" shaped fibers, (3) crura fornix, (4) olfactory bulb, and (5) olfactory tract

Internal Capsule: The internal capsule is a group of fibers located medial to the lentiform nucleus (Figs. 8.9 and 8.15). It can be subdivided into five portions: anterior limb, frontocerebellar fibers; genu, corticonuclear tract; posterior limb, corticospinal tract; retrolenticular portion, auditory and visual radiations; sublenticular portion, auditory and visual radiations.

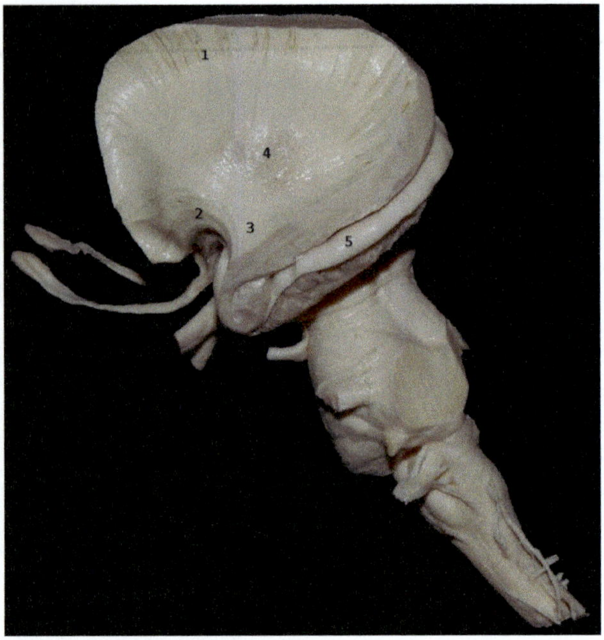

Fig. 8.12 Dissection of white matter related to the central core from lateral to medial (1). Corona radiata, (2) uncinate fasciculus, (3) inferior fronto-occipital fasciculus, (4) lentiform nucleus, and (5) crura fornix

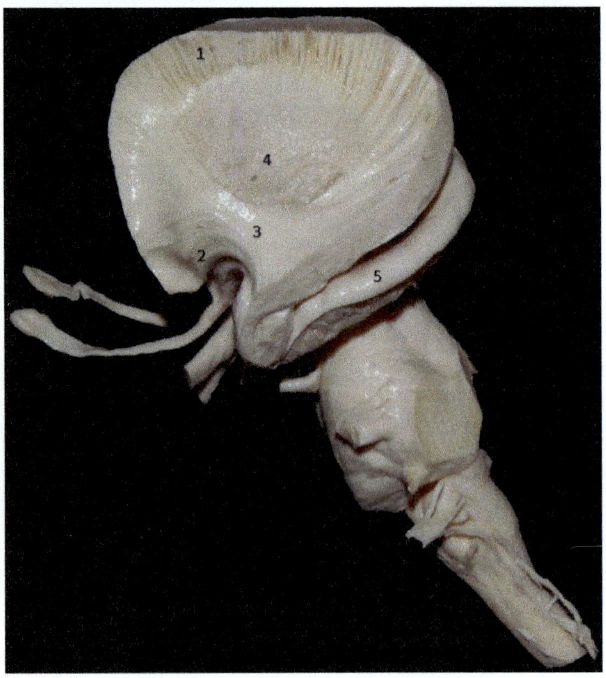

Fig. 8.13 Dissection of white matter related to the central core from lateral to medial (1). Corona radiata, (2) uncinate fasciculus, (3) inferior fronto-occipital fasciculus, (4) lentiform nucleus, and (5) crura fornix

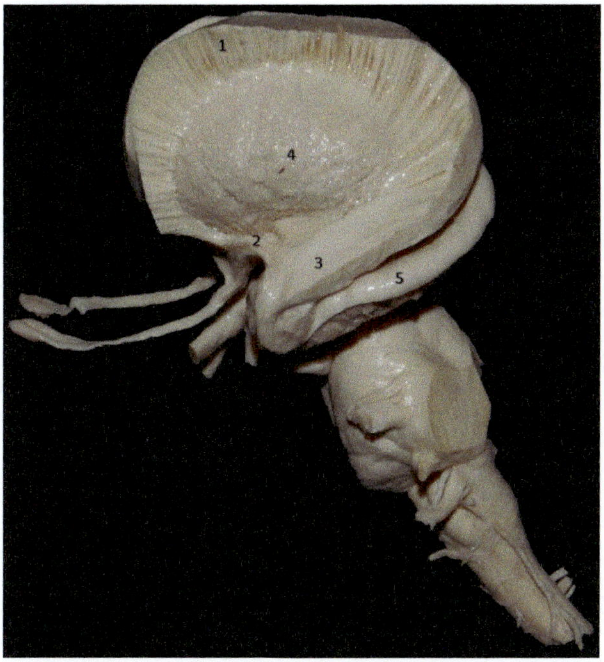

Fig. 8.14 Dissection of white matter related to the central core from lateral to medial (1). Corona radiata, (2) uncinate fasciculus, (3) inferior fronto-occipital fasciculus, (4) lentiform nucleus, and (5) crura fornix

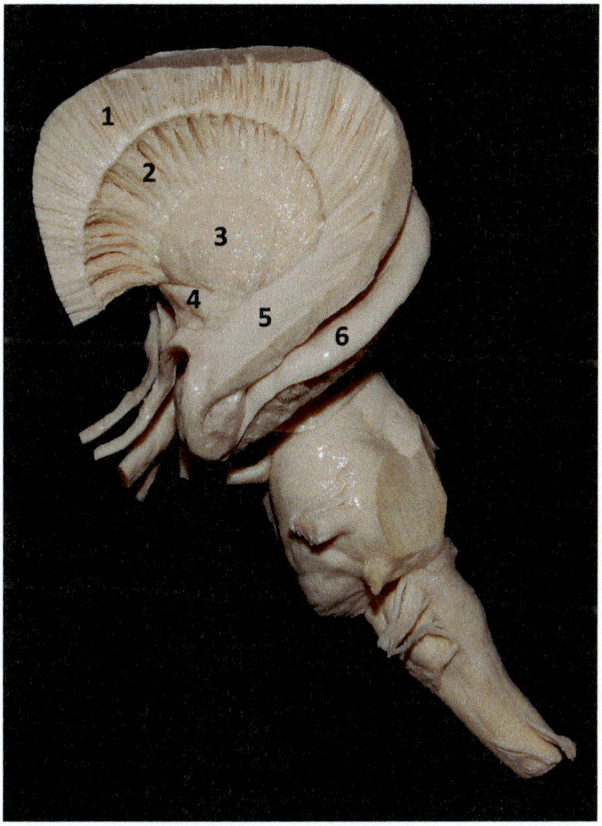

Fig. 8.15 Dissection of the white matter related to the central core from lateral to medial (1). Corona radiata, (2) internal capsule, (3) lentiform nucleus, (4) anterior commissure, (5) inferior fronto-occipital fasciculus, and (6) crura fornix

8.5 Caudate Nucleus

The head of the caudate nucleus constitutes the lateral wall of the anterior horn of the lateral ventricle. The caudate nucleus is located on the upper surface of the thalamus and corresponds to the lateral wall of the ventricular body (Fig. 8.9). The tail of the caudate nucleus surrounds the pulvinar of the thalamus posteriorly and laterally and then runs along the roof of the inferior horn of the lateral ventricle.

The putamen and caudate nuclei comprise the striatum, an important input area for the basal nuclei. Posteriorly, they are separated from the internal capsule by fibers, while their anterior surfaces are continuous below the anterior and inferior edges of the internal capsule, forming the ventral striatum, which corresponds to the nucleus accumbens.

8.6 Thalamus

The thalamus is a gray matter structure of the diencephalon located above the brainstem and has various functions in human physiology. It consists of several nuclei with different functions, ranging from the retransmission of sensory and motor signals to the regulation of consciousness and alertness. It forms the lateral wall of the third ventricle, while its posterior surface forms part of the floor of the body of the lateral ventricle (Fig. 8.7). Subsequently, the thalamus was limited to the posterior limb of the internal capsule. Anterolaterally, it limits the head of the ventral and caudate nuclei, together with the subthalamus and hypothalamus.

The thalamus is divided into the medial, lateral, superior, inferior, anterior, and posterior surfaces. The lateral surface is convex and located below the caudate nucleus and above the posterior segment of the internal capsule. The posterior surface, also known as the pulvinar, is divided by the fornix into an ependymal surface (ventricular surface) and an extraventricular or cisternal surface related to the quadrigeminal cistern (Fig. 8.16). The medial surface forms the lateral wall of the third ventricle. The upper surface is divided by the thalamic medullary stria into medial and lateral halves. The lateral half is related to the caudate nucleus and constitutes the floor of the lateral ventricle, while the medial half is related to the choroidal tissue and the fornix. The lower surface is located above the midbrain. The anterior surface is divided into the medial and lateral halves. The lateral half is related to the head of the caudate nucleus, while the medial half forms the posterior limit of the foramen of Monro.

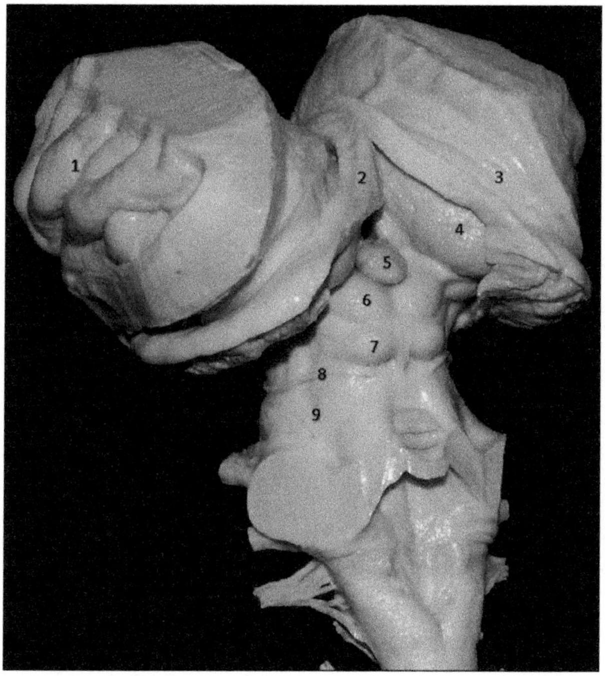

Fig. 8.16 The thalamus is a "head" above the brain stem and has different functions in human physiology (1). Insular lobe, (2) crura fornix, (3) ventricular part of the pulvinar, (4) cisternal part of the pulvinar, (5) pineal gland, (6) left superior colliculus, (7) left inferior colliculus, (8) left cranial nerve IV (trochlear nerve), and (9) interpeduncular sulcus

Bibliography

1. Chaddad-Neto F, Silva da Costa MD. Surgical anatomy of the central Core of the brain. In: Microneuroanatomy and surgery. Cham: Springer; 2022.
2. Tanriover N, Rhoton-Jr AL, Kawashima M, Ulm AJ, Yasuda AJ. Microsurgical anatomy of the insula and the sylvian fissure. Neurosurg. 2004;100:891–922.
3. Choi CY, Han SR, Yee GT. Central core of the cerebrum. Lee CH J Neurosurg. 2011;114:463–9.
4. Costa M, Braga VL, Yağmurlu K, Centeno RS, Cavalheiro S, Chaddad-Neto F. A technical guide for fiber tract dissection of the internal capsule. Turk Neurosurg. 2018;28(6):934–9.
5. Goiri MAA, de Amorim BL, Sarti THM, da Costa MDS, Chaddad-Neto F. Building a micro-neurosurgical laboratory in Latin America: challenges and possibilities. Surg Neurol Int. 2021;12:573. Published 2021 Nov 23. https://doi.org/10.25259/SNI_978_2021
6. Ahumada-Vizcaino JC, Wuo-Silva R, Hernández MM, Chaddad-Neto F. The art of combining neuroanatomy and microsurgical skills in modern neurosurgery. Front Neurol. 2023;13:1076778. Published 2023 Jan 12. https://doi.org/10.3389/fneur.2022.1076778

Chapter 9
Dissecting the Brainstem

9.1 Introduction

Surgery for intrinsic brainstem lesions poses a significant challenge. The feasibility of such a procedure has remained controversial for years. The surgical removal of focal gliomas, cavernous malformations, or hemangioblastomas within the brainstem has caused heated discussions in scientific meetings and academic literature. The primary challenge stems from the intricate anatomy of the brainstem, which contains a dense concentration of nuclei and fibers in a small sectional area, resulting in a high likelihood of morbidity after manipulation. Therefore, undergoing training in microneurosurgical skills and acquiring comprehensive anatomical knowledge are crucial for individuals planning to conduct surgery on brainstem lesions. Awareness of the primary safe entry zones on the brainstem is critical for reducing morbidity in cases where lesions do not extend to the pial or ependymal surface. Such zones denote entry points and trajectories where eloquent structures and perforators are sparse and where a neurotomy would cause the least possible damage. The Microneurosurgical Anatomy Lab provides an optimal environment to acquire the necessary skills and confidence to effectively manage brainstem lesions while also receiving training from experts in the field. For didactic purposes, the brainstem anatomy will be divided into three separate structures: the midbrain, pons, and medulla (Fig. 9.1). Consequently, each structure will be divided into different perspectives and surfaces to better visualize and understand the three-dimensional view and the anatomical relationships.

F. Chaddad-Neto, M. D. S. da Costa, *Microneuroanatomy and Lab*,
https://doi.org/10.1007/978-3-031-91026-5_9

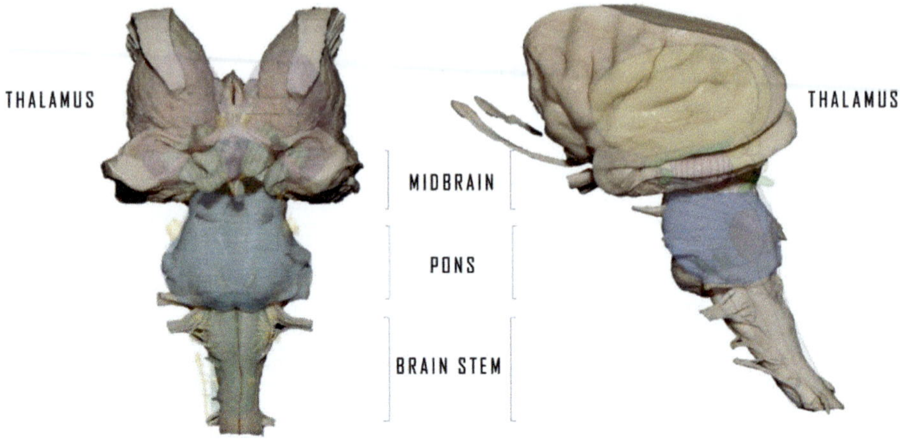

Fig. 9.1 Anterior and lateral view of the brainstem. Thalamus is projected in yellow in the right and lateral image

9.2 Midbrain

The midbrain, also referred to as the mesencephalon, constitutes a small portion of the brainstem situated between the diencephalon and the pons. Understanding the thalamus as the "head" of the brainstem creates a conceptual continuum between the midbrain and the thalamus. Macroscopically distinguishing the subthalamus from the midbrain proves challenging. Hence, it is important to remember that the midbrain lies directly beneath the thalamus or the medial geniculate body. In the laboratory, an oblique cut is made below the medial geniculate body, enabling the observation and study of the internal division of the midbrain.

The midbrain is divided into the tectum and peduncle by an imaginary line that traverses the aqueduct. Furthermore, the peduncle is subdivided into the base of the peduncle and tegmentum by the substantia nigra. The tectum is separated from the peduncle by an imaginary line that traverses the mesencephalic aqueduct. Anterior to this line lies the peduncle, while posterior to this line lies the tectum. Additionally, the midbrain's external configuration facilitates its classification into the following three distinct surfaces: anterior, lateral, and posterior (Fig. 9.2).

The anterior surface is characterized by a midline depression known as the interpeduncular fossa and a bilateral prominence known as the cerebral peduncles. Within the interpeduncular fossa, the posterior perforated substance can be discerned, along with the emergence of the third nerve. The latter delimits the medial border of the cerebral peduncles (Fig. 9.3).

The base of the cerebral peduncles is formed by the projection fibers originating from the cortex. This structure can be conceptually divided into thirds: the medial

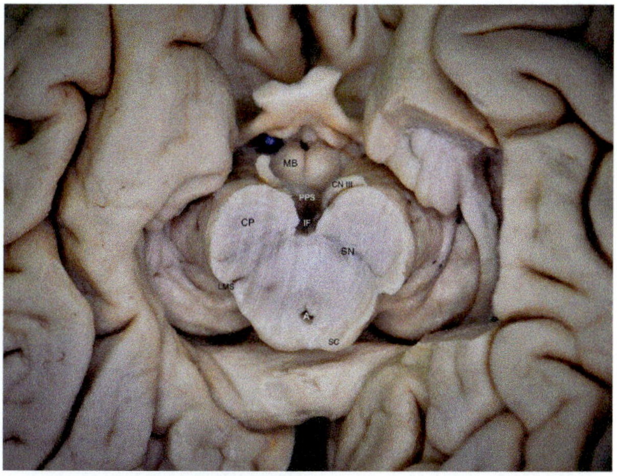

Fig. 9.2 Inferior view of the midbran: *A* aqueduct, *CN III* third cranial nerve, *CP* cerebral peduncle, *IF* interpeduncular fossa, *MB* mamillary body, *LMS* lateral mesencephalic sulcus, *PPS* posterior perforated substance, *SC* superior colliculi, *SN* substantia nigra

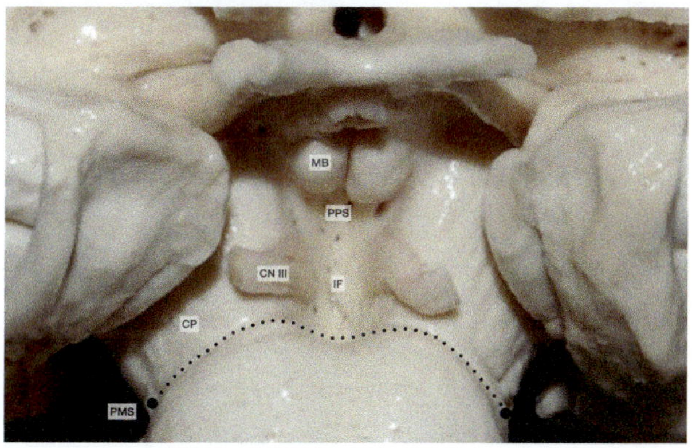

Fig. 9.3 Anterior view of the midbrain. *CN III* third cranial nerve, *CP* cerebral peduncle, *IF* interpeduncular fossa, *MB* mamillary body, *PMS* pontomesencephalic sulcus, *PPS* posterior perforated substance. (Photo by Richard Párraga)

third contains the corticopontine fibers, the middle third contains the corticospinal tract and corticopontine fibers, and the lateral third contains the temporo-parieto-occipito-pontine fibers.

The lateral surface consists of the lateral mesencephalic sulcus, which extends continuously to the interpeduncular sulcus (IPS) below the fourth nerve (Fig. 9.4). Notably, the lateral mesencephalic sulcus serves as a landmark, indicating the presence of the medial lemniscus internally.

On the posterior surface, the quadrigeminal plate is visible. It is divided into a superior portion (superior colliculi) and an inferior portion (inferior colliculi). Below the inferior colliculi lies the fourth nerve, which serves as an important landmark for approaching the lateral and posterior surfaces (Fig. 9.5).

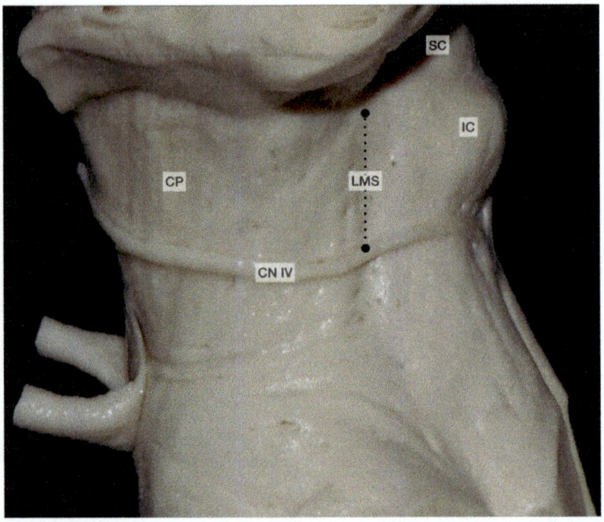

Fig. 9.4 Lateral view of the midbrain. *CN IV* fourth cranial nerve, *CP* cerebral peduncle, *IC* inferior colliculi, *LMS* lateral mesencephalic sulcus, *SC* superior colliculi. (Photo by Richard Párraga)

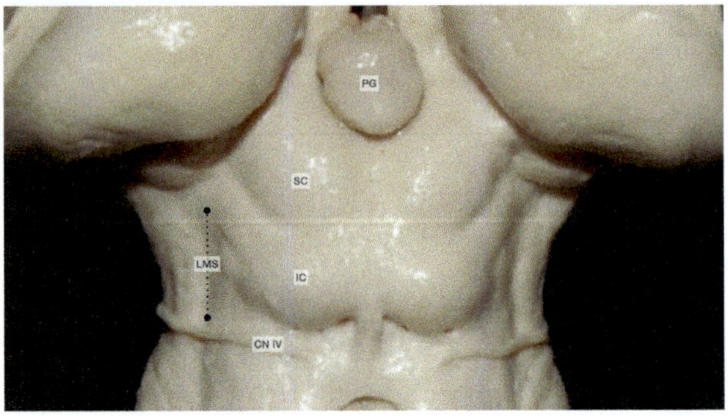

Fig. 9.5 Posterior surface of the midbrain. *CN IV* fourth cranial nerve, *IC* inferior colliculi, *LMS* lateral mesencephalic sulcus, *SC* superior colliculi, *PG* pineal gland. (Photo by Richard Párraga)

9.3 Safe Entry Zones of the Midbrain

The safe entry zones (EZ) for surgical procedures in the midbrain have been strategically identified to ensure precision and minimize damage. These zones are key access points for medical interventions and research purposes. Here, we outline three main safe entry zones within the midbrain:

9.3.1 Perioculomotor Zone

The perioculomotor entry zone provides access to lesions in the ventral midbrain. It is bordered medially by cranial nerve (CN) III and laterally by the corticospinal tract. The optic tract serves as the superior limit, while the pontomesencephalic sulcus marks the inferior limit. Upon entry through this corridor, the structures situated beyond the frontopontine fibers include the substantia nigra, medial lemniscus, and red nucleus. Instruments must be maneuvered in a rostrocaudal fashion to avoid injury to the CN III and corticospinal tract and must not be advanced beyond the substantia nigra (Fig. 9.6).

9.3.2 Lateral Mesencephalic Sulcus Zone

The lateral mesencephalic sulcus entry zone is commonly used to access the midbrain tegmentum. The anterior limit corresponds to the temporo-parieto-occipitopontine fibers, the anteromedial limit to the substantia nigra, and the posterior limit to the lateral and medial lemniscus. The medial geniculate body and pontomesencephalic sulcus serve as the superior and inferior limits, respectively. At the deepest part, the red nucleus can be found. These boundaries are critical when using this entry zone; anteroposterior dissection must be avoided to prevent damage to these structures (Fig. 9.7).

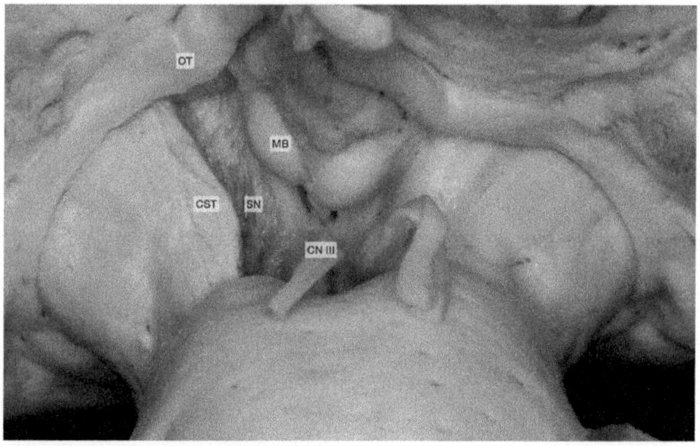

Fig. 9.6 Perioculomotor zone. *CN III* third cranial nerve, *CST* corticospinal tract, *OT* optic tract, *SN* substantia nigra. (Photo by Juan Leonardo Serrato Ávila)

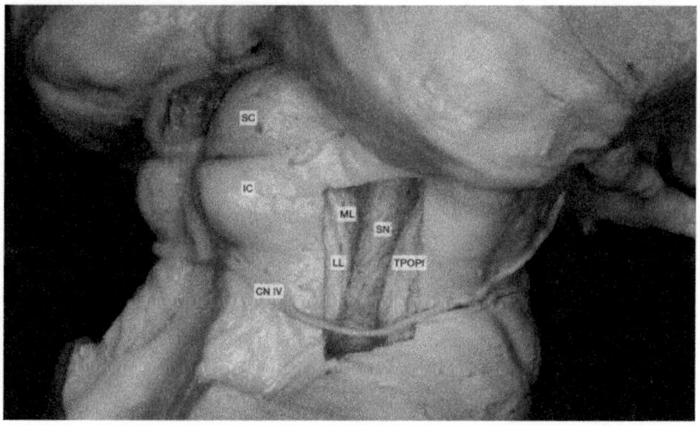

Fig. 9.7 Lateral mesencephalic sulcus zone. *CN IV* fourth cranial nerve, *IC* inferior colliculi, *LL* lateral lemniscus, *ML* medial lemniscus, *SC* superior colliculi, *SN* substantia nigra, *TPOPf* temporo-parieto-occipito-pontine fibers. (Photo by Juan Leonardo Serrato Ávila)

9.3.3 Supracollicular and Infracollicular Zones

The supracollicular and infracollicular zones are commonly used to access the lesions in the midbrain tectum. The supracollicular zone is used for lesions located in the upper half of the quadrigeminal plate, while the infracollicular zone is chosen for lesions situated in the lower half.

The supracollicular entry zone is limited anteriorly by the aqueduct and the periaqueductal gray matter, superiorly by the posterior and habenular commissures, and inferiorly by the superior colliculus. This entry zone must be approached toward the aqueduct to minimize the rostrocaudal movements of the instruments (Fig. 9.8).

The infracollicular entry zone is limited anteriorly by the anterior wall of the aqueduct, superiorly by the inferior colliculus, and inferolaterally by the apparent origin of CN IV. The superior medullary vellum lies between the superior cerebellar peduncle and below the EZ. Similar to the supracollicular entry zone, dissection in the infracollicular entry zone should be directed toward the aqueduct to avoid damage to the aforementioned structures (Fig. 9.9).

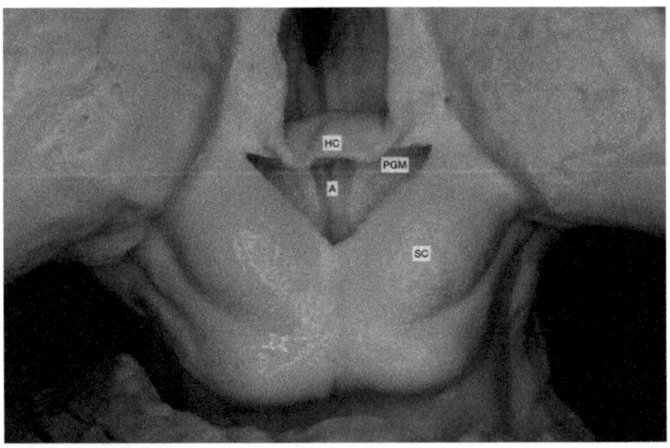

Fig. 9.8 Supracollicular zone. *A* aqueduct, *HC* habenular commissure, *PGM* periaqueductal gray matter, *SC* superior colliculi. (Photo by Juan Leonardo Serrato Ávila)

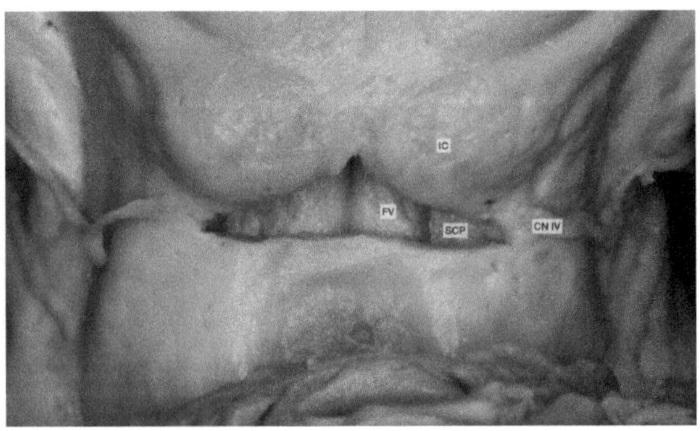

Fig. 9.9 Infracollicular zone. *CN IV* fourth cranial nerve, *FV* fourth ventricle, *IC* inferior colliculi, *SCP* superior cerebellar peduncle. (Photo by Juan Leonardo Serrato Ávila)

9.4 Pons

The pons is located between the midbrain and medulla. It is delimited superiorly by the pontomesencephalic sulcus and inferiorly by the pontomedullary sulcus. It has three surfaces: anterior, lateral, and posterior. The anterior and lateral surfaces are separated from the posterior one by the interpeduncular sulcus, which is the inferior continuation of the lateral mesencephalic sulcus (Fig. 9.10).

The posterior surface is limited superiorly by the inferior colliculi and fourth nerve and inferiorly by the lateral recess of the fourth ventricle.

In the lateral surface, the emergence of the trigeminal nerve is observable (Figs. 9.11 and 9.12). This nerve serves as a critical landmark when accessing lesions through the anterolateral, lateral, and posterolateral approaches. It delineates three safe entry zones: peritrigeminal, epitrigeminal, and lateral pontine zones.

The posterior surface corresponds to the upper half of the floor of the fourth ventricle, separated from the medulla by the stria medullaris. The anatomic structures identifiable on this surface include the median sulcus, medial eminence, facial colliculus, sulcus limitans, and locus coeruleus (Fig. 9.13). The facial colliculus

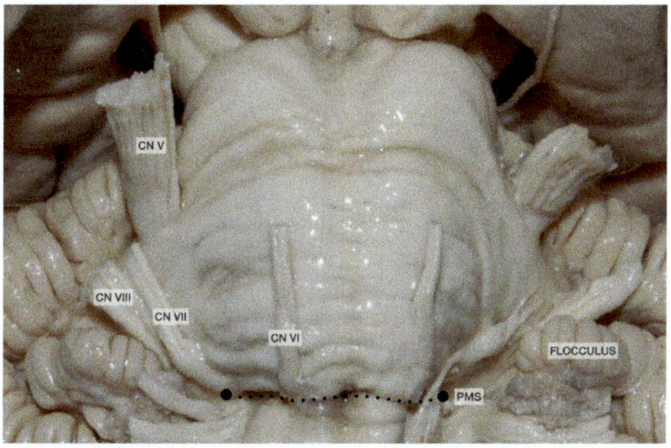

Fig. 9.10 Anterior view of the pons. *CN V* fifth cranial nerve, *CN VI* sixth cranial nerve, *CN VII* seventh cranial nerve, *CN VIII* eighth cranial nerve, *PMS* pontomedullary sulcus. (Photo by Richard Párraga)

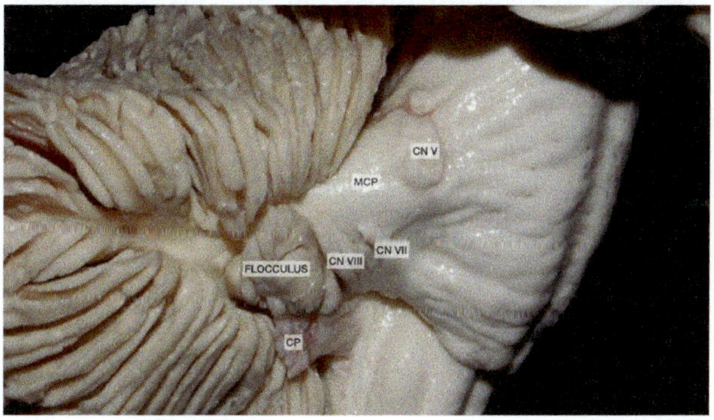

Fig. 9.11 Lateral view of the pons. *CN V* fifth cranial nerve, *CN VII* seventh cranial nerve, *CN VIII* eighth cranial nerve, *CP* choroid plexus, *MCP* middle cerebellar peduncle. (Photo by Richard Párraga)

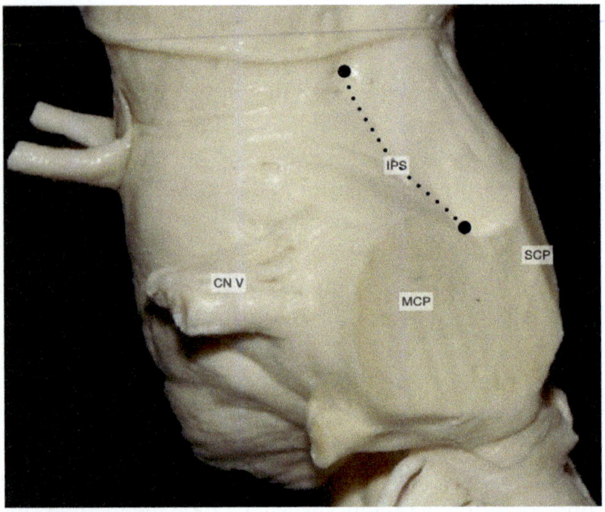

Fig. 9.12 Lateral view of the pons (cerebellum resected). *CN V* fifth cranial nerve, *IPS* interpeduncular sulcus, *MCP* middle cerebellar peduncle, *SCP* superior cerebellar peduncle. (Photo by Richard Párraga)

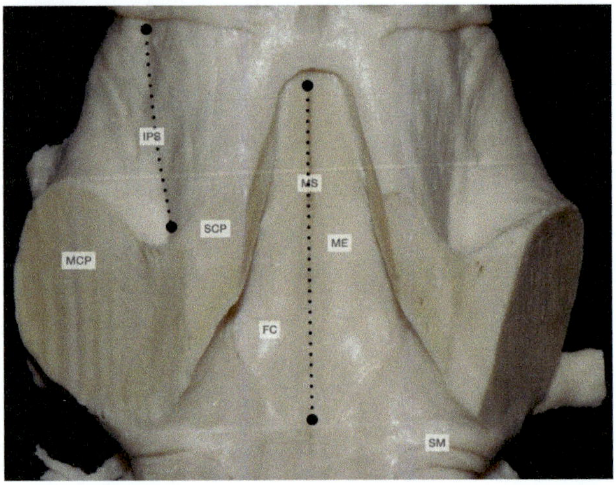

Fig. 9.13 Posterior view of the pons (cerebellum resected). *FC* facial colliculus, *ME* medial eminence, *MS* median sulcus, *IPS* interpeduncular sulcus, *MCP* middle cerebellar peduncle, *SCP* superior cerebellar peduncle, *SM* stria medullaris. (Photo by Richard Párraga)

serves as the primary landmark on this surface, facilitating access to the pons via the suprafacial and infrafacial zones.

Efficient and precise access to specific regions of the brainstem is crucial for surgical procedures and targeted interventions. The identification of safe entry zones ensures that neurosurgeons can navigate with accuracy while minimizing the risk of damage to critical neural structures. Here, we highlight several distinct safe entry zones in the pons:

9.5 Supratrigeminal Zone

The supratrigeminal entry zone is located below CN III, lateral to the midline, and medial to the corticospinal tract. At the deepest part of the entry zone, the medial lemniscus serves as the boundary. Extending dissection laterally risks compromising the corticospinal tract. Therefore, the rostrocaudal movements of instruments are advisable (Fig. 9.14).

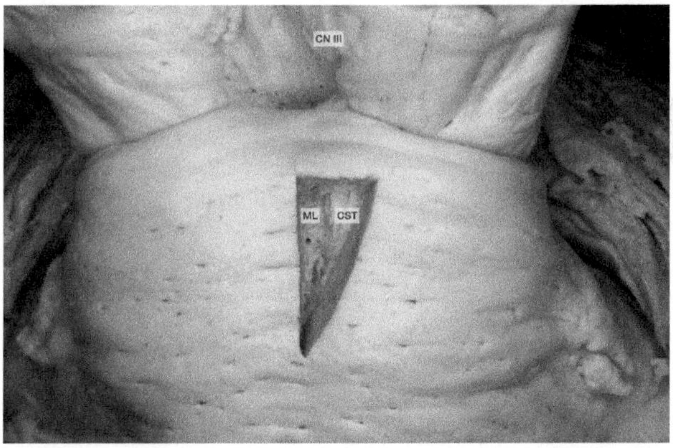

Fig. 9.14 Supratrigeminal zone. *CN III* third cranial nerve, *CST* corticospinal tract, *ML* medial lemniscus. (Photo by Juan Leonardo Serrato Ávila)

9.6 Peritrigeminal Zone

The peritrigeminal zone is situated between CN V and CN VII. The trigeminospinal tract, lateral lemniscus, and medial lemniscus represent the medial boundaries. The rostral limit matches the intrapontine segment of CN V, while the caudal limit matches the IPS of CN VII. The corticospinal tract marks the ventral limit, while the dorsal cochlear nucleus represents the dorsocaudal limit (Fig. 9.15).

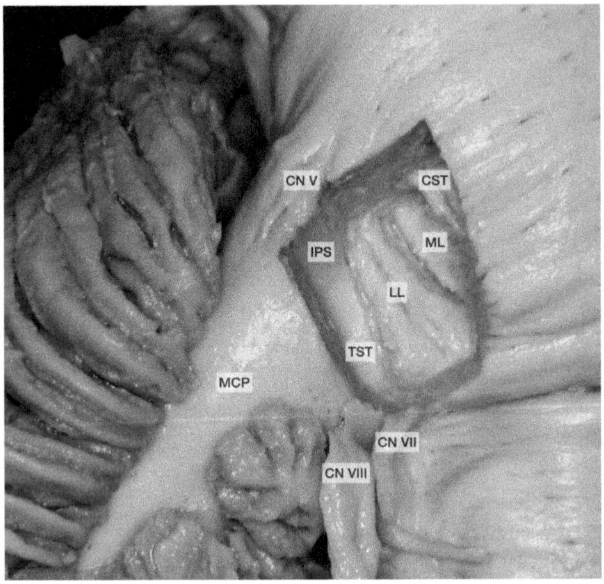

Fig. 9.15 Peritrigeminal zone. *CN V* fifth cranial nerve, *CN VII* seventh cranial nerve, *CN VIII* eighth cranial nerve, *CST* corticospinal tract, *IPS* intrapontine segment of *CN V LL lateral lemniscus*, *MCP* middle cerebellar peduncle, *ML* medial lemniscus, *TST* trigeminospinal tract. (Photo by Juan Leonardo Serrato Ávila)

9.7 Epitrigeminal Zone

Above the apparent origin of CN V, the epitrigeminal zone can be found, bounded anteromedially by the lateral and medial lemniscus and anteriorly by the corticospinal tract. Inferior extension must be avoided to prevent injury to the intrapontine segment of CN V.

9.8 Lateral Transpeducular Zone

The lateral transpeduncular zone is situated within the middle cerebellar peduncle, ventral to the cerebellar hemisphere. It traverses above the intrapontine segment of CN V toward the dorsolateral pons. The boundaries include the corticospinal tract anteriorly, the lateral and medial lemniscus anteromedially, the cerebellar cortex posteriorly, and the intrapontine segment of CN V inferiorly (Fig. 9.16).

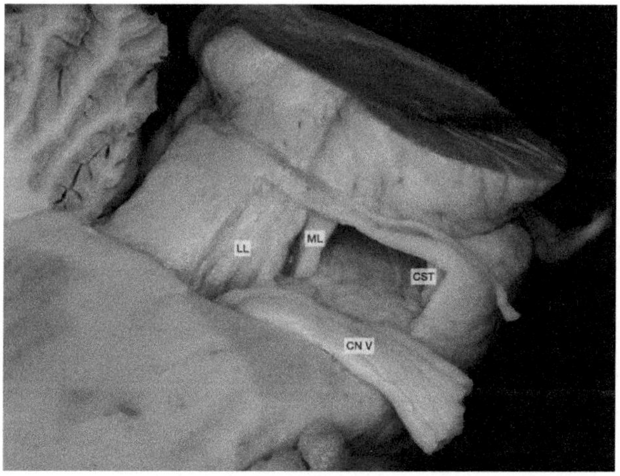

Fig. 9.16 Epitrigeminal and lateral transpeduncular zone. *CN V* fifth cranial nerve, *CST* corticospinal tract, *LL* lateral lemniscus, *ML* medial lemniscus. (Photo by Juan Leonardo Serrato Ávila)

9.9 Suprafacial and Infrafacial Entry Zones

The suprafacial and infrafacial entry zones are corridors used to reach the pons tegmentum through the fourth ventricle. The suprafacial zone is chosen for lesions situated above the facial colliculus, while the infrafacial zone is used for lesions situated below it.

The suprafacial entry zone is located in the upper half of the floor of the fourth ventricle. Its boundaries include the middle longitudinal fasciculus medially and the central tegmental tract and the trigeminal mesencephalic tract laterally, corresponding to the surface with the sulcus limitans. The superior limit is marked by the apparent origin of CN IV and the frenulum veli, while the inferior limit is marked by the superior segment of intrapontine CN VII, which corresponds with the superior aspect of the facial colliculus. During the approach, the movements of instruments are preferably made in the rostrocaudal axis due to the proximity from the middle longitudinal fasciculus and central tegmental tract (Fig. 9.17).

In relation to the infrafacial entry zone, its medial limit is the middle longitudinal fasciculus, while its lateral limit is the corticospinal tract. The superior limit is the inferior segment of intrapontine CN VII (an inferior aspect of the facial colliculus), while the inferior limit is the superior border of the hypoglossal trigone. Similar to the suprafacial zone, it is preferable to work in the rostrocaudal axis and consider the medial lemniscus as the anterior limit (Fig. 9.18).

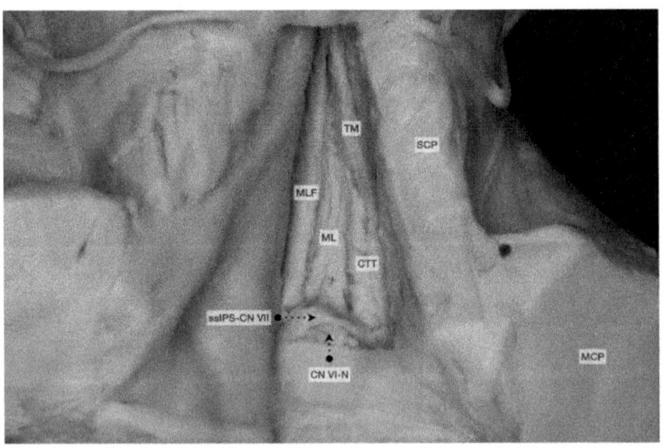

Fig. 9.17 Suprafacial zone. *CN VI-N* nucleus of the sixth cranial nerve, *CTT* central tegmental tract, *MCP* middle cerebellar peduncle, *ML* medial lemniscus, *MLF* middle longitudinal fasciculus, *SCP* superior cerebellar peduncle, *ssIPS-CN VII* superior segment of intrapontine CN VII, *TM* trigeminal mesencephalic. (Photo by Juan Leonardo Serrato Ávila)

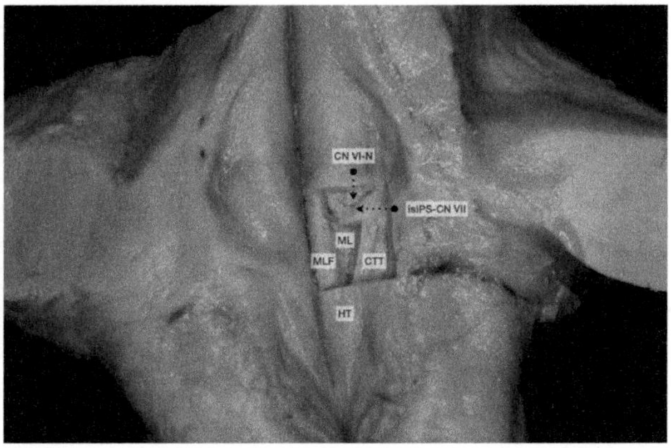

Fig. 9.18 Infrafacial zone. *CN VI-N* nucleus of the sixth cranial nerve, *CTT* central tegmental tract, *HT* hypoglossal triangle, *isIPS-CN VII* inferior segment of intrapontine, *CN VII ML* medial lemniscus, *MLF* middle longitudinal fasciculus. (Photo by Juan Leonardo Serrato Ávila)

9.10 Medulla

The medulla, situated between the pons and the spinal cord, is the lower portion of the brainstem. Its superior part is demarcated by the pontomedullary sulcus, while three anatomical landmarks are used to define the inferior limit: decussation of the pyramids, first dentate ligament insertion, and the ventral root of the first spinal cervical nerve.

The medulla is divided into three surfaces: anterior, lateral, and posterior. The anterior surface is oriented toward the clivus. It has two columns called pyramids, which are separated by the anterior medial fissure in the midline (Fig. 9.19).

The lateral surface contains two eminences known as the olives, delimited anteriorly by the preolivary sulcus and posteriorly by the retroolivary sulcus. The hypoglossal nerve emerges from the preolivary sulcus, while the glossopharyngeal, vagus, and accessory nerves emerge from the retroolivary sulcus (Fig. 9.20). The surgical entry zones in the anterolateral medulla are the preolivary sulcus, between the hypoglossal and first spinal cervical nerve; retroolivary sulcus; and transolivary zone.

The posterior surface can be divided into the superior or intraventricular part, corresponding to the lower half of the floor of the fourth ventricle and the inferior cerebellar peduncle. The inferior part is formed by the gracile tubercle medially and cuneate tubercle laterally. In the intraventricular part, the striae medullaris is established by the superior limit, and the hypoglossal and vagal triangles are localized from medial to lateral, respectively. At the inferior limit, the obex is located (Fig. 9.21).

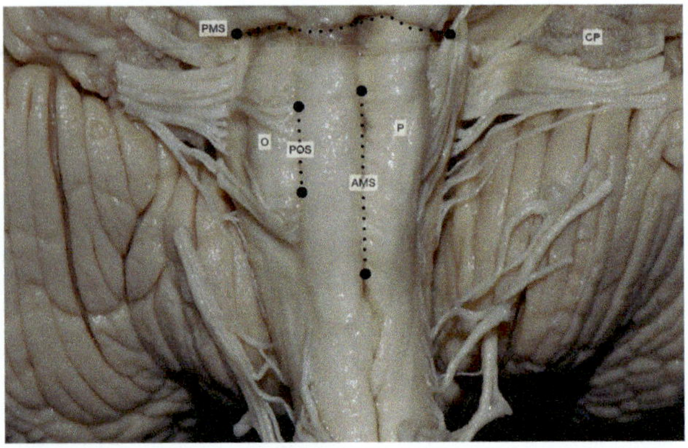

Fig. 9.19 Anterior view of the medulla. *AMS* anterior medial sulcus *CP* choroid plexus, *O* olive, *P* pyramid, *PMS* pontomedullary sulcus, *POS* preolivary sulcus. (Photo by Richard Párraga)

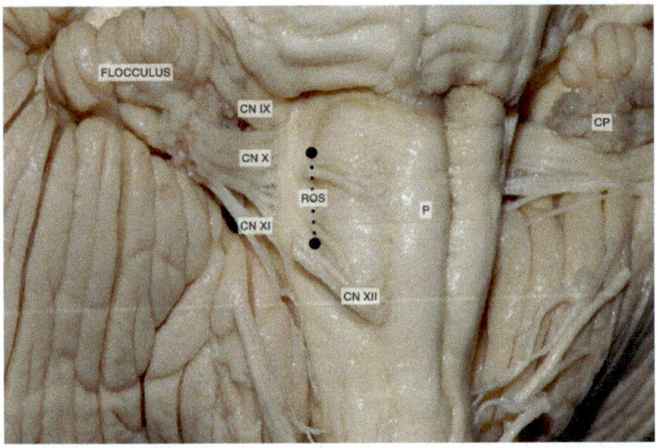

Fig. 9.20 Anterolateral view of the medulla. *CN IX* ninth cranial nerve, *CN X* tenth cranial nerve, *CN XI* eleventh cranial nerve, *CN XII* 12th cranial nerve, *CP* choroid plexus, *P* pyramid, *ROS* retroolivary sulcus. (Photo by Richard Párraga)

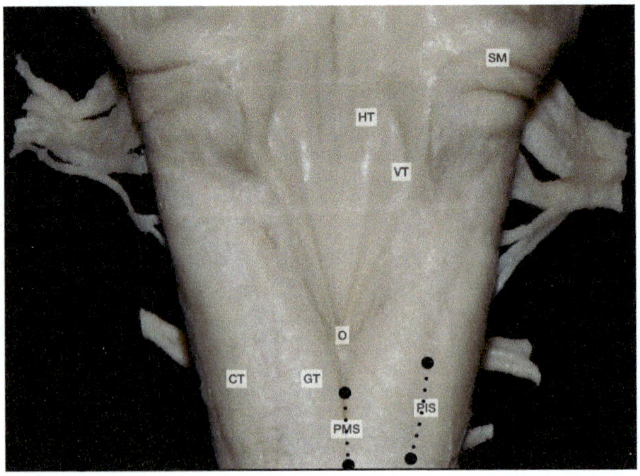

Fig. 9.21 Posterior view of the medulla. *CT* cuneate tubercle, *GT* gracile tubercle, *HT* hypoglossal triangle, *O* obex, *PIS* posterior intermediate sulcus, *PMS* posterior median sulcus, *SM* stria medullaris, *VT* vagal triangle. (Photo by Richard Párraga)

9.11 Anterolateral (Preolivary) Sulcus

The preolivary sulcus is located between the caudal roots of the hypoglossal and the rostral C1 rootlets; this corridor is not commonly used due to the proximity of the corticospinal tract and its decussation.

9.12 Transolivary Zone

The transolivary zone is used to access the lateral medulla via the olive. The medial lemniscus limits this entry zone in its medial, superior, and inferior aspects and the corticospinal tract anteriorly. Its posterior limit corresponds to the anterolateral pathway, composed of the spinocerebellar and spinothalamic tracts. When operating through this zone, the rostrocaudal axis should be used to avoid inadvertent entry into the corticospinal tract or anterolateral pathway (Fig. 9.22).

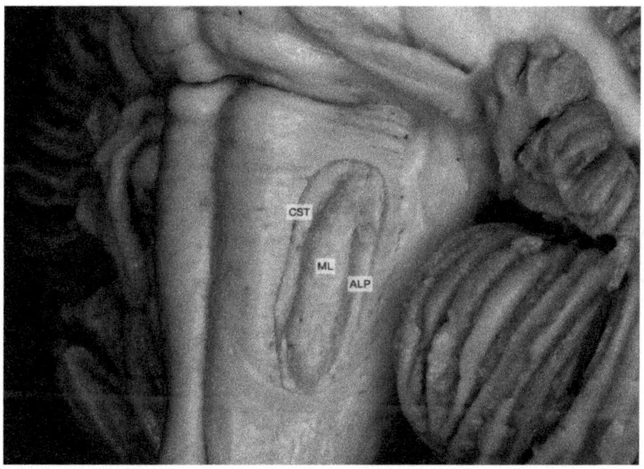

Fig. 9.22 Transolivay zone. *ALP* anterolateral pathway, *CST* corticospinal tract, *ML* medial lemniscus. (Photo by Juan Leonardo Serrato Ávila)

9.13 Retroolivary Sulcus

As mentioned previously, the retroolivary sulcus is located between the olive and inferior cerebellar peduncle. It is situated ventral to the glossopharyngeal and vagus rootlets.

9.14 Posterior Entry Zones

The posterior median sulcus is located inferior to the obex in the midline and provides access to lesions in this region, similar to the intramedullary spinal cord pathologies. The posterior intermediate sulcus, located between the gracile and cuneate fasciculi, and the posterior lateral sulcus, positioned laterally to the cuneate fasciculus, are other zones to access the dorsal medulla.

9.15 Conclusion

Brainstem surgery remains controversial despite advances in neuroimaging and neuromonitoring. Fortunately, pathologies in this highly dense anatomical region tend to displace structures, creating windows for safe resections. It is crucial to return to the laboratory, understand the internal configuration of the brainstem through specimen dissection, and perform approaches to improve exposition while minimizing the manipulation of the surrounding tracts and nucleus.

Bibliography

1. Serrato-Avila JL, Paz Archila JA, Costa MDS da, Rocha PR, Marques SR, de Moraes LOC, et al. Microsurgical approaches to the cerebellar interpeduncular region: qualitative and quantitative analysis. J Neurosurg 2022;136(5):1410–1423.
2. Serrato-Avila JL, Archila JAP, da Costa MDS, Biol PRR, Marques SR, de Moraes LOC, et al. Microsurgical anatomy of the cerebellar interpeduncular entry zones. World Neurosurg. 2022;166:e933–48.
3. Cavalcanti DD, Preul MC, Kalani MYS, Spetzler RF. Microsurgical anatomy of safe entry zones to the brainstem. J Neurosurg. 2016;124(5):1359–76.
4. Yagmurlu K, Rhoton AL Jr, Tanriover N, Bennett JA. Three-dimensional microsurgical anatomy and the safe entry zones of the brainstem. Neurosurgery. 2014;10 Suppl 4(4):602–19; discussion 619-20.
5. Kocer IB, Demiralin MO, Erturk M, Arslan D, Sengul G. Microsurgical anatomy of safe entry zones on the ventrolateral brainstem: a morphometric study. Neurosurg Rev. 2022;45(2):1363–70.
6. Hebb MO, Spetzler RF. Lateral transpeduncular approach to intrinsic lesions of the rostral pons. Neurosurgery. 2010;66(3 Suppl Operative):26–9; discussion 29.

7. Cavalheiro S, Yagmurlu K, da Costa MDS, Nicácio JM, Rodrigues TP, Chaddad-Neto F, et al. Surgical approaches for brainstem tumors in pediatric patients. Childs Nerv Syst. 2015;31(10):1815–40.
8. Kalani MYS, Yağmurlu K, Spetzler RF. The interpeduncular fossa approach for resection of ventromedial midbrain lesions. J Neurosurg. 2018;128(3):834–9.
9. Matsushima K, Yagmurlu K, Kohno M, Rhoton AL. Anatomy and approaches along the cerebellar-brainstem fissures. J Neurosurg. 2016;124(1):248–63.
10. Párraga RG, Possatti LL, Alves RV, Ribas GC, Türe U, de Oliveira E. Microsurgical anatomy and internal architecture of the brainstem in 3D images: surgical considerations. J Neurosurg. 2016;124(5):1377–95.
11. Graffeo CS, Srinivasan VM, Scherschinski L, Benner D, Karahalios K, Devia DA, et al. Expanding the reach of the trans–middle cerebellar peduncle approach: pontine cavernous malformations, tissue transgression beyond the safe entry zone, and the invisible triangle. J Neurosurg. 2023;140:1–13.
12. Cavalheiro S, Serrato-Avila JL, Párraga RG, Da Costa MDS, Nicácio JM, Rocha PR, et al. Interpeduncular sulcus approach to the posterolateral pons. World Neurosurg. 2020;138:e795–805.
13. Serrato-Avila JL, Paz Archila JA, Silva da Costa MD, Riechelmann GS, Rocha PR, Marques SR, et al. Three-dimensional quantitative analysis of the brainstem safe entry zones based on internal structures. World Neurosurg. 2022;158:e64–74.
14. Serrato-Avila JL, Paz Archila JA, Monroy-Sosa A, et al. Resection of the quadrangular lobule of the cerebellum to increase exposure of the cerebellomesencephalic fissure: an anatomical study with clinical correlation. J Neurosurg. 2023;140(4):1160–8. Published 2023 Oct 6. https://doi.org/10.3171/2023.7.JNS222838

Chapter 10
Dissection of the Cerebellum and Fourth Ventricle

10.1 Cerebellum

The dissection and anatomical study of the cerebellum and fourth ventricle present significant challenges, requiring a great deal of dedication and patience. Mastering the anatomy of the cerebellum and fourth ventricle is critical for improving the outcomes of posterior fossa surgery.

10.2 Superficial Anatomy of the Cerebellum

After following the steps outlined for preparing the anatomical specimen in the previous chapters, we will proceed with the examination and analysis of cerebellar surfaces.

In our laboratory training, we first examined the three cerebellar surfaces: tentorial, suboccipital, and petrous. After identifying the hemispheric, vermian, and brainstem structures, we meticulously removed the arachnoid membrane and attached blood vessels (Fig. 10.1).

The dissection of the arachnoid membrane must be performed under microscopic guidance with X6–X40 magnification, using specialized microsurgical tools such as micro-pincers and a no. 11 scalpel blade. The use of surgical microscopes and delicate instruments is essential to minimize trauma to the surrounding tissues, mirroring real surgical scenarios. Although conducted in a laboratory setting, this surgical procedure serves to refine microsurgical skills and prepare students for future clinical dissections.

This stage demands meticulous attention and time, providing students with a realistic simulation of the entire surgical process of opening the arachnoid membrane. Maintaining hydration of the surface with water sprays during dissection

F. Chaddad-Neto, M. D. S. da Costa, *Microneuroanatomy and Lab*,
https://doi.org/10.1007/978-3-031-91026-5_10

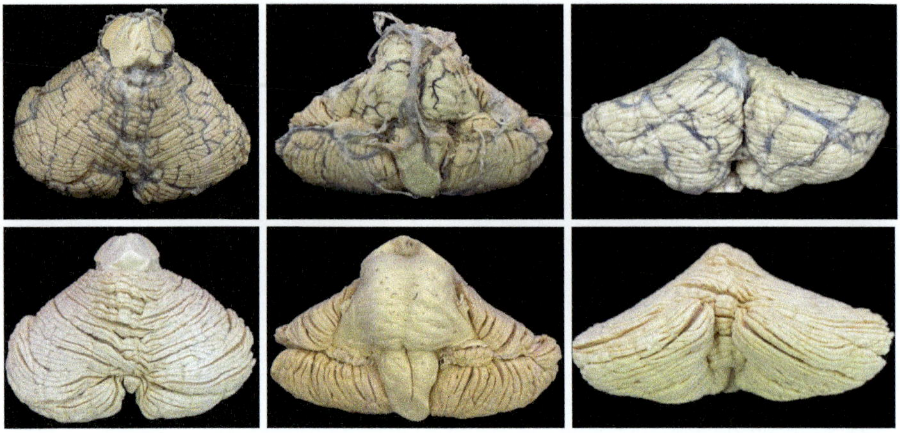

Fig. 10.1 Superior images displaying the tentorial, petrous, and suboccipital surfaces (from left to the right), prior to the vessel and arachnoid removal. The inferior series of images display the same specimens after the vessel and arachnoid removal; no damage is noted on the cerebellar surfaces

ensures that the membrane is less adherent to the parenchyma, thereby reducing the risk of traumatic injuries.

10.3 Surface Analysis

The cerebellum was divided into three surfaces. Each must be carefully analyzed, and its structure must be identified before the dissection process begins. The cerebellum is composed of the vermis, located in the center; right cerebellar hemisphere; and left cerebellar hemisphere. The cerebellar surface is marked by the sulci and gyri, which help distinguish different functional regions.

10.4 Tentorial Surface

The tentorial surface derives its name from its proximity to and contact with the tentorium of the cerebellum and is located just below it (Figs. 10.2 and 10.3). On this surface, the transition between the vermis and hemispheres is more gradual compared with the suboccipital surface; however, the vermian structures and their corresponding structures in the hemispheres remain discernible.

The culmen (vermis) corresponds to the quadrangular lobe (hemisphere). The hemisphere is separated inferiorly by the primary fissure into the declive lobule (vermis) and simple lobule (hemisphere). The simple lobe is separated inferiorly from the folium (vermis) and the superior semilunar lobe (hemisphere) by the postclival fissure (Table 10.1 and Fig. 10.4).

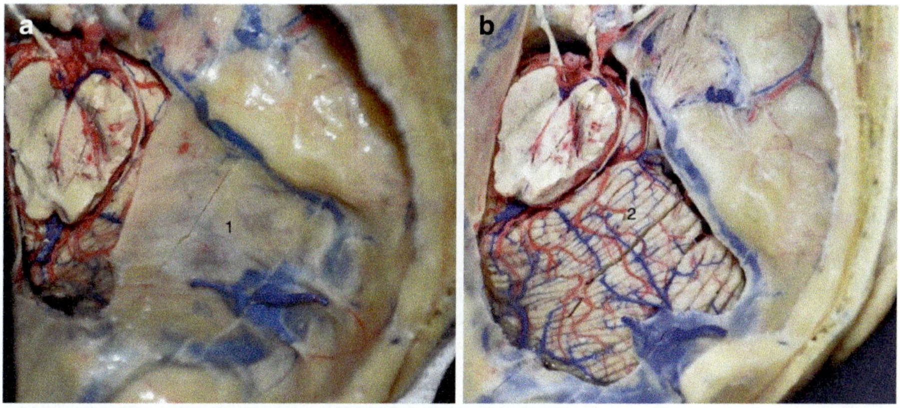

Fig. 10.2 Axial image after brain removal. The brainstem was maintained at the level of the midbrain. (**a**) The tentorial membrane (number 1) covers a significant portion of the posterior fossa, with its sole opening at the tentorial notch. (**b**) Upon tentorium removal, the tentorial surface of the cerebellum can be observed (number 2)

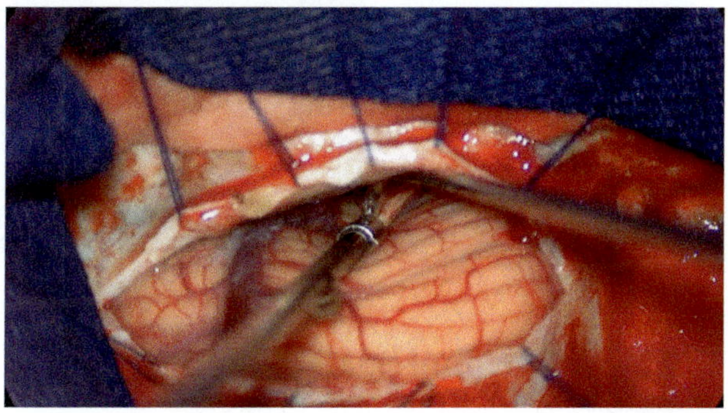

Fig. 10.3 Suboccipital craniotomy exposing the tentorial surface of the cerebellum

Table 10.1 Cerebellar vermis and hemisphere correlation in the tentorial surface

Vermis	Hemisphere
Culmen	Quadrangular lobule
Primary fissure	
Declive	Simple lobule
Post-clival fissure	
Folium	Superior semilunar lobule

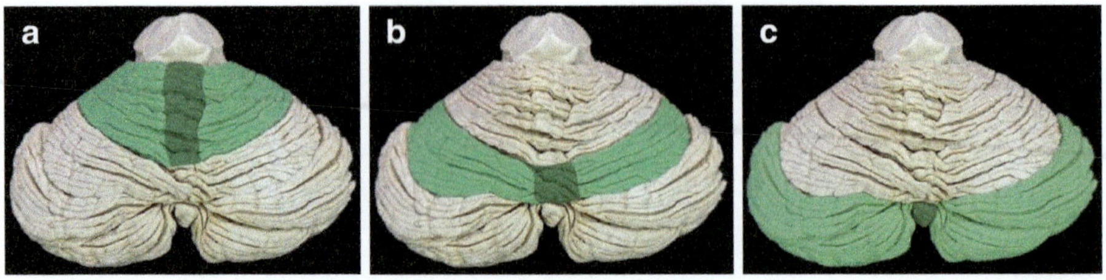

Fig. 10.4 Schematic representation of the structures of the vermis and cerebellar hemispheres of the tentorial surface. (**a**) Quadrangular lobe (light green) and culmen (dark green). (**b**) Simple lobule (light green) and declive lobule (dark green). (**c**) Superior semilunar lobule (light green) and folium (dark green)

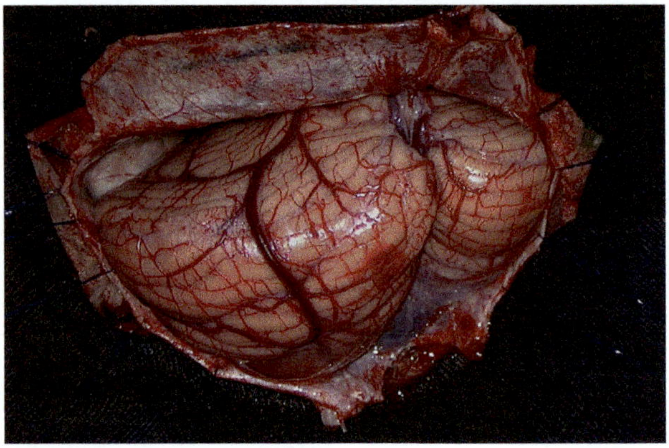

Fig. 10.5 Suboccipital craniotomy exposing the tentorial and suboccipital surface of the cerebellum

10.5 Suboccipital Surface

The suboccipital surface is located just below the transverse sinuses and medially to the sigmoid sinuses. This surface is exposed during wide bilateral suboccipital craniotomies (Fig. 10.5), making detailed anatomical knowledge crucial.

We identified the posterior cerebellar notch, a deep median vertical sulcus where the falx cerebelli rests. The cerebellar vermis lies within the sulcus and is separated from the cerebellar hemispheres by the vermian-hemispheric fissures.

We identified the vermian and hemispheric cerebellar structures and the fissures that separated them (Table 10.2 and Fig. 10.6).

The tonsils are prominent lower structures located in the inferomedial portion of the suboccipital surface.

Table 10.2 Cerebellar vermis and hemisphere correlation in the suboccipital surface

Vermis	Hemisphere
Folium	Superior semilunar lobule
Horizontal fissure	
Tuber	Inferior semilunar lobule
Prebiventral fissure	
Pyramid	Biventral lobule
Tonsilobiventral fissure	
Uvula	Tonsil

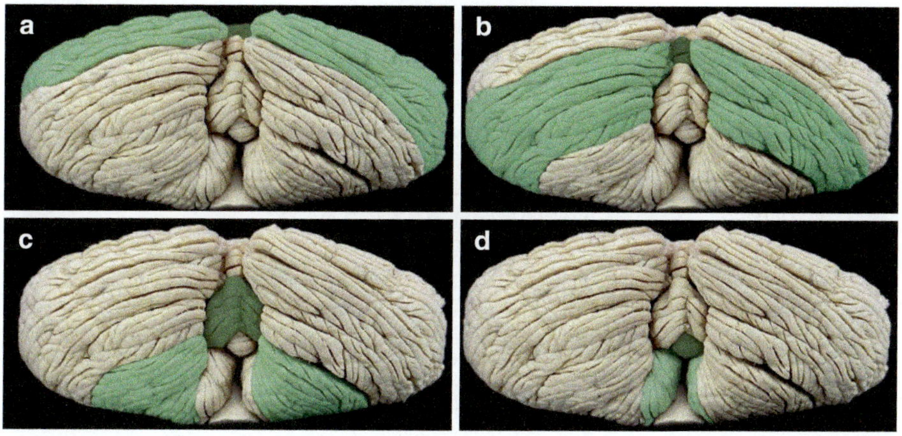

Fig. 10.6 Schematic representation of the structures of the vermis and cerebellar hemispheres in the suboccipital surface. (**a**) Superior semilunar lobule (light green) and folium (dark green). (**b**) Inferior semilunar lobule (light green) and tuber (dark green). (**c**) Biventral lobule (light green) and pyramid (dark green). (**d**) Tonsils (light green) and uvula (dark green)

10.6 Petrous Surface

The petrous surface, also known as the anterior surface, is found on the posterior surface of the petrous portion of the temporal bone. It has a deep longitudinal groove called the anterior cerebellar notch, where the brainstem and the fourth ventricle meet. The surface is accessed and retracted using lateral suboccipital (retrosigmoid) approaches to expose the cerebellopontine angle (Fig. 10.7).

During the initial examination, the cerebellopontine fissure, also known as the cerebellopontine angle, was observed, which is a V-shaped fissure with its upper and lower lips converging toward the lateral apex. This is where the horizontal (or petrous) fissure originates, extending toward the suboccipital surface and dividing it into upper and lower halves.

The fourth ventricle is the median structure of this surface, and the related vermian structures include the lingula, central lobe, culmen, and nodules. Among these structures, only the lingula has no hemispheric counterparts.

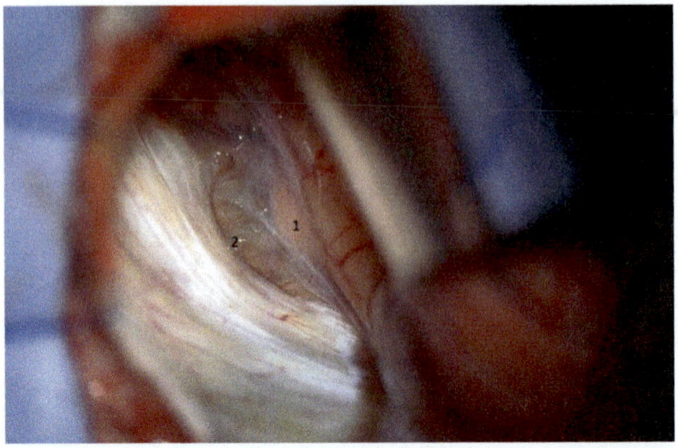

Fig. 10.7 Retrosigmoid craniotomy showing the petrous surface of the cerebellum. After the correct spatulation of the petrous surface, the flocculus (1) and the jugular foramen (2) are exposed

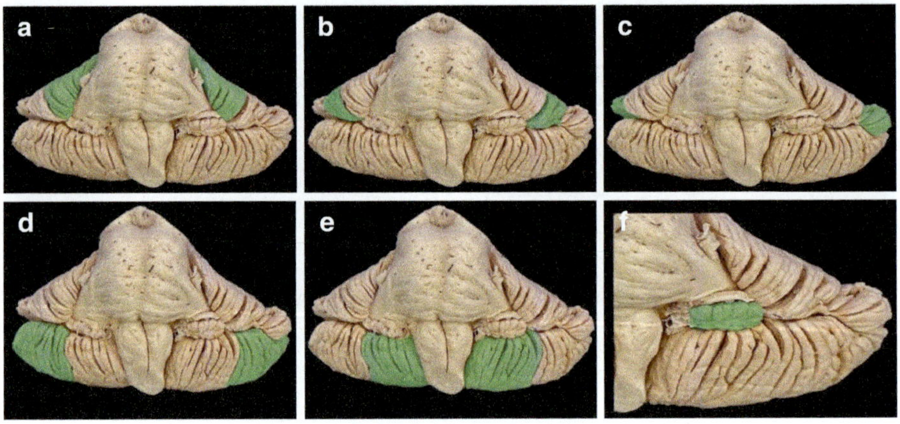

Fig. 10.8 Schematic representation of the structures of the cerebellar hemispheres on the petrosal surface. (**a**) Quadrangular lobule. (**b**) Simple lobule. (**c**) Superior semilunar lobule. (**d**) Inferior semilunar lobule. (**e**) Biventral lobule. (**f**) Floccule

The main landmarks of this surface are the flocculus and choroid plexus, which extend laterally to the foramen of Luschka. This is the only surface where the flocculus can be observed. The identification of the choroid plexus at this surface is straightforward and crucial during surgery, as locating the choroid plexus allows for the subsequent identification of the flocculus positioned superior to it. This, in turn, facilitates the identification of the brainstem exit of the cochlear and facial nerve complex, located anterior and superior to the flocculus (Fig. 10.8).

10.7 Dissection of the Tentorial Surface

Following the completion of the first stage, sequential dissections are performed. Prior knowledge of the structures being dissected is essential as the direction of the movement of spatulas and dissectors must be parallel to the direction of the fibers.

The opposite direction can lead to structural damage and the loss of anatomical pieces.

The cerebellum is divided into two identical portions through a longitudinal cut in the midline.

The first step in tentorial surface dissection is to locate the junction between the quadrangular and simple lobules. The postclival fissure serves as the posterior limit for this stage of resection. Using delicate movements, always following the direction of the fibers to be studied (in this case, from lateral to medial), the cortex of the quadrangular lobule is removed.

Dissection begins with gentle rocking movements from bottom to top and from lateral to medial. The goal is to completely remove the cortex of the quadrangular lobe while ensuring that the lower limit of the folia is respected (Fig. 10.9). Great care must be taken at this stage to avoid cutting too deeply and damaging the specimen. The cerebellar folia are resected en bloc to prevent fragmentation.

After removing the cortex, the insertions of the leaves, known as "U" fibers, which have a wavy formation, are observed (Fig. 10.9a). This layer is removed to clearly visualize the superior, middle, and inferior cerebellar peduncles (ICPs) (Fig. 10.9b).

The anterior half of the dentate nucleus (DN) is located just below the ICP, making a direct connection with the fibers of the superior cerebellar peduncle (SCP). When the fibers are carefully removed from the ICP, the gray matter belonging to the DN can be visualized (Fig. 10.9c–d).

The middle cerebellar peduncle (MCP) is easily identifiable by its voluminous cortico-ponto-cerebellar fibers appearing on the lateral border of the pons and extending posteriorly toward the cerebellar hemisphere. A smaller subset of these fibers was identified as crossing posteriorly to the DN.

The interpeduncular sulcus is an inferior projection of the lateral mesencephalic sulcus, which separates the SCP from the MCP. The SCP fibers run anteroposteriorly and superiorly to inferiorly from the midbrain toward the DN. Its medial edges connect to the superior medullary velum, forming the upper half of the lateral wall of the fourth ventricular roof. Its connection to the DN is covered by the ICP, which must be dissected to fully expose the connection between the DN and the SCP.

The fibers of the ICP run perpendicular to the fibers of the other peduncles, following a path from the bulb to the contralateral cerebellum and crossing over the nodule. Some fibers may remain in the ipsilateral hemisphere, converging on the cerebellar vermis. These fibers run from lateral to medial directions and from inferior to superior directions, emerging from the interpeduncular sulcus and passing over the SCP fibers anterior to the DN.

After removing the ICP, the fibers of the fastigial-bulbar tract can be observed immediately below it; following the dissection, the fibers of the SCP connected to the hilum of the DN can be reached.

The DN is the largest among the cerebellar nuclei. Its prominent bulge over other structures serves as a guide during dissection. It has a triangular shape, with its base facing posteriorly and its apex (known as the hilum) directed toward the SCP. It is surrounded by a layer of fibers called the Fleece of Stilling or the external capsule of the DN, which connects it to the cerebellar lobules. This layer is removed to

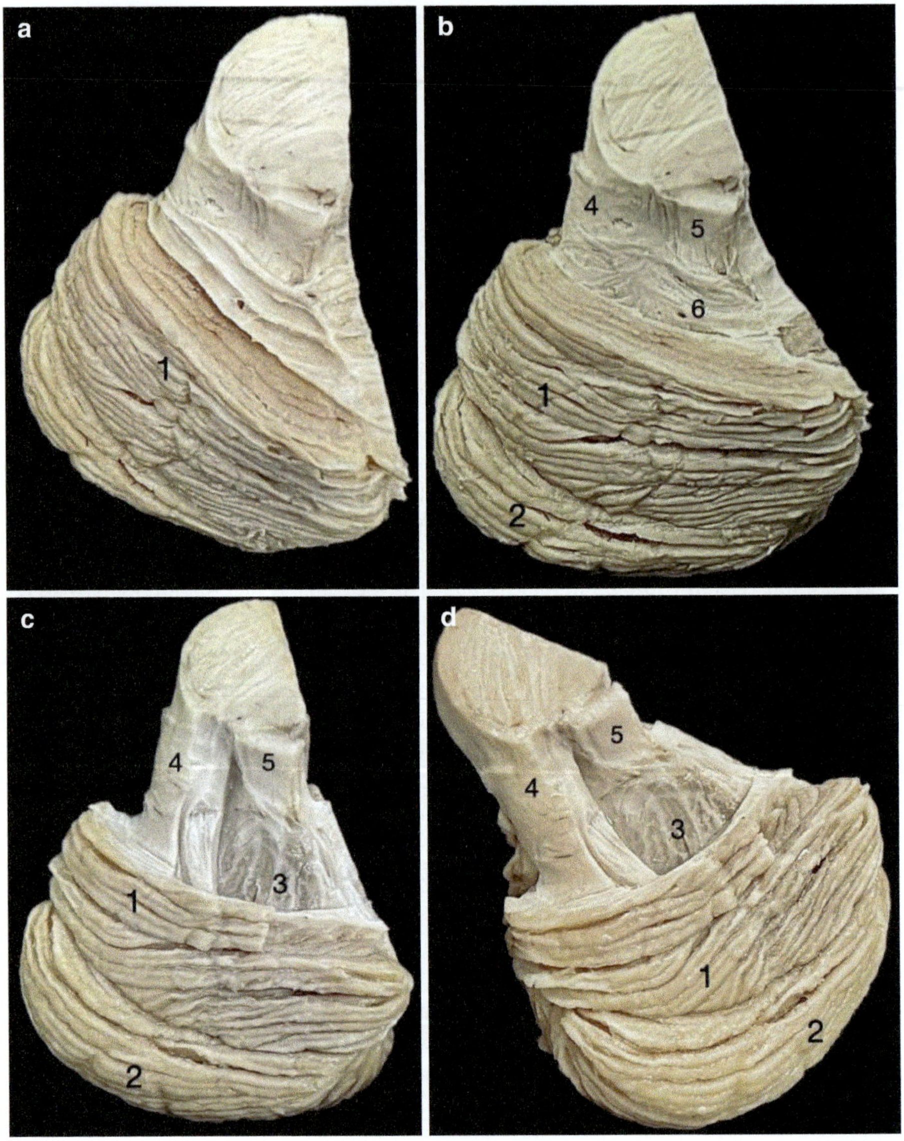

Fig. 10.9 Steps in dissecting the cerebellum. (**a**) Upon removal of the cortical part of the quadrangular lobe, the "U-" shaped fibers can be visualized. The posterior limit of this dissection is the simple lobule (number 1). (**b**) Following the removal of the "U" fibers, the fibers of the inferior cerebellar peduncle, which follow a path from lateral to medial, toward the vermis and contralateral cortex can be observed. At this stage, the middle (4) and superior (5) cerebellar peduncles can also be clearly visualized. (**c** and **d**) After cautious removal of the inferior cerebellar peduncle, the anterior half of the dentate nucleus can be seen (3), projecting its fibers toward the superior cerebellar peduncle. Legends: 1, simple lobule; 2, superior semilunar lobule; 3, dentate nucleus; 4, middle cerebellar peduncle; 5, superior cerebellar peduncle; 6, inferior cerebellar peduncle

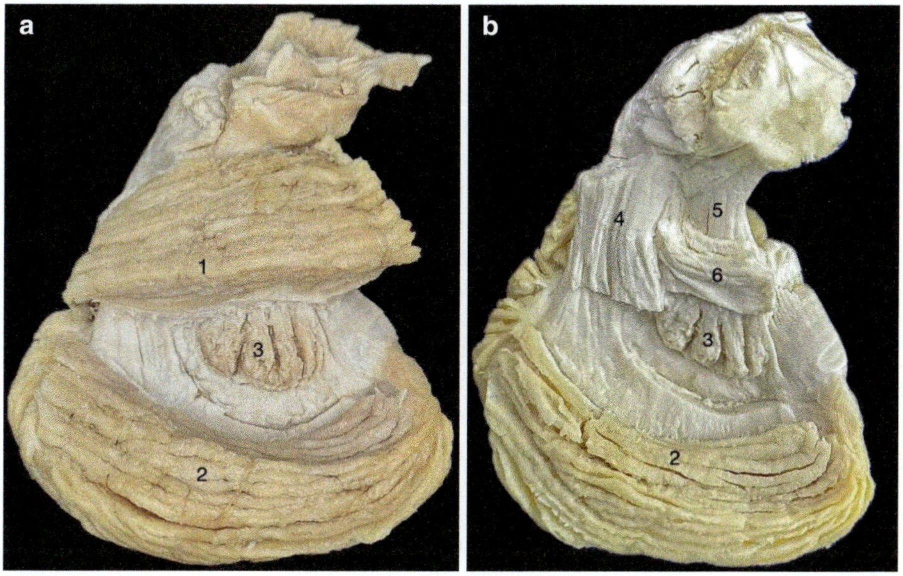

Fig. 10.10 (**a**) The dissection begins by removing the simple lobe. This allows visualization of the posterior half of the dentate nucleus (3), which is not covered by the inferior cerebellar peduncle (6). The dentate nucleus occupies approximately the two anterior thirds of the simple lobule, with the posterior third being formed by fibers projecting from the middle cerebellar peduncle (4). (**b**) After removing the quadrangular lobe (1), the cerebellar peduncles become visible with greater precision. Legend: 1, quadrangular lobule; 2, superior semilunar lobule; 3, dentate nucleus; 4, middle cerebellar peduncle; 5, superior cerebellar peduncle; and 6, inferior cerebellar peduncle

better expose the nuclei. Akakin et al. described a technique to better delineate contours, which involved attaching a cotton ball soaked in an alcohol solution to a low-speed motor drill.

Alternatively, an initial approach to dissection could involve removing the simple lobe while adhering to the aforementioned movements. In this case, the quadrangular lobe serves as the anterior limit, while the superior semilunar lobe serves as the posterior limit.

When the simple lobe is removed, the posterior half of the DN is exposed, which is not covered by ICP fibers. In the posterior region, the DN is bordered laterally, superiorly, and inferiorly by the MCP fibers. Following careful dissection, this stage is concluded by removing the quadrangular lobe, which exposes the origin and projections of the cerebellar peduncles (Fig. 10.10).

As the cerebellum has a central nucleus of gray matter surrounded by a set of white fibers, this region (DN and SCP) is considered the central cerebellar core.

10.8 Dissection of the Suboccipital Surface

This stage is of fundamental importance as it involves visualization of the surface during classic median suboccipital craniotomy. We observed that the structures on this surface had more prominent and easily identifiable sulci.

Initially, the tonsils, which have a single peduncle on their superomedial margins, are dissected. All other surfaces were freed and prepared for mobilization. The dissection of all free edges precedes the removal of the tonsillar peduncle "en bloc." In surgical approaches, tonsil removal does not allow for the visualization of the superolateral recess of the fourth ventricle.The cerebellar tonsils overlay their medial surface, forming a median structure called a vallecula. Its upper margin is juxtaposed with the inferior medulla and tela choroidea to create a telovelotonsillar fissure. The biventral lobe and bulb are located laterally and anteriorly, respectively (Fig. 10.11).The uvula has a vermian counterpart. It has a longitudinal shape and is located immediately below the pyramid, posterior to the nodules.Resection of the biventral lobe, immediately lateral to the tonsil, is essential for clear visualization of the aforementioned structures. Following resection, the MCP fibers covering the

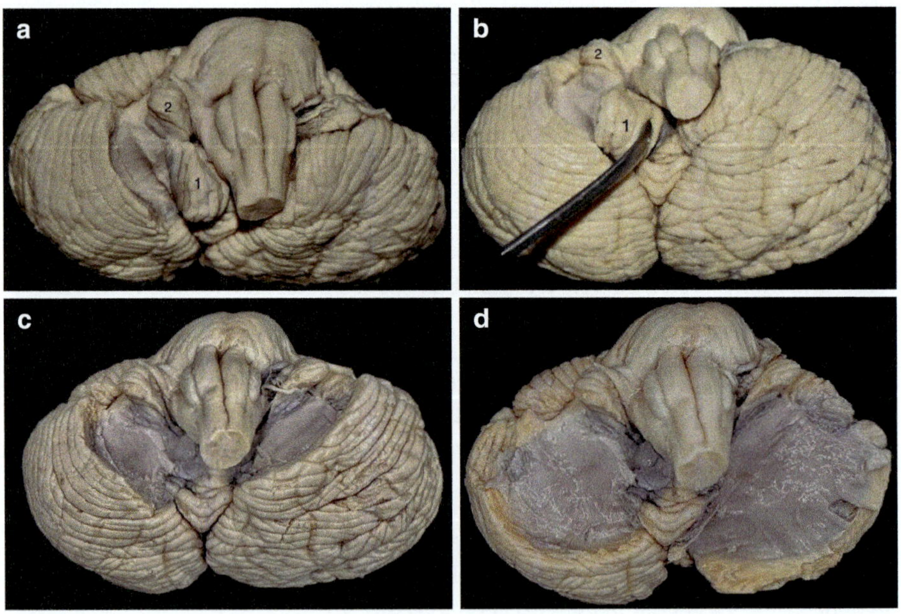

Fig. 10.11 Dissection of the suboccipital surface of the cerebellum. (**a**) The biventral lobe is carefully removed to mobilize and expose the limits of the tonsil (1). (**b**) By mobilizing the tonsil laterally, the vallecula just medial to the tonsillar is exposed. Above the tonsil, the flocculus (2) is visible. (**c**) Bilateral removal of the biventral lobes is continued, exposing the posterolateral limits of the fourth ventricle and visualizing the posterior part of the brain stem. (**d**) The dissection concludes with the removal and meticulous dissection of the inferior semilunar lobes until the lower edge of the dentate nucleus is reached

DN become visible (Fig. 10.11). The DN can be visualized using two approaches. The first approach involves direct visualization following tentorial surface resection, aiming to connect its superior and inferior borders.Alternatively, beginning dissection from the suboccipital surface involves the careful removal of the MCP fibers until the DN becomes visible. At this stage, color changes indicate the presence of gray matter in the DN.In the final stage of dissection of this surface, the inferior vermian structures are exposed. A midline incision is made using a no. 11 blade, passing through the tubercle, pyramid, uvula, and nodule (Fig. 10.11).

10.9 Dissection of the Petrous Surface

In this context, some important anatomical landmarks that aid surgeons or even anatomists in navigating this complex topography safely are discussed. These structures act as checkpoints for safe navigation of the posterior fossa. The trochlear nerve serves as the boundary between the midbrain and the pons in the posterior fossa. Above it lies the midbrain roof with the quadrigeminal lamina and the lateral mesencephalic sulcus. Below the trochlear nerve, the pons with the SCP, superior medullary vellum, and interpeduncular sulcus can be found (Fig. 10.12).

The SCP is a direct continuation of the midbrain, the middle cerebellar peduncle of the pons, and the ICP of the bulb; only the middle cerebellar peduncle is not a part of the fourth ventricle. If one were to assign the "degrees of importance" to the peduncles, the SCP would certainly be of greater clinical importance due to its role in transmitting the fibers of the DN, as described in the above paragraphs on cerebellum anatomy.

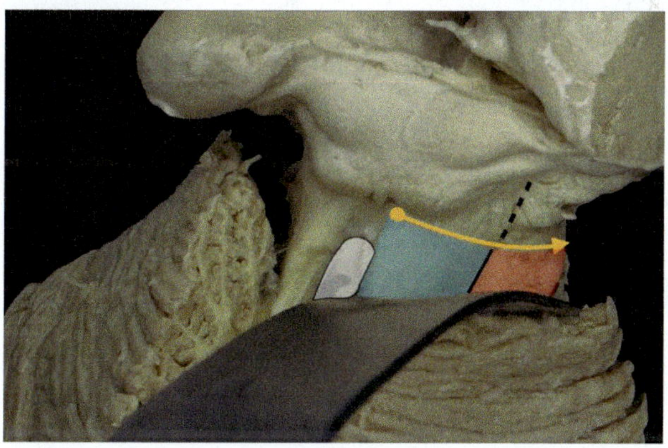

Fig. 10.12 Superior and posterior view of the brainstem. The trochlear nerve (yellow line) is the primary landmark of the posterior fossa. A continuous sulcus on the lateral surface of the midbrain changes its name when it crosses behind the fourth nerve. This is referred to as the lateral mesencephalic sulcus (dotted black line). Below it lies the interpeduncular sulcus (black line), which separates the SCP (blue area) from the middle cerebellar peduncle (red area)

10.10 Fourth Ventricle

The fourth ventricle is a tent-shaped structure positioned posterior to the brainstem and anterior to the cerebellum. It has a roof divided into upper and lower halves, two sidewalls, and a floor.

The upper half of the fourth ventricle roof is composed of the SCP, the superior medullary velum, and the língula; the lower half of the fourth ventricle roof is composed of the inferior medullary velum, tela choroidea, choroid plexus, and the nodule. The meeting point of the lower and upper halves of the fourth ventricle roof is called the fastigium (Fig. 10.13).

The lateral recess of the fourth ventricle and its lateral opening are bordered by the superior, middle, and inferior cerebellar peduncles; rhomboid lip; and flocculus. The flocculus communicates with the nodule via the flocculus peduncle or the inferior medullary velum, which is the bilateral communication of the fourth ventricle with the CP angle through the foramen of Luschka.

The fourth ventricular floor has a rhomboid shape, divided by a junctional zone located between the two lateral recesses, where the medullary striae projects horizontally. The functional zone divides the floor of the fourth ventricle into two triangles: a larger upper triangle with its apex facing the cerebral aqueduct, posterior to the pons, and a smaller lower triangle with its apex facing the obex, posterior to the medulla oblongata (Fig. 10.14).

Both the triangles and the junctional zone are divided longitudinally into two symmetrical halves by the median sulcus. Bilaterally, it has a second depression called the sulcus limitans, and the space between these two depressions is called the

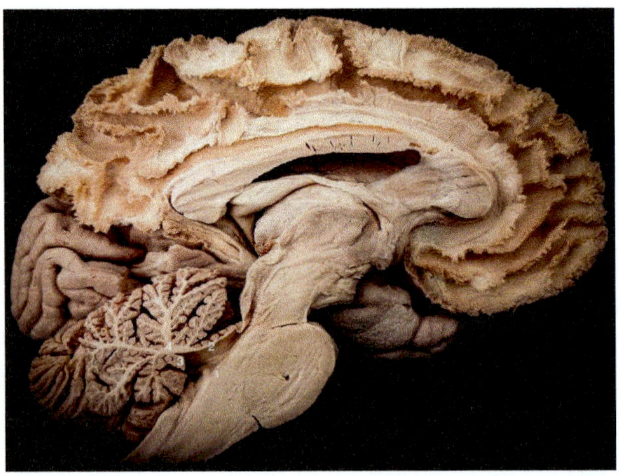

Fig. 10.13 Lateral view of a cadaveric specimen after dissection of the vascular structures, arachnoid membranes, and choroid plexus, revealing the structures that make up the fourth ventricle. (1) Floor of the fourth ventricle. (2) Lingula (component of the upper half of the fourth ventricle roof). (3) Nodule (component of the lower half of the fourth ventricle roof). (4) Fastigium (the meeting point of the lower and upper halves of the fourth ventricle roof)

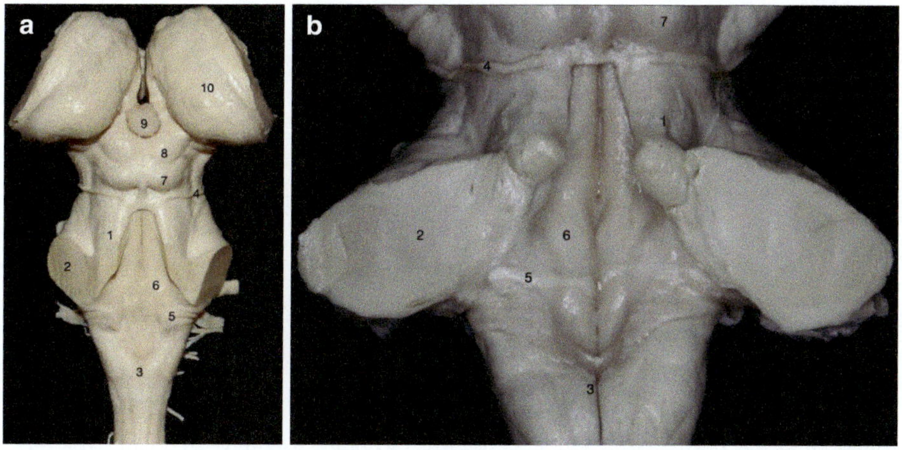

Fig. 10.14 Posterior view of a cadaveric specimen after meticulous dissections of the IV ventricle. (1) Superior cerebellar peduncle, (2) middle cerebellar peduncle, (3) obex, (4) cranial nerve IV, (5) striae medullaris, (6) facial colliculus, (7) inferior colliculus, (8) superior colliculus, (9) pineal gland, and (10) thalamus

medial eminence. The vestibular area is located lateral to the sulcus limitans, followed by the cochlear tubercle. The sulcus limitans divides the motor nuclei medially and the sensory nuclei laterally (Fig. 10.14).

The motor structures in the brainstem are medially positioned. In the medial eminence, the facial colliculus can be found, which is formed by the fibers of the facial nerve (CN VII) surrounding the nucleus of the abducens nerve (CN VI) in the shape of the knee. The number of striae medullaris can vary from one to four. They originate in the median sulcus of the fourth ventricle and run toward the vestibular area; they are the primary anatomical reference for finding the facial follicle, which is located immediately above them (Fig. 10.14).

Below the medullary striae lies two triangles delimited by the median sulcus of the fourth ventricle and the limiting sulcus, and another between the limiting sulcus and the ICP. The medial nerve is called the hypoglossal nerve trigone, while the lateral triangle is called the vagus nerve trigone. Inferiorly, the area postrema and obex are located (Fig. 10.14).

10.10.1 Dissection of the Fourth Ventricle

To benefit most from fourth ventricle dissection, students should possess both basic knowledge of the relevant anatomy and skills in microsurgical techniques.

Standard fourth ventricle approaches generally require similar positioning and exposure. The patient may be placed in either prone or sitting position. A midline suboccipital craniotomy is performed, which may sometimes be extended to include a C1 laminectomy if necessary.

10.11 Telovelar Approach

The telovelar approach involves exposing the cerebello-medullary fissure and incising the tela choroidea and inferior medullary velum. This approach provides access from the obex to the aqueduct and the lateral recesses of the fourth ventricle. Importantly, it avoids splitting the vermis, thereby reducing the risk of cerebellar mutism and other cerebellar deficits.

10.12 Tonsil Retraction/Resection

Depending on the required exposure, either retraction or resection of the cerebellar tonsils may be performed, which generally provides adequate exposure for most procedures. However, resection may be necessary to create a wider corridor to the cerebral aqueduct and lateral recess (Fig. 10.15).

The cerebellar tonsils are gently retracted to visualize the cerebello-medullary fissures. This fissure is a natural cleavage plane found between the cerebellar tonsil and medulla. Dissecting the spaces around the tonsils allows for the retraction of the tonsils and uvula, providing a sufficient view of the ventricular wall without splitting the vermis (Figs. 10.16 and 10.17).

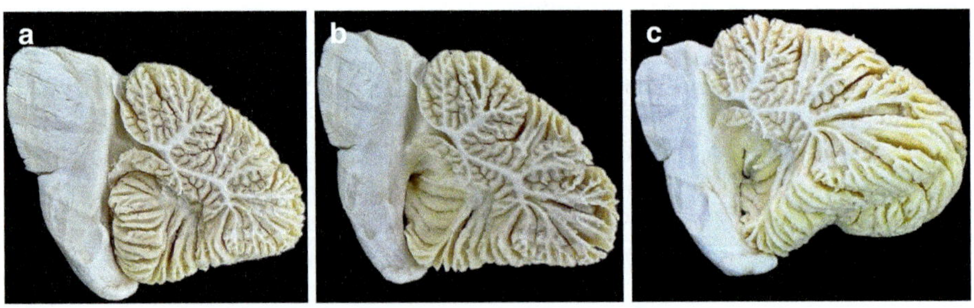

Fig. 10.15 Midline section of the brainstem and cerebellum, showing the upper and lower limits of the fourth ventricle after removal of the arachnoid membrane. (**a**) The cerebellar tonsil is connected superolaterally by the peduncle of the tonsil to its counterpart, the uvula, in the cerebellar vermis. (**b**) After removing the tonsil, the inferior medullary velum and the tela choroidea, which form the inferior portion of the roof of the fourth ventricle, can be visualized. (**c**) The superolateral aspect of the fourth ventricle is visualized after tonsil removal. Therefore, tonsillectomy may be performed in cases of cerebellar lesions affecting the superolateral aspect of the fourth ventricle

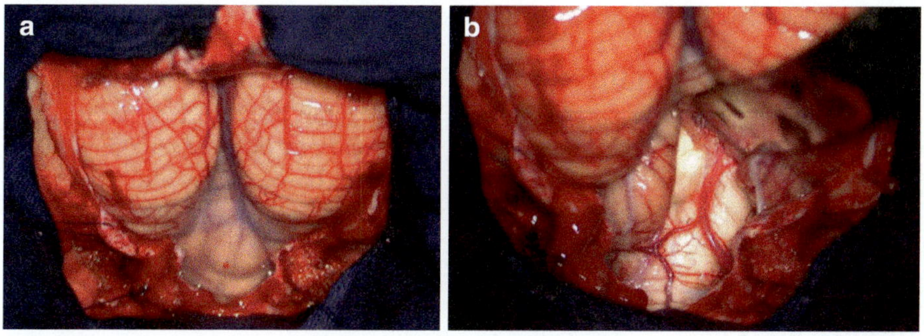

Fig. 10.16 (**a**) Median suboccipital craniotomy for surgical access to the fourth ventricle. A suboccipital craniotomy can be performed with the patient in the semi-sitting or lateral decubitus position, with the side of interest facing downward to facilitate access to the cerebellar tonsils and the surrounding structures. (**b**) Depending on the required exposure, either retraction or resection of the cerebellar tonsils may be performed. Tonsillar retraction generally provides adequate exposure for most procedures, but resection may be necessary to create a wider corridor to the cerebral aqueduct and lateral recess

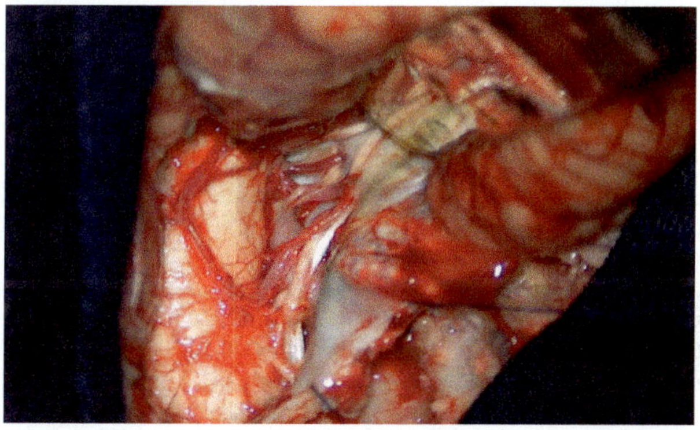

Fig. 10.17 A wide suboccipital craniotomy is performed. When the neurosurgeon requires a wider corridor to access the cerebral aqueduct or superolateral recess, tonsil resection may be helpful. This figure presents a resection of the right tonsil, showing the superolateral aspect of the fourth ventricle

10.13 Transvermian Approach

The transvermian cerebellar surgical approach is used to access the fourth ventricle via an incision through the inferior cerebellar vermis. This approach provides direct access to the entire rostrocaudal length of the fourth ventricle floor from the aqueduct to the obex and allows for a modest increase in the operating angle when accessing the rostral half of the fourth ventricle. However, it does not expose the lateral and superolateral recesses or foramen of Luschka, which are accessible via the telovelar approach.

One of the significant risks associated with the transvermian approach is the potential for postoperative complications, including gait ataxia and dysarthria, due to the disruption of the cerebellar vermis. In clinical practice, the choice between the transvermian and telovelar approaches should be based on specific anatomical and pathological considerations of the lesion.

Bibliography

1. Rhoton AL Jr. Rhoton's cranial anatomy and surgical approaches. Oxford, UK: Oxford University Press; 2019.
2. Dang DD, Rechberger JS, Leonel LCPC, et al. Anatomical step-by-step dissection of midline suboccipital approaches to the fourth ventricle for trainees: surgical anatomy of the telovelar, transvermian, and superior transvelar routes, surgical principles, and illustrative cases. J Neurol Surg B Skull Base. 2023;85(2):172–88. https://doi.org/10.1055/a-2018-4745.
3. Akakin A, Peris-Celda M, Kilic T, Seker A, Gutierrez-Martin A, Rhoton A Jr. The dentate nucleus and its projection system in the human cerebellum: the dentate nucleus microsurgical anatomical study. Neurosurgery. 2014;74(4):401–25. https://doi.org/10.1227/NEU.0000000000000293.
4. Aydin I, Hanalioglu S, Peker HO, et al. The tonsillouvular fissure approach: access to dorsal and lateral aspects of the fourth ventricle. World Neurosurg. 2018;114:e1107–19. https://doi.org/10.1016/j.wneu.2018.03.157.
5. Tanriover N, Ulm AJ, Rhoton AL Jr, Yasuda A. Comparison of the transvermian and telovelar approaches to the fourth ventricle. J Neurosurg. 2004;101(3):484–98. https://doi.org/10.3171/jns.2004.101.3.0484.
6. Matsushima T, Rutka J, Matsushima K. Evolution of cerebellomedullary fissure opening: its effects on posterior fossa surgeries from the fourth ventricle to the brainstem. Neurosurg Rev. 2021;44(2):699–708. https://doi.org/10.1007/s10143-020-01295-2.
7. Tomasello F, Conti A, Cardali S, La Torre D, Angileri FF. Telovelar approach to fourth ventricle tumors: highlights and limitations. World Neurosurg. 2015;83(6):1141–7. https://doi.org/10.1016/j.wneu.2015.01.039.
8. Goiri MAA, de Amorim BL, Sarti THM, da Costa MDS, Chaddad-Neto F. Building a microneurosurgical laboratory in Latin America: challenges and possibilities. Surg Neurol Int. 2021;12:573. Published 2021 Nov 23. https://doi.org/10.25259/SNI_978_2021
9. Biondi-Soares LG, Párraga RG, Apaza-Tintaya RA, et al. Mapping Anatomical Landmarks of the Cerebellum Central Core: Enhancing Precision in Surgical Interventions for Cerebellar Lesions. Cerebellum. 2025;24(4):87. Published 2025 Apr 24. https://doi.org/10.1007/s12311-025-01841-y
10. Serrato-Avila JL, Paz Archila JA, Monroy-Sosa A, et al. Resection of the quadrangular lobule of the cerebellum to increase exposure of the cerebellomesencephalic fissure: an anatomical study with clinical correlation. J Neurosurg. 2023;140(4):1160–8. Published 2023 Oct 6. https://doi.org/10.3171/2023.7.JNS222838
11. Cavalheiro S, Yagmurlu K, da Costa MD, et al. Surgical approaches for brainstem tumors in pediatric patients. Childs Nerv Syst. 2015;31(10):1815–40. https://doi.org/10.1007/s00381-015-2799-y

Chapter 11
Supratentorial Arterial Vascularization

Intracranial vascularization is formed by two arterial systems: the anterior circulation (also known as the carotid system) and the posterior circulation (also known as the vertebrobasilar system). These systems are interconnected by an anastomosis, with the most significant being the posterior communicating artery and, occasionally, the persistent embryological arteries. The carotid system is divided into internal and external circulations, which interconnect through anastomoses along their respective pathways.

A comprehensive understanding of the supratentorial vascular anatomy is essential for neurosurgeons owing to the high prevalence of pathologies within the supratentorial intracranial compartment and the complexities associated with their surgical management.

11.1 ICA Origin and Segments

The right common carotid artery originates in the neck from the brachiocephalic trunk, while the left common carotid artery arises from the aortic arch in the thorax. Typically, the common carotid artery bifurcates at the level of the fourth cervical vertebra, which aligns with the upper border of the thyroid cartilage and the angle of the mandible. Less commonly, they bifurcate at the C5 or C6 level. This gives rise to the internal carotid artery (ICA) and external carotid artery (ECA). The ICA is further divided into segments based on its anatomical location and branches.

The cervical segment is the first and longest segment. This segment begins at the bifurcation of the common carotid artery and extends through the neck before entering the skull. It ascends through the carotid sheath alongside the internal jugular vein and vagus nerve, typically without giving rise to any branches. Knowledge of its anatomical relationships and the ability to expose this segment are vital for performing procedures such as carotid endarterectomy for occlusive disease, high-flow

F. Chaddad-Neto, M. D. S. da Costa, *Microneuroanatomy and Lab*,
https://doi.org/10.1007/978-3-031-91026-5_11

bypass, and proximal control of vascular pathologies, including paraclinoid aneurysms. After cutting through the skin, subcutaneous tissue, and platysma muscle, the sternocleidomastoid muscle, covered by the superficial cervical fascia, is then exposed. By incising the superficial cervical fascia medial to the medial border of the sternocleidomastoid muscle and reflecting it posteriorly, the carotid artery becomes visible within the carotid sheath. This approach allows for the identification of its bifurcation, with the ICA discernable by its posterolateral position relative to the ECA and the absence of collaterals. Laterally, it is connected to the internal jugular vein and posterior to the vagus nerve (Fig. 11.1).

The second ICA segment is the petrous segment, which begins at the external opening of the carotid canal in the petrous part of the temporal bone at the skull base (Fig. 11.2). This segment is divided into two portions along its course from posterolateral to anteromedial: a shorter vertical portion and a longer horizontal portion, which turns upward above the fibrocartilage-filled foramen lacerum. This portion is closely associated with the Gasser's ganglion (which is separated by a thin layer of bone in approximately 60% of cases). The ganglion is located lateral to the mandibular division of the trigeminal nerve, posterior to the tensor tympani muscle and eustachian tube (both covered by bone), and underneath the thin bony layer inferior to the greater superficial petrosal nerve (GSPN). It gives rise to two collateral branches: the caroticotympanic artery at the level of the carotid canal and the vidian

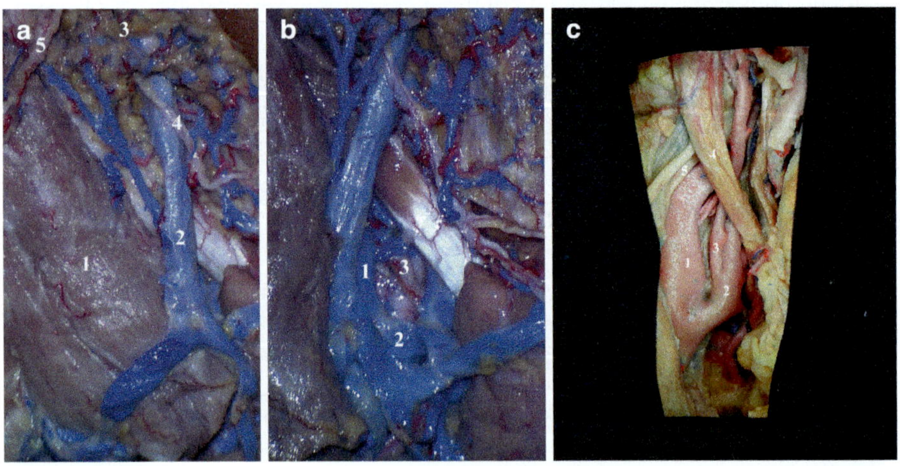

Fig. 11.1 (**a**) Right lateral aspect of the cervical region. After dissecting the platysma, the following structures are visible: the sternocleidomastoid muscle (1), external jugular vein and its tributaries (2), parotid gland (3), facial nerve (4), and great auricular nerve (5). (**b**) In a deeper plane, after retracting the anterior edge of the sternocleidomastoid muscle and opening the carotid sheath, the Farabeuf's triangle is observed. This triangle is formed by the internal jugular vein (1), facial vein (2), and hypoglossal nerve (3), with its content being the bifurcation of the common carotid artery. (**c**) The bifurcation of the common carotid artery is exposed. The internal carotid artery, in its cervical segment (1), is positioned posterolaterally to the external carotid artery (2), which gives off collateral branches at the cervical level, such as the ascending pharyngeal artery (3). The posterior belly of the digastric muscle (4) and vagus nerve (5) can also be observed

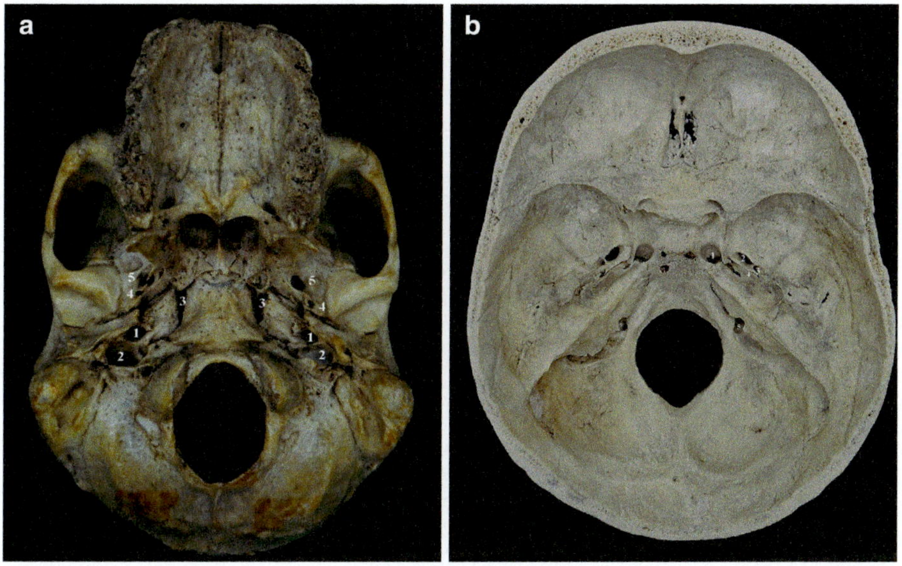

Fig. 11.2 (**a**) Carotid canal (1) is viewed from the exocranium along with key anatomical landmarks such as the jugular foramen (2), foramen lacerum (3), foramen spinosum (4), and foramen ovale (5). (**b**) Endocranial view showing significant anatomical landmarks associated with the petrosal segment, such as the foramen lacerum (1), foramen ovale (2), foramen spinosum (3), bony groove for the greater petrosal superficial nerve (4), and jugular foramen (5)

artery. To expose this segment, the middle fossa must be accessed first to separate the two dural sheets. An incision is initially made at the most lateral end of the superior orbital fissure, corresponding to the meningo-orbital band, which is the most superficial dural band connecting the frontotemporal dura to the periorbita. This meningeal band provides a well-defined cleavage plane between the endosteal and meningeal sheets. Blunt dissection of these two layers is then performed from anterior to posterior using a dissector. Once the middle fossa is completely exposed, landmarks such as the GSPN, trigeminal nerve, ganglion, foramen spinosum, and ovale are used to identify the horizontal segment of the petrous ICA, if not visible upon elevating the dura. The GSPN and its trajectory serve as important anatomical landmarks for guiding the initial dissection, as it runs anteromedially above the horizontal portion. Finally, to expose the horizontal portion, the middle fossa floor is drilled posterior and medial to the GSPN, lateral to the lateral margin of V3, and 5–10 mm medial to the foramen spinosum (Fig. 11.3).

The third segment of the ICA is known as the lacerum. This short vertical segment extends from above the foramen lacerum and ends at the level of the petrolingual ligament, crossing the lateral surface. Both the lacerum segment and petrolingual ligament are located medial to the trigeminal ganglion (Fig. 11.4). The petrolingual ligament serves as the posteroinferior attachment of the lateral wall of the cavernous sinus and spans from the lingula of the sphenoid bone anteriorly to the petrous apex posteriorly. In the laboratory setting, exposing this segment requires

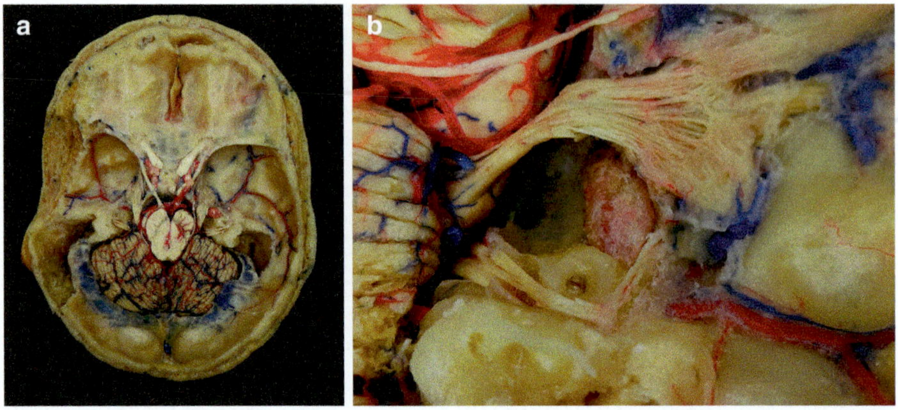

Fig. 11.3 (**a**) Superior view of the middle fossa following bone removal and exposure of the petrous segment of the internal carotid artery (ICA) (1) and anterior clinoidectomy. The following structures are visible: trigeminal nerve (2), Gasser's ganglion (3), middle meningeal artery entering through the foramen spinosum (4), greater superficial petrosal nerve (5), facial nerve (6), cochlea (7), trochlear nerve (8), oculomotor nerve (9), optic nerve (10), supraclinoid ICA (11), and pituitary stalk (12). (**b**) Superior and lateral view, focusing on the horizontal portion of the petrous segment of the ICA after drilling the middle fossa bone

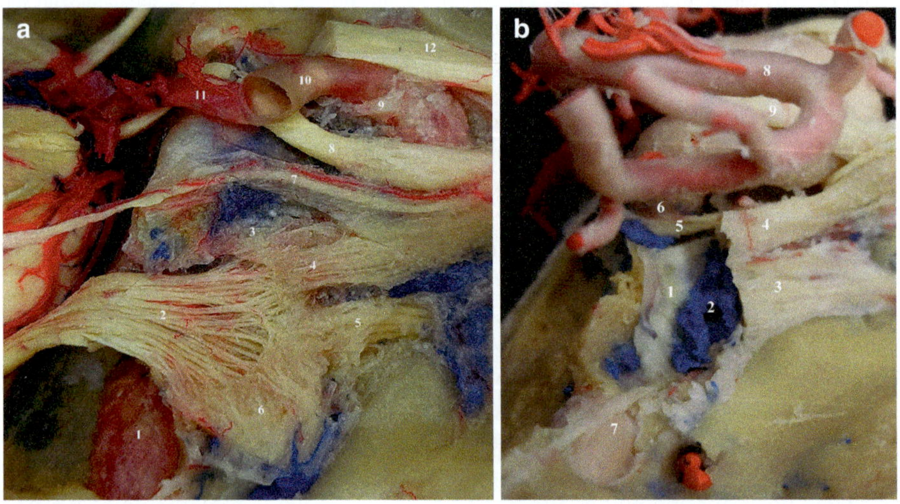

Fig. 11.4 (**a**) The trigeminal ganglion covers the lacerum segment of the internal carotid artery (ICA): (1) Petrous segment of the ICA (2). Trigeminal ganglion (3). Superior margin of the petrolingual ligament (4). V1 (5). V2 (6). V3 (7). Trochlear nerve (8). Oculomotor nerve (9). Distal dural ring (10). Supraclinoid ICA (11). Posterior communicating artery (12). Optic nerve. (**b**) After detaching the trigeminal ganglion and roots, the petrolingual ligament is exposed: (1) Petrolingual ligament (2). Cavernous sinus (3). V1 (4). Oculomotor nerve (5). Abducens nerve (6). Intracavernous carotid (7). Petrous carotid (8). Middle cerebral artery (9). Optic nerve

detaching the trigeminal ganglion and the proximal portion of its branches. The superior margin of the petrolingual ligament is located approximately aligned with a line extending backward along the upper edge of V2, parallel to the abducens nerve.

The fourth segment of the ICA is the cavernous segment and, similar to the previous segments, is extradural (Fig. 11.5). The upper margin of the petroligual ligament marks the anatomical boundary at which the ICA transitions to the intracavernous ICA. This segment is situated between the dura mater layers forming the cavernous sinus and situated in the carotid groove on the side of the sphenoid bone. It is composed of five portions: a posterior ascending portion, an anteriorly curving segment known as the posterior bend, a horizontal portion, the anterior bend, and the anterior ascending portion. The meningohypophyseal trunk originates

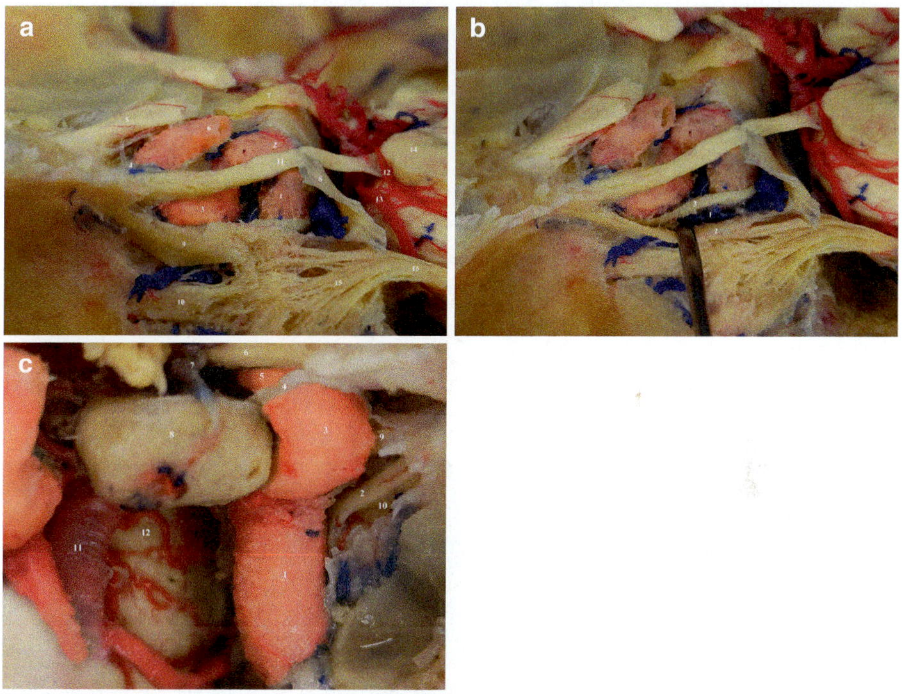

Fig. 11.5 (**a**) Dissection of the medial layer of the lateral wall of the cavernous sinus exposes the cavernous segment of the internal carotid artery (ICA): (1) Posterior ascending portion (2). Posterior bend (3). Horizontal portion (4). Proximal dural ring (5). Optic nerve (6). Supraclinoid ICA (7). Pituitary stalk (8). Posterior wall of the cavernous sinus (9). V1 (10). V2 (11). Oculomotor nerve (12). Posterior cerebral artery (13). Superior cerebellar artery (14). Cerebral peduncle. (15) Trigeminal ganglion. (16) Trigeminal nerve. (**b**) Mobilization of the ophthalmic nerve exposes the abducens nerve in its intracavernous portion: (1) Cavernous sinus (2). V1 (3). Abducens nerve. (**c**) Endoscopic view following the dissection and exposure of the ICA segments through a transclival approach: (1) Paraclival carotid artery (lacerum segment/posterior ascending portion) (2). Abducens nerve (3). Parasellar carotid artery (anterior ascending portion/clinoidal segment) (4). Distal dural ring (5). Supraclinoid ICA (6). Optic nerve (7). Pituitary stalk (8). Pituitary gland (9). Oculomotor nerve (10). V1 (11). Basilar trunk (12). Pons

from the posterior bend; this trunk gives rise to the dorsal meningeal artery, the inferior hypophyseal artery, and the artery of Bernasconi and Cassinari. The horizontal portion gives rise to the inferolateral trunk and, distally, to the medial branches (<10% of cases) known as McConnell's capsular arteries, which supply the pituitary gland capsule. This segment is exposed in the laboratory just before the middle fossa peeling. It can be observed between the cranial nerves contained within the inner layer of the lateral wall of the cavernous sinus (III, IV, and ophthalmic division of V) and medial to the intracavernous abducens nerve.

Between the proximal and distal dural rings lies the fifth part of the ICA, known as the clinoid segment. This segment is extradural and extracavernous (Fig. 11.6). The proximal dural ring marks the true upper limit of the cavernous sinus. It is a projection of the membrane that covers the oculomotor nerve (carotid-oculomotor membrane) and surrounds the ICA by 360°, but not as tightly as the proximal ring, allowing numerous venous channels from the cavernous sinus to pass through. By contrast, the distal dural ring is a medial extension of the dura mater that covers the upper surface of the anterior clinoid process and surrounds the ICA by 360°, adhering strongly. The anterior genu of the ICA may be classified as extradural, extracavernous, intracavernous, or intradural depending on the position of the carotid-oculomotor membrane. This segment is critical for the treatment of paraclinoid and cavernous aneurysms. To expose this segment, anterior clinoidectomy, a vital procedure for treating aneurysms and tumors in this region, must be performed.

Above the distal dural ring are the intradural portion of the ICA and supraclinoid ICA (Fig. 11.7).

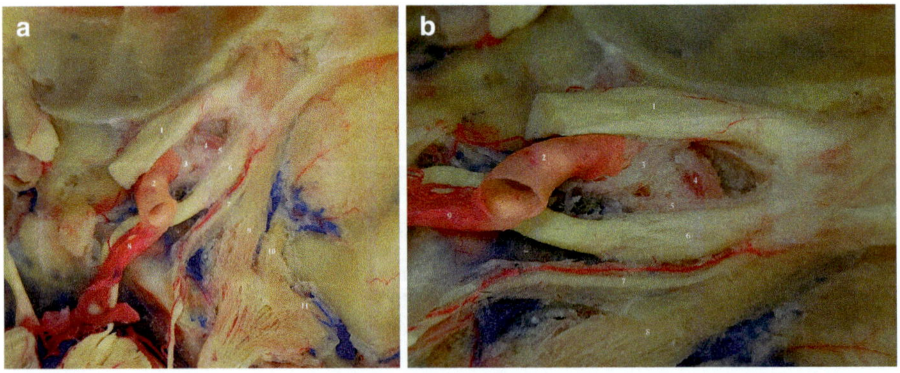

Fig. 11.6 (**a**) Superior view of the clinoidal segment of the internal carotid artery (ICA) following an anterior clinoidectomy: (1) Optic nerve (2). Supraclinoid ICA (3). Distal dural ring (4). Clinoidal segment (5). Proximal dural ring (carotid-oculomotor membrane) (6). Oculomotor nerve (7). Trochlear nerve (8). Posterior communicating artery (9). V1 (10). V2 (11). V3. (**b**) Lateral view of the clinoidal segment: (1) Optic nerve (2). Supraclinoid ICA (3). Distal dural ring (4). Clinoidal segment (5). Proximal dural ring (carotid-oculomotor membrane) (6). Oculomotor nerve (7). Trochlear nerve (8). V1 (9). Posterior communicating artery

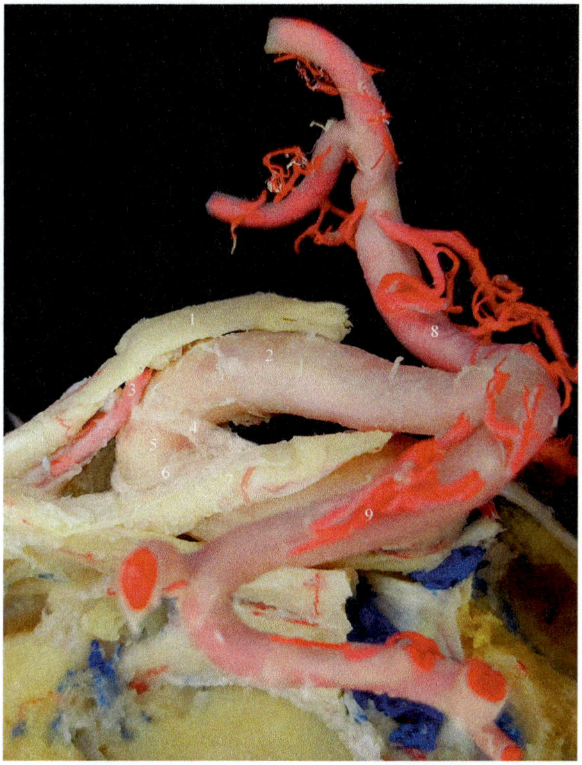

Fig. 11.7 Supraclinoid internal carotid artery (ICA). (1) Optic nerve (2). Supraclinoid ICA (3). Ophthalmic artery (4). Distal dural ring (5). Clinoidal segment (6). Proximal dural ring (7). Oculomotor nerve (8). Anterior cerebral artery. (9) Middle cerebral artery

Students should be able to name each segment of the ICA and identify its anatomical limits. All of these segments are extradural and give rise to branches that supply the extradural structures and extra-axial lesions. These segments are listed as follows:

1. The cervical segment extends from the common carotid artery bifurcation to the external opening of the carotid canal.
2. The petrous segment extends from the external opening of the carotid canal to the lateral margin of the trigeminal nerve.
3. The lacerum segment extends from the lateral margin of the trigeminal nerve to the superior margin of the petrolingual ligament.
4. The cavernous segment extends from the superior margin of the petrolingual ligament to the proximal dural ring.
5. Clinoid segment extends from the proximal to the distal dural ring.

11.2 Supraclinoid ICA

Once the ICA passes through the distal dural ring, the supraclinoid segment is formed. This segment extends superiorly, posteriorly, and laterally to the end and bifurcates immediately below the anterior perforated substance. The distal dural ring delineates the sixth portion of the ICA and ophthalmic segment anteriorly. This segment gives rise to the ophthalmic and superior hypophyseal arteries. Once the ICA is positioned inferolateral to the optic nerve, the ophthalmic artery originates in the superior, anterior, and medial walls of the ICA and follows the optic nerve in the inferolateral portion of the optic canal. In a small percentage of patients, the ophthalmic artery may originate extradurally from the clinoid segment. The meningo-orbitory artery serves as the primary collateral vessel of the ophthalmic artery. Additionally, the superior hypophyseal artery arises from the ophthalmic segment of the ICA and usually presents as one or two branches larger in diameter than the other perforators from the medial face of this segment. These branches supply the pituitary gland, stalk, surrounding nerves, and optic chiasm.

The seventh ICA segment is the communicating segment, which extends from the origin of the posterior communicating artery (PComA) in the posterior and medial aspects to the origin of the anterior choroidal artery (AChA) in the posterior and lateral aspects. Finally, the eighth segment extends from the origin of the AChA

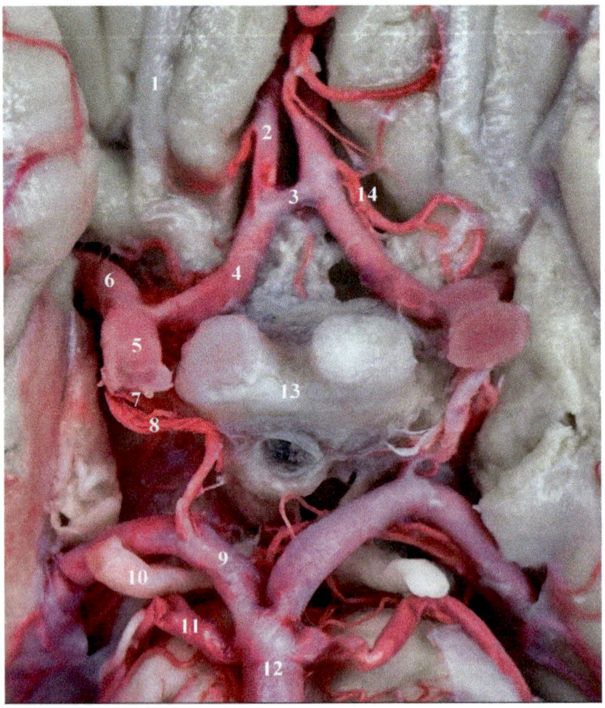

Fig. 11.8 Basal view of the circle of Willis (1). Olfactory nerve (2). A2 segment of the anterior cerebral artery (ACA). (3) Anterior communicating artery. (4) A1 segment of the ACA (5). Supraclinoid internal carotid artery. (6) Middle cerebral artery (7). Anterior choroidal artery (8). Posterior communicating artery (9). Posterior cerebral artery (10). Oculomotor nerve (11). Superior cerebellar artery (12). Basilar trunk (13). Optic chiasm (14). Recurrent artery of Heubner

to the ICA bifurcation into the anterior cerebral artery (ACA) and middle cerebral artery (MCA) (Fig. 11.8).

11.3 ICA and Basal Cisterns

The basal cisterns are cerebrospinal fluid reservoirs enclosed by the arachnoidal trabeculae attached to the skull base. These cisterns have a large capacity (Fig. 11.9). All ICA branches extend from the carotid cistern to other cisterns. Therefore, they are all included in at least two cisterns (Fig. 11.10).

The first intracranial ICA branch is the ophthalmic artery, which extends from the carotid to the ophthalmic cistern. The superior hypophyseal artery extends from the carotid cistern to the inferior half of the optic chiasm.

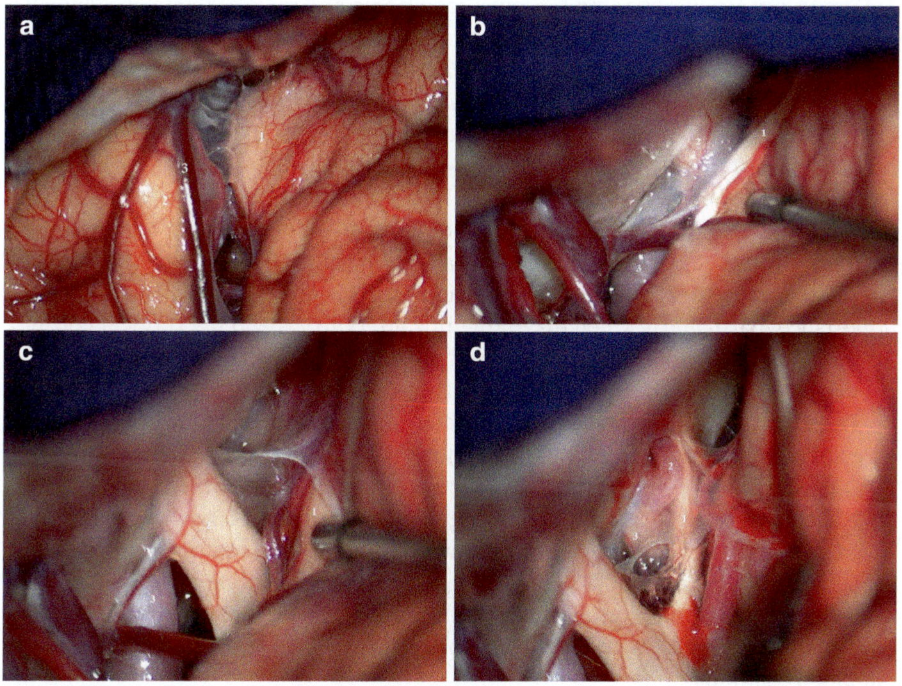

Fig. 11.9 Operative view of the arachnoid cisterns during a transsylvian approach following a left pterional craniotomy (**a**) Lateral arachnoid membrane of the Sylvian cistern, extending from the inferior frontal gyrus (1), to the superior temporal gyrus (2), and superficial Sylvian vein (3). (**b**) Olfactory, chiasmatic, and carotid cisterns and their respective contents: olfactory tract (1), optic nerve (2), and supraclinoid internal carotid artery (3). (**c**) Opening of the cisterns at the level of the gyrus rectus (1) with exposure of the optic nerve (2) and supraclinoid ICA (3). (**d**) View of the contralateral chiasmatic and carotid cisterns containing the optic nerve (1), ophthalmic artery (2), and supraclinoid ICA (3)

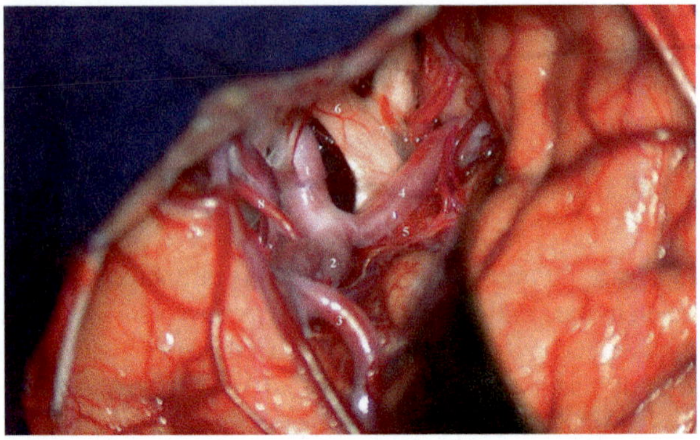

Fig. 11.10 Operative view after cisternal dissection (1). Supraclinoid internal carotid artery. (2) M1 (middle cerebral artery [MCA]) (3). M2 (MCA) (4). A1 (anterior choroidal artery) (5). Anterior lenticulostriate arteries (6). Optic nerve (7). Optic chiasm (8). Temporopolar artery (early branch)

The PComA penetrates the Lliequist membrane and reaches the interpeduncular cistern, where it joins the posterior cerebral artery (PCA). The perforators of this artery, known as the anterior thalamoperforating arteries, originate from its superior surface and typically from its proximal half and supply the internal capsule, optic tract, thalamus, posterior perforated substance, and floor of the third ventricle. The premammillary artery is a significant vessel with three potential patterns according to the posterior circulation supply: adult, hypoplastic, and fetal. The fetal pattern is responsible for the vascularization of the circulation distal to the P1 segment of the PCA, while the adult and hypoplastic patterns do not contribute to the posterior circulation, regardless of the artery's diameter. This information is of paramount importance, particularly when dissecting this artery to expand the surgical corridor. Typically, the PComA courses superomedially to the third nerve. In fetal pattern, the nerve courses above or lateral to the oculomotor nerve.

The AChA extends from the carotid cistern to the lower end of the choroidal fissure at the inferior choroidal point and enters the temporal horn. The cisternal segment initially runs along the medial surface of the anterior segment of the uncus and continues superiorly to the posterior segment of the uncus below the optic tract. Upon entering the temporal horn, the intraventricular segment anastomoses with branches from the lateral posterior choroidal artery. Perforating branches typically arise from the cisternal segment and supply the optic tract, uncus, lateral geniculate body, and anterior perforated substance, providing blood to the internal capsule and the globus pallidus.

Both the PComA and the AChA originate from the inferior ICA surface. However, the PComA courses medially, while the AChA courses laterally.

Digital subtraction angiography is a dynamic imaging technique that enables a detailed examination of the cerebral vascular system. The different segments and their respective branches are easily identifiable on the angiogram. The beginning of the supraclinoid ICA is marked by the origin of the ophthalmic artery, which is the first branch to extend anteriorly. Although the distal dural ring anatomically marks

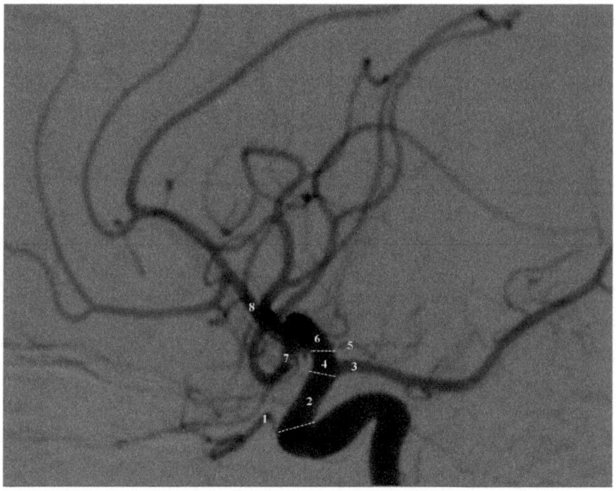

Fig. 11.11 Lateral view of a digital subtraction angiography of the left internal carotid artery: (1) Ophthalmic artery (2). Ophthalmic segment (3). Posterior communicating artery (4). Communicating segment (5). Anterior choroidal artery (6). Choroidal segment (7). Middle cerebral artery (8). Anterior cerebral artery

the beginning of this segment, it is not visible on angiography. The second branch visible on the angiogram is the PComA. The origin of this artery marks the distal end of the ophthalmic segment and the beginning of the communicating segment, which concludes at the origin of the AChA. Finally, the choroidal segment runs from the origin of the AChA to the bifurcation of the ICA where it splits into two terminal branches, the ACA and MCA (Fig. 11.11).

11.4 Basal Surface

The bifurcation of the ICA is situated below the anterior perforated substance. From its posterior wall, a group of anterior perforating arteries emerges. The recurrent artery of Heubner is closely associated with the ICA bifurcation. Typically, this artery passes superiorly to the ICA bifurcation; however, it may also travel anteriorly or posteriorly. The two terminal branches of the ICA give rise to perforating arteries known as the lenticulostriate arteries. Perforating arteries arising from the A1 segment are called medial lenticulostriate arteries, while those arising from the M1 segment are called lateral lenticulostriate arteries.

The A1 segment extends from the carotid cistern to the superior half of the optic chiasma cistern. It is easily identifiable as it passes superiorly to the optic chiasm. Its anterior wall does not give rise to lenticulostriate arteries, making it a safe zone for dissection. The anterior communicating artery (ACA) is situated above the optic chiasm within the cistern of the lamina terminalis and gives rise to small branches that supply adjacent structures, such as the anterior hypothalamus. In approximately

2%–13% of cases, it gives rise to a median callosal artery, which is involved in embryological development. A persistent medial callosal artery supplies the fornix, frontal lobe, corpus callosum, septum pellucidum, and septal region.

The M1 segment, also known as the sphenoid segment, extends from the bifurcation of the ICA above the anterior segment of the uncus to the deep portion of the Sylvian cistern. It courses from medial to lateral and is parallel to the lesser sphenoid wing, which is oriented obliquely from medial to lateral and from inferior to superior. The posterior wall of the M1 segment gives rise to the lenticulostriate arteries.

11.5 Lateral Surface

11.5.1 Lateral Surface: Dissection of the Sylvian Fissure

The Sylvian fissure is a cisternal space that serves as a transition zone between the basal cisterns and the subarachnoid space of the cerebral convexity. The MCA traverses this fissure. To access its proximal portions, the fissure must be opened, either partially or along its entire length, depending on the nature, topography, and size of the pathology, as well as the surgeon's experience.

For optimal access to the Sylvian fissure, the patient's head should be rotated 15°–20° with lateral flexion of the neck. This position aligns the Sylvian fissure parallel to the surgeon's line of sight. To access aneurysms of the ACA, carotid bifurcation, and MCA, approximately 20° of deflection is necessary. At the Sylvian fissure, the initial structure that can be identified is the superficial Sylvian vein. At the frontoparietal and temporal cortical areas, the M4 segment of the MCA is visible. This segment begins where the MCA makes a 90° turn from the opercular face

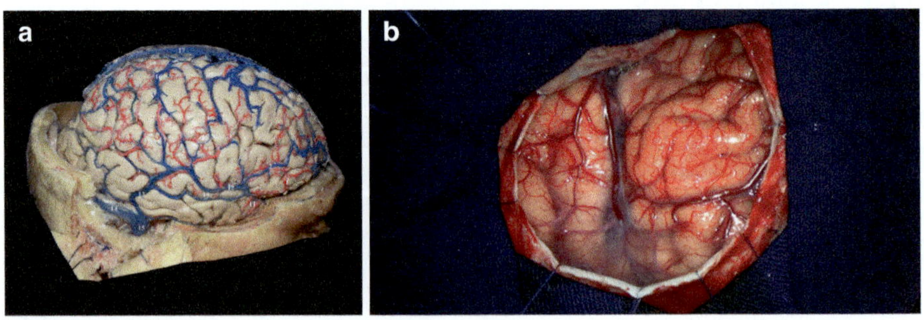

Fig. 11.12 (**a**) Superolateral surface of the brain supplied by the branches of the M4 segment and the superficial venous system: (1) Orbitofrontal (2). Prefrontal (3). Precentral (4). Central (5). Anterior parietal (6). Posterior parietal (7). Angular (8). Temporo-occipital (9). Posterior temporal (10). Medial temporal (11). Anterior temporal (12). Superficial Sylvian vein (13). Vein of Labbé (14). Transverse sinus. (15) Sigmoid sinus. (16) Vein of Trolard. (17) Superior sagittal sinus. (**b**) Operative view of the superolateral surface of the brain following a left pterional approach

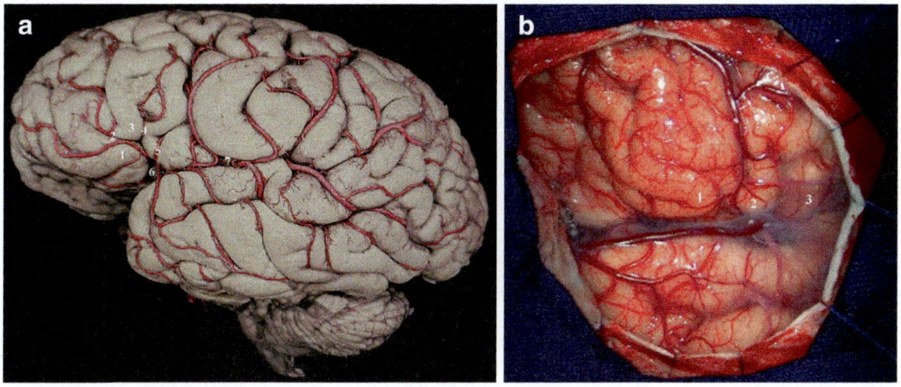

Fig. 11.13 (a) Sylvian fissure: (1) Pars orbitalis (2). Horizontal ramus (3). Pars triangularis (4). Ascending ramus (5). Pars opercularis (6). Anterior Sylvian point (7). Posterior ramus. (b) Operative view of the left Sylvian fissure after a left pterional approach: (1) Pars orbitalis (2). Pars triangularis (3). Pars opercularis. *Anterior Sylvian point

of the frontal, parietal, and temporal lobes to the lateral surface of the brain within the Sylvian fissure. Twelve branches of the M4 segment can be identified, each radiating into 12 distinct regions of the superolateral cerebral cortex. These branches, listed from front to back, are the orbitofrontal, prefrontal, precentral, central, anterior parietal, posterior parietal, angular, temporo-occipital, posterior temporal, medial temporal, anterior temporal, and temporopolar (Fig. 11.12).

The opening of the Sylvian fissure typically begins at the anterior Sylvian point, where the space between the frontal and temporal lobes is wider owing to the retraction of the *pars triangularis* of the inferior frontal gyrus (Fig. 11.13).

To open the fissure, cutting instruments (no. 11 scalpel and microscissors) are used, with bipolar instruments also available to assist in the opening. High-magnification microscopy is recommended for identifying small vessels and differentiating between arteries and veins. The superficial part of the Sylvian fissure should be opened using a fine aspirator with an atraumatic tip, preferably 5 French, with low suction pressure. This approach helps expose the structures while keeping the surgical field clean (Fig. 11.14).

Dissection is typically performed on the frontal side of the superficial Sylvian vein, leaving the vein adjacent to the temporal lobe, as it usually drains into the sphenoparietal sinus at the tip of the temporal lobe. In some patients, this vein predominantly drains into the frontal veins and superior sagittal sinus. In these patients, the dissection is performed on the temporal side of the superficial Sylvian vein (Fig. 11.15).

Dissection is continued by separating the frontal lobe from the temporal lobe. During this process, the posterior orbital gyrus is separated from the *planum polar* of the temporal lobe, allowing the identification of the MCA in its M3 or opercular portion and M2 or insular portion. The M3 segment is formed by multiple branches that supply the opercular face of the frontal, parietal, and temporal lobes. It

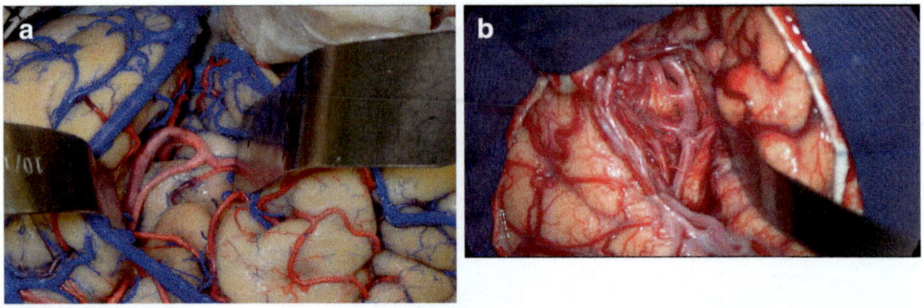

Fig. 11.14 (**a**) Anatomical representation of the left Sylvian fissure (**b**) Operative view of a left Sylvian fissure opened

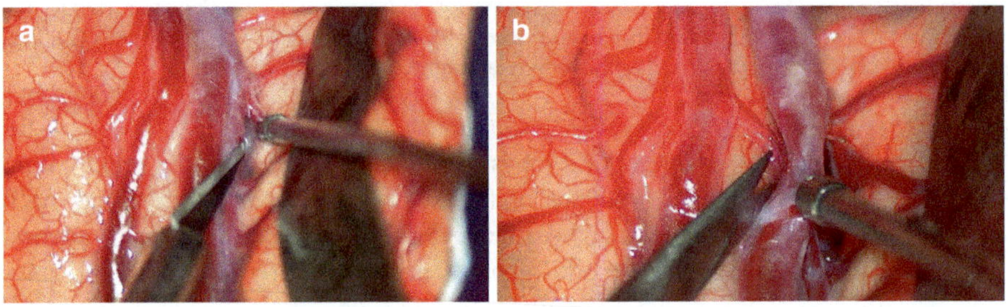

Fig. 11.15 (**a**) Dissection of the frontal side of the superficial Sylvian vein. (**b**) Dissection of the temporal side of the superficial Sylvian vein

originates where the middle cerebral artery makes a 90° turn from the insular surface toward the opercular portion of the Sylvian fissure, at the limiting sulci of the insula. The M3 segment extends until it transitions into the M4 portion on the surface of the Sylvian fissure. The M2 segment begins when the MCA makes a 90° turn, shifting the direction from anterior to posterior at the limen of the insula, located at the Sylvian vallecula (the boundary between the sphenoidal and operculoinsular compartments of the Sylvian cistern). It ends when the MCA makes another 90° turn at the level of the frontoparietal and temporal opercula, shifting from a medial to lateral direction and transitioning into the M3 segment (Fig. 11.16). At this stage, the dissection proceeds medially along the direction of the M1 or sphenoidal portion, which extends from the ICA bifurcation at the carotid cistern, adjacent to the medial end of the Sylvian fissure. This portion runs beneath the anterior perforated substance and posterior to the division of the olfactory tract into the medial and lateral olfactory striae. The M1 segment travels in a medial to lateral direction beneath the anterior perforated substance and extends 1 cm parallel and posterior to the lesser wing of the sphenoid. It enters the sphenoidal compartment of

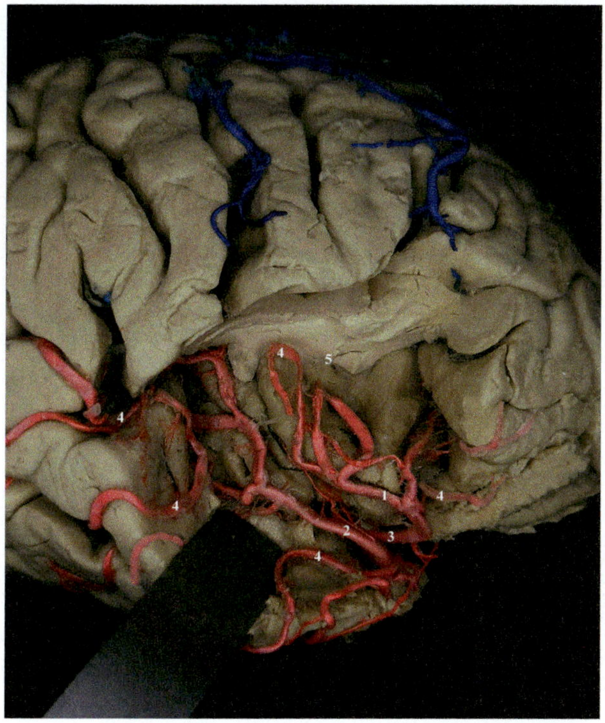

Fig. 11.16 (**a**) Right middle cerebral artery segmentation. After dissection of the Sylvian fissure and resection of the frontal operculum, the M1 segment (3) can be observed rotating 90 degrees posteriorly at the level of the limen of the insula, giving rise to M2 segment with its frontal (1) and temporal branches (2). These branches further give rise to the M3 branches (4), which rotate 90 degrees laterally, crossing the superior (5) and inferior limiting sulcus of the insula

the Sylvian cistern above the anterior segment of the uncus and terminates at the limen of the insula. Typically, the MCA bifurcates just before the M1–M2 transition point into an upper or frontal trunk and an inferior or temporal trunk. Although this bifurcation can occur at the beginning of the M1 segment, it can be categorized into pre- and post-bifurcation. Sylvian bifurcation occurs in 80% of patients, division occurs in three branches in 10% of the patients, and multiple branches develop in the other 10% of the patients. Collateral branches, known as early branches, emerge from the anterior face of M1 and supply the adjacent frontal and temporal cortices. The posterior branches, known as the lateral lenticulostriate arteries, are smaller in caliber, more numerous, and significant. They extend toward the anterior perforated substance, providing crucial blood supply to the basal ganglia and internal capsule (Fig. 11.17).

The M1 trajectory is followed until the cisterns of the base are exposed and identified from lateral to medial:

- The Sylvian cistern begins at the level of the rhinal sulcus of the temporal lobe, bordering the carotid cistern, and extends outward into the convexity, culminating in the posterior part of the insula. Its large extension results in the formation of two compartments. The sphenoidal compartment extends from the origin of

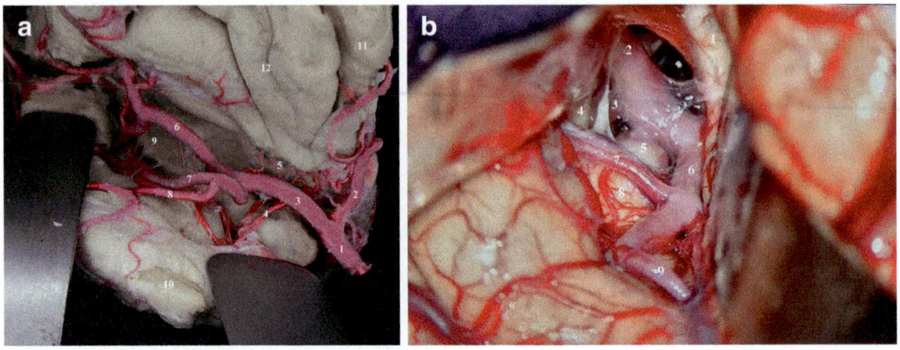

Fig. 11.17 (**a**) Anterior view of the sphenoidal compartment of the Sylvian cistern: (1) internal carotid artery (ICA) bifurcation (2). Anterior cerebral artery. (3) Pre-bifurcation M1 segment (4). Temporopolar artery. (5) Lateral lenticulostriate arteries. 6) Frontal branch of the post-bifurcation M1 segment (7). Temporal branch of the post-bifurcation M1 segment (8). Anterior temporal artery (9). Limen of the insula (10). Temporal pole (11). Gyrus rectus (12). Orbital gyri. (**b**) Operative view of the transsylvian access for microsurgical treatment of a choroidal segment aneurysm: (1) Optic nerve (2). ICA (3). posterior communicating artery (4). Oculomotor nerve (5). Aneurysm (6). M1 (7). Early branch (8). Anterior segment of the uncus (9). M2

the Sylvian cistern to the limen of the insula. This compartment is parallel to the lesser wing of the sphenoid and is thus axially oriented. The operculoinsular compartment is the widest part of the cistern. It is situated sagittally perpendicular to the first compartment and formed by the juxtaposed faces of the opercula. This compartment is visible on the surface through the Sylvian fissure. The Sylvian cistern contains the Sylvian artery with its branches and Sylvian veins.

- Carotid cistern: The medial wall is composed of the medial carotid membrane, which separates it from the chiasmatic cistern. The lateral wall is formed by the arachnoid, which joins the anterior segment of the uncus and orbital gyri. The anterior wall is formed by the arachnoid bridging the olfactory trigone, lateral border of the optic chiasm, and anterior part of the uncus. The superior wall is the central part of the anterior perforated substance, while the inferior wall is formed by the outer arachnoidal membrane, which faces the dura mater over the posterior clinoid process and the cavernous sinus. It houses the carotid artery, which gives rise to the superior hypophyseal, posterior communicating, and anterior choroidal arteries.
- Cistern of the lamina terminalis: The arachnoid membrane forming the superior aspect of the cistern extends from the anterior edge of the optic chiasm and the superior aspect of the optic nerves upward to the posterior part of the rectus gyri, constituting the external boundary of the olfactory stria compartment. The anterior surface or floor of the compartment corresponds to the superior aspect of the chiasm, while the inferior surface corresponds to the lamina terminalis. The cistern extends from the chiasm to the anterior commissure above the genu of the corpus callosum. Laterally, by marking the entrance site of the anterior cerebral artery (A1 segment) into the cistern, an arachnoid arch can be identified. This arch extends from the area of the olfactory tubercle to the junction of the optic

nerve and the chiasm. In this cistern, the A1 segments, anterior communicating artery and its hypothalamic branches, precallosal artery, origin of the A2 segments, two fronto-orbital arteries, anterior cerebral veins, and communicating vein are positioned deeper position relative to the arteries. Additionally, the frontopolar artery forms the pericallosal cistern boundary.

- Chiasmatic cistern: This cistern can be observed through the interoptic space and has a triangular shape, with its apex oriented backward or downward when the patient is in a dorsal position. The base is located along a line connecting both optic nerves from their homonymous canals. The lateral aspect is enclosed by the medial carotid membrane, a septum that separates it from the carotid cistern. The anterior wall or floor is formed by the sellar diaphragm, bordered by two bony landmarks: the tuberculum sellae anteriorly and the dorsum sellae posteriorly. The posterior or inferior aspect is defined as the Liliequist membrane, while the posterior-superior or upper aspect comprises the interoptic space and optic nerve. A pituitary stalk is observed in this cistern.

The above description outlines a dissection approach from distal to proximal, which is typically preferred in most patients. However, when the frontoparietal and temporal opercula are tightly adhered, the dissection should start from proximal to distal, beginning in the carotid cistern up to the Sylvian cistern. This allows for the identification of the branches of the middle cerebral artery before returning to dissect the superficial portion of the Sylvian fissure, thereby minimizing the risk of injury to the pial and cortical surfaces of the frontal and temporal lobes. In such cases, the structures mentioned above can be observed from the proximal and medial to the distal and lateral directions.

During the dissection of the Sylvian fissure, veins running parallel to the fissure and those crossing from the frontal lobe to the temporal lobe may be encountered. When preserving the vessels, if any veins hinder the progress, only those crossing the fissure should be coagulated and cut, while those parallel to it should be left intact. Self-retaining retractors are only used to maintain the brain position once a space is opened or to separate the orbital part of the frontal lobe, which occasionally covers the Sylvian fissure, and are not used for traction (Fig. 11.18).

Highlighting the crucial role of the surgeon's safety, skill, and microsurgical practice is essential when opening a Sylvian fissure, making laboratory practice important. This information enables surgeons to accurately identify each structure in an anatomical specimen in the laboratory.

11.5.2 Dissection of the Temporal Lobe to Expose the Temporal Horn of the Lateral Ventricle

The temporal lobe is also located below the Sylvian fissure on the lateral surface of the brain. In the laboratory, dissection can be performed at the level of the middle temporal gyrus, which projects parallel to the floor of the temporal fossa. This

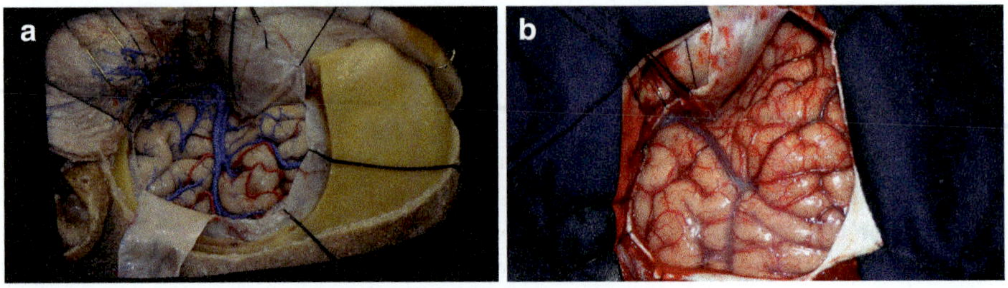

Fig. 11.18 Anatomical representation (**a**) and operative view (**b**) of the superficial Sylvian veins parallel to the Sylvian fissure exposed by the fronto-orbito-zygomatic approach

approach provides access to the temporal horn of the lateral ventricles located inferolateral to the thalamus. Structures related to the limbic system and mesial temporal region can be identified. Such dissection is particularly relevant in procedures like amygdalohippocampectomy in patients with epilepsy secondary to tumors in this region or mesial temporal sclerosis. Entry into the temporal horn can also be achieved via the superior temporal gyrus with a downward projection or the inferior temporal gyrus with an upward projection.

The temporal horn extends from the atrium to the posterior surface of the amygdala. Dissection is performed 3 cm from the temporal pole. Once the temporal horn is accessed, the head, body, and tail of the hippocampus can be identified. In a prepared specimen, the tip of the temporal horn is located 11 mm from the limen of the insula.

The boundary between the head and body of the hippocampus is marked by the inferior choroidal point, situated above the hippocampus. The head of the hippocampus is devoid of the choroid plexus and terminates at this point. It also presents digitations resembling feline paws and connects anteriorly with the amygdala, which can be visible in the anterior wall of the temporal horn. Additionally, the uncal recess of the temporal horn, the ventricular extension following the curvature of the hippocampal head, can be observed. This recess corresponds to the uncal apex on the medial surface. The choroidal fissure between the thalamus and the fimbria of the fornix can be observed above the hippocampus, terminating at the inferior choroidal point. Transverse hippocampal veins are visible on the floor of the temporal horn. Lateral to the hippocampus is the collateral eminence, an impression in the ventricle of the collateral sulcus on the basal surface of the temporal lobe.

Upon opening the choroidal fissure at the level of the temporal horn between the thalamus and the fimbria of the fornix, entry is made into the basal cisterns. At the inferior choroidal point, the anterior and posterior lateral choroidal arteries are observed, along with the inferior ventricular, transverse hippocampal, amygdaloid body, and inferior choroidal veins. These vessels enter the ambient cistern, which can be visualized from this position, and connect the basal vein of Rosenthal. Behind the inferior choroidal point, the lateral geniculate body of the thalamus is visible. On the cisternal side, the inferior choroidal point delineates the boundary between the crural cistern anteriorly and the ambient cistern posteriorly.

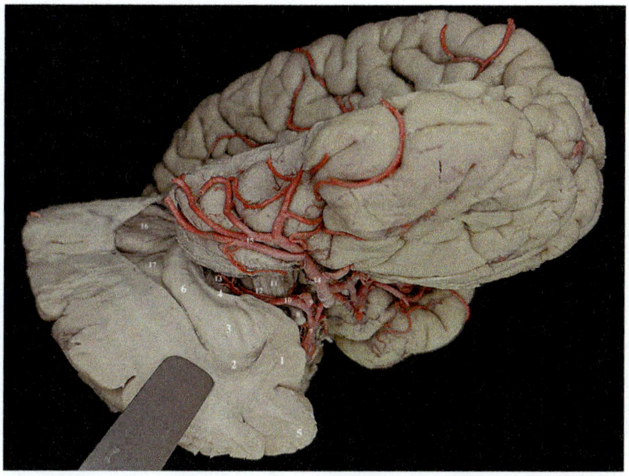

Fig. 11.19 Opening of the temporal choroidal fissure achieved by sectioning the temporal stem and exposing the temporal horn and atrium of the right lateral ventricle. The following structures can be visualized: (1) Amygdala (2). Uncal recess (collateral eminence) (3). Head of the hippocampus (4). Fimbria (fornix) (5). Temporal pole (6). Body of the hippocampus (7). Basilar trunk (8). Oculomotor nerve (9). Posterior communicating artery (10). Posterior cerebral artery (11). Cerebral peduncle (12). Medial posterior choroidal artery (13). Lateral posterior choroidal artery (14). M1. (15) M2. (16) Calcar avis. (17) Collateral trigone

The roof of the temporal horn is closely related to the internal capsule, where the sublenticular part is located, transmitting optic and acoustic radiation and contributing to the formation of the temporal stem.

Medial to the temporal horn of the lateral ventricle, above the hippocampus, and between it and the thalamus, lies the choroidal fissure. Upon opening, choroidal telangiectasia is observed. Upon removal, the posterior cerebral artery, basal vein in the ambient cistern, and fourth cranial nerve in the posterior portion of the cistern under the thalamus are visible. Enlarging this opening by removing the amygdala anteriorly, as in a transamygdalar approach, allows the visualization of the structures in the crural and interpeduncular cisterns. Through this window, the cisternal portion of the anterior choroidal artery can be observed. This artery arises from the carotid artery and courses near the optic tract along the roof of the crural cistern until it reaches the inferior choroidal point, where it enters the lateral ventricle. Additionally, the third cranial nerve, the origin of the PCA, and the medial posterior choroidal artery, which typically begins at the P1 segment within the interpeduncular cistern, can be seen. These structures pass around the brainstem and traverse the ambient and quadrigeminal cisterns to reach the tela choroidea on the roof of the third ventricle.

In the laboratory, temporal disconnection can be performed by opening the choroidal fissure along the temporal horn and sectioning through the temporal stem (Fig. 11.19). These techniques facilitate the release of the temporal lobe, thereby exposing the structures of the crural and ambient cisterns.

Thus, the walls of the temporal horn are formed as follows, and each structure can be identified (Fig. 11.20):

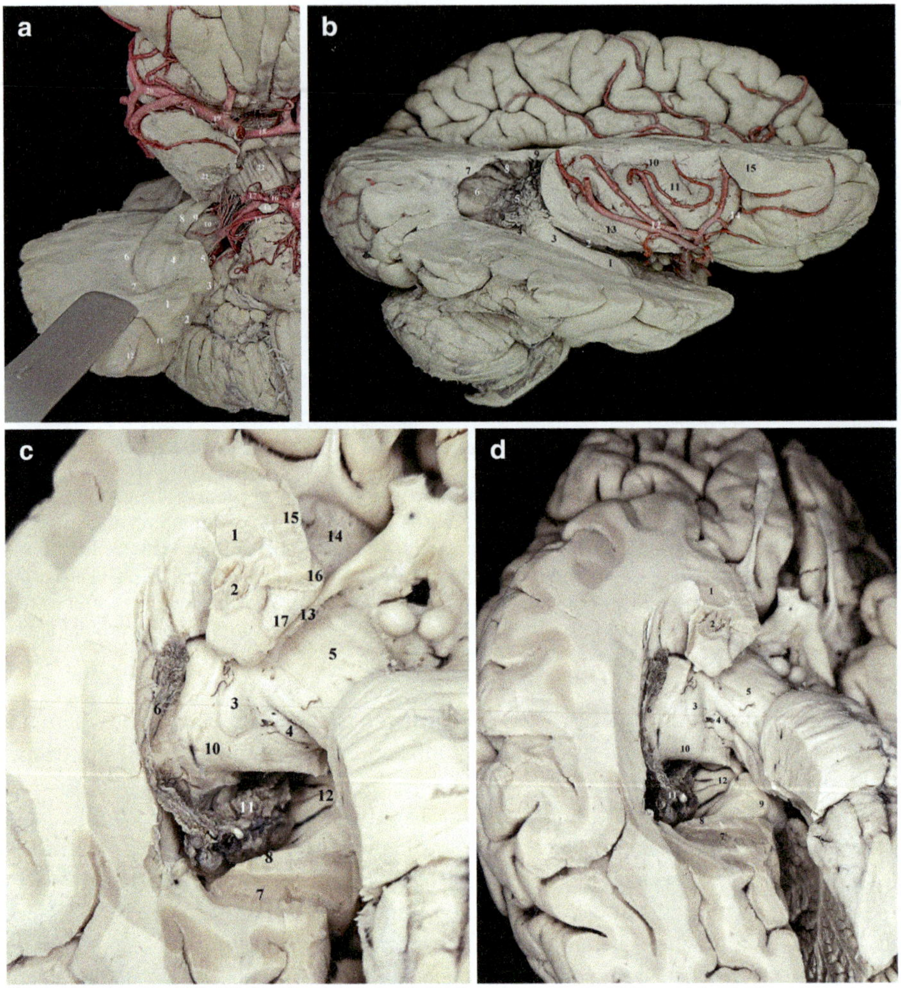

Fig. 11.20 Temporal horn and atrium structures. (**a**) Anterior view: (1) Amygdala (2). Anterior segment of the uncus (3). Uncal apex (4). Head of the hippocampus (5). Posterior segment of the uncus (6). Collateral eminence (7). Uncal recess (8). Fimbria (fornix) (9). Fimbriodentate sulcus (10). Parahippocampal gyrus (11). Rhinal sulcus (12). Temporal pole (13). Superior cerebellar artery (14). Oculomotor nerve. (15) Basilar trunk. (16) Posterior cerebral artery. (17) Posterior communicating artery. (18) A1. (19) M1. (20) M2. (21) Temporal stem (sectioned). (22) Cerebral peduncle. (**b**) Lateral view after resection of the superior and middle temporal gyri and opening of the choroidal fissure by sectioning the temporal stem: (1) Head of the hippocampus (2). Choroidal plexus (3). Body of the hippocampus (4). Collateral trigone (5). Glomus (6). Calcar avis (7). Tapetum (8). Bulb of the corpus callosum (forceps major) (9). Body of the corpus callosum (10). Superior limiting sulcus (11). Insula (12). M2 (13). Inferior limiting sulcus (14). Anterior limiting sulcus. (15) Pars orbitalis. C and D) Inferior view after resection of the parahippocampal gyrus and floor of the temporal horn: (1) Amygdala (2). Head of the hippocampus (3). Lateral geniculate body (4). Medial geniculate body (5). Cerebral peduncle (6). Choroidal plexus (7). Calcarine sulcus (8). Calcar avis (9). Splenium of the corpus callosum (10). Pulvinar (thalamus) (11). Glomus (12). Bulb of the corpus callosum (13). Optic tract (14). Anterior perforate substance. (15) Anterior segment of the uncus. (16) Uncal apex. (17) Posterior segment of the uncus

- Anterior to the amygdala. It is located below the globus pallidus, and behind and below the M1 segment of the MCA, corresponding to the anterior segment of the uncus.
- The floor is formed medially by the hippocampus and the fimbria of the fornix, and laterally by the collateral eminence.
- The roof is formed medially to laterally by the inferior surface of the thalamus, stria terminalis, tail of the caudate nucleus, and tapetum of the corpus callosum.
- The lateral wall is formed by the tapetum of the corpus callosum.
- The medial wall is formed by the choroidal fissure and choroid plexus.

Bibliography

1. Bouthillier A, van Loveren HR, Keller JT. Segments of the internal carotid artery: a new classification. Neurosurgery. 1996;38(3):425–33.
2. Rhoton AL Jr. Roton cranial anatomy and surgical approaches. Oxford University Press; 2019.
3. Chaddad-Neto F, Da Costa MD. Microneuroanatomy and surgery: a practical anatomical guide. Springer; 2022.
4. Ahumada-Vizcaino JC, Wuo-Silva R, Hernández MM, Chaddad-Neto F. The art of combining neuroanatomy and microsurgical skills in modern neurosurgery. Front Neurol. 2023;13:1076778.
5. Osawa S, Rhoton AL Jr, Tanriover N, Shimizu S, Fujii K. Microsurgical anatomy and surgical exposure of the petrous segment of the internal carotid artery. Neurosurgery. 2008;63(4 Suppl 2):210–38; discussion 239.
6. Seoane E, Rhoton A, de Oliveira ED. Microsurgical anatomy of the dural collar (carotid collar) and rings around the clinoid segment of the internal carotid artery. Neurosurgery. 1998;42:869–84; discussion 884.
7. Türe U, Yaşargil MG, Al-Mefty O, Yaşargil DC. Arteries of the insula. J Neurosurg. 2000;92(4):676–87.
8. Tanriover N, Rhoton AL Jr, Kawashima M, Ulm AJ, Yasuda A. Microsurgical anatomy of the insula and the sylvian fissure. J Neurosurg. 2004;100(5):891–922.
9. Microneurosurgery YM. In: microsurgical anatomy of the basal cisterns and vessels of the brain, diagnostic studies, general operative techniques, and pathological considerations of intracranial aneurysms, vol. 1. New York: George Thieme Verlag; 1984. p. 1.
10. Yasargil MG, Kasdaglis K, Jain KK, Weber HP. Anatomical observations of the subarachnoid cisterns of the brain during surgery. J Neurosurg. 1976;44(3):298–302.
11. Inoue K, Seker A, Osawa S, Alencastro LF, Matsushima T, Rhoton AL Jr. Microsurgical and endoscopic anatomy of the supratentorial arachnoidal membranes and cisterns. Neurosurgery. 2009;65(4):644–64; discussion 665.
12. Chaddad-Neto F, Campos Filho JM, Dória-Netto HL, Faria MH, Ribas GC, Oliveira E. The pterional craniotomy: tips and tricks. Arq Neuropsiquiatr. 2012;70(9):727–32.
13. Goiri MAA, de Amorim BL, Sarti THM, da Costa MDS, Chaddad-Neto F. Building a microneurosurgical laboratory in Latin America: challenges and possibilities. Surg Neurol Int. 2021;12:573. Published 2021 Nov 23. https://doi.org/10.25259/SNI_978_2021

Chapter 12
Dissecting the Brain Vein System

12.1 Introduction

Microsurgery in neurosurgery involves the intricate handling of vessels: arteries and veins. The arteries are generally more predictable, as their exact pathway, branches, and areas of perfusion are well studied. By contrast, the veins are more complex. Neurosurgeons must exercise caution when operating on veins, as certain veins can be safely sacrificed, while others require preservation. The ability to accurately determine this distinction is critical to the success of the procedure. Therefore, a precise understanding of the anatomical structure of the surgical site, including the veins relevant for surgical approach, is essential for achieving optimal patient outcomes. This chapter aimed to deepen the understanding of cerebral venous anatomy.

12.2 Anatomical Description

The cerebral venous system can be classified as superficial or deep. The superficial venous system drains the cortical surface (Fig. 12.1), while the deep venous system drains the neural structures surrounding the ventricles and basal cisterns. The superficial system is easily distinguishable. It drains into the superficial dural sinuses, such as the superior sagittal sinus, transverse sinus, sphenoparietal sinus, and superior and inferior petrosal sinus. Meanwhile, the deep system drains into the vein of Galen.

F. Chaddad-Neto, M. D. S. da Costa, *Microneuroanatomy and Lab*,
https://doi.org/10.1007/978-3-031-91026-5_12

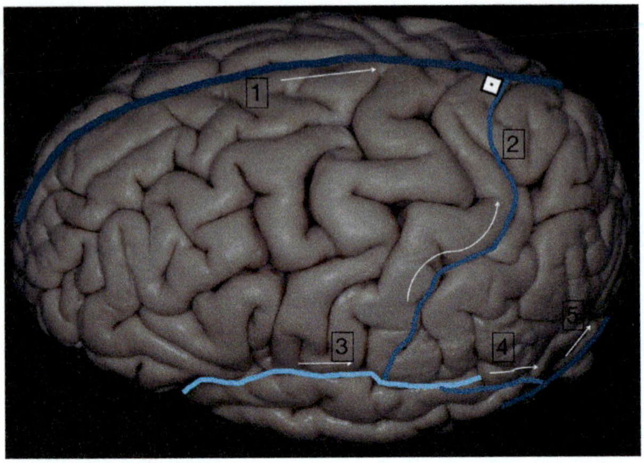

Fig. 12.1 This schematic drawing illustrates the middle cerebral vein (3) draining into the superior sagittal sinus (1) through the superior anastomotic vein (vein of Trolard (2) at a right angle and into the transverse sinus (5) through the inferior anastomotic vein (vein of Labbé (4))

12.3 Superficial Venous System

12.3.1 Venous Sinuses and Group

The venous sinuses are large channels situated between the two layers of the dura mater, which covers the brain, and are lined by a thin layer of the vascular endothelium. They receive blood from the veins of the brain, drain it into the jugular veins, and return it to the general circulation. Some venous sinuses, although not all, are associated with bone structures and in may be located within channels carved into the bones. Venous sinuses can be classified as even or odd. The odd venous sinuses include the superior and inferior longitudinal, straight, basilar, and suboccipital sinuses. The paired venous sinuses include the cavernous, sphenoparietal, sphenobasal, and sphenopetrosus sinuses; the superior and inferior petrosal sinuses; the transverse sinuses; the medial and lateral tentorial sinuses; and the sigmoid sinuses.

The torcula Herophilus or Herophilus' press is a venous confluence where the transverse, straight, and superior longitudinal sinuses converge. It is formed by the unfolding of the dural leaves and is situated on the anterior face of the internal occipital protuberance, which is externally marked in the midline by the external occipital protuberance.

The superficial veins are divided into four groups according to the venous sinus into which they drain: superior sagittal group (superior longitudinal sinus), sphenoid group (sphenoid and cavernous sinuses), tentorial group (superior petrosal sinuses and transverse sinus), and falcinal group (inferior longitudinal sinuses and straight sinus).

The superior sagittal group consists of veins that drain the superior longitudinal sinus. It includes the veins from the superior part of the medial surface; the lateral surface of the frontal, parietal, and occipital lobes; and the anterior part of the orbital surface of the frontal lobe.

The sphenoid group is composed of venous bridges that drain into the sinuses and run along the inner surface of the sphenoid bone. It drains the frontal, parietal, and temporal regions adjacent to the Sylvian fissures. These veins drain into the sphenoparietal or cavernous sinuses.

The tentorial group is composed of veins that drain into the tentorium sinuses (superior petrosal and transverse sinuses). These veins drain the lateral surface of the temporal lobe and occipital-temporal surface.

The falcine group consists of veins that drain into the inferior sagittal sinus or the straight sinus, either directly or through the internal cerebral vein or the basal vein of Rosenthal. These veins drain the cortical area of the limbic lobe and pericallosal cortex, including the parahippocampal gyrus, uncus, cingulate gyrus, paraterminal gyrus, paraolfactory gyrus, and the upper part of the midbrain.

12.3.2 Superior Longitudinal Sinus or Superior Sagittal Sinus

Managing the dural sinuses, especially the superior sagittal sinus (SSS), presents a significant challenge even for experienced neurosurgeons.

The superior sagittal sinus (Fig. 12.2) is divided into three sections based on distinct craniometric landmarks relevant for surgical planning and techniques. The anterior third extends from its origin to the bregma, where the coronal and sagittal sutures meet. The middle third is located between the bregma and the lambda, the junction of the lambdoid and sagittal sutures. The posterior third spans from the lambda to the confluence of the sinuses, near the external occipital protuberance.

The superior sagittal sinus begins above the foramen cecum and extends posteriorly through the channel of the superior longitudinal sinus, which is carved into the internal table of the skull. It has a triangular shape with an upper base and a lower vertex that connects to the falx cerebri. This sinus can communicate with the foramen cecum through the veins of the nasal cavity.

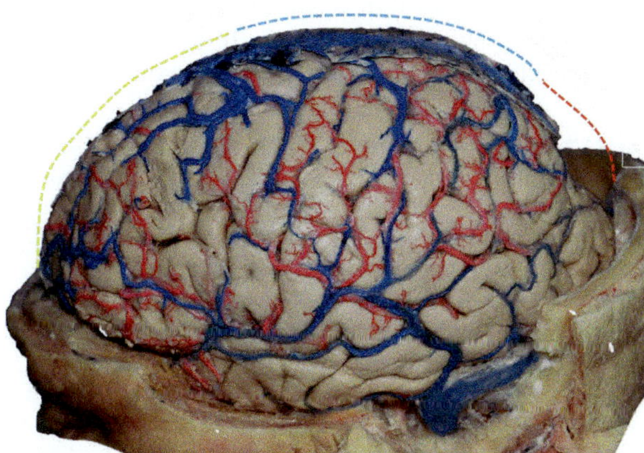

Fig. 12.2 The superior sagittal sinus is divided into three portions: the anterior third (1, yellow) extends to the bregma, the middle third (2, blue) extends from the bregma to the lambda, and the posterior third (3, red) extends from the lambda to the confluence of the sinuses

The superior sagittal sinus drains the anterior part of the inferior surface of the frontal lobe and the superior regions of the lateral and medial surfaces of the frontal, parietal, and occipital lobes.

The veins from each cortical area connect to the superior sagittal sinus. The veins arising near the frontal pole course posteriorly in the same direction as the blood flow within the sinus. Conversely, veins arising from the posterior part of the frontal lobe travel forward and enter the sinus in a direction opposite to the flow within the sinus. In contrast, veins from the intermediate frontal areas join the sinus at an approximately right angle. The terminal ends of the parietal and occipital veins pass anteriorly and enter the superior sagittal sinus at an angle opposite to the direction of the flow. Most of the posterior veins run anteriorly and slightly inferiorly, entering the lower margin of the sinus.

Dilated venous spaces, called lacunae, are located in the dura mater, adjacent to the superior longitudinal sinus. The veins are more numerous and voluminous in the parietal area, while they are fewer in number and smaller in size in the frontal and occipital areas.

The lacunae predominantly contain meningeal veins. The veins leading to the superior longitudinal sinus pass below the lacunae. Arachnoid granulations appear as evaginations on the floor and walls of the lacunae.

Neurosurgical procedures that involve the incision of the falx cerebri, such as those for parasagittal meningiomas, can be safely performed within the "safe zone" identified for the anterior superior sagittal sinus. However, this approach is not applicable to the posterior portion owing to the higher incidence of venous plexuses.

12.3.3 Inferior Longitudinal Sinus or Inferior Sagittal Sinus

The inferior sagittal sinus (Fig. 12.3) is formed by the unfolding of dural sheets constituting the falx cerebri. It is located at the caudal end of the falx cerebri and superior to the corpus callosum. It extends from the middle of the falx to the straight sinus. The importance of the inferior sagittal sinus during the surgery is due to its proximity to the cingulate gyrus. In an interhemispheric approach, the procedure involves entering a subdural space that extends to the inferior edge of the inferior

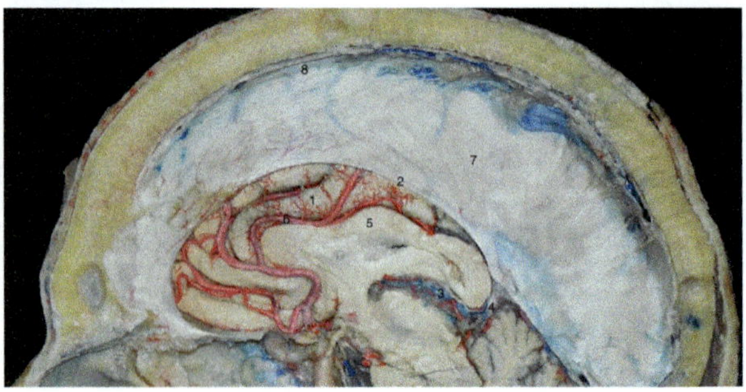

Fig. 12.3 (1) Cingulum gyrus, (2) inferior sagittal sinus, (3) internal cerebral vein, (4) cerebral vein of Galen, (5) corpus callosum, (6) pericallosal artery, (7) falx cerebral, and (8) superior sagittal sinus

longitudinal sinus. Within this space lies the supracallosal cistern, positioned between the left and right cingulate gyri. The "lateral wall" of this supracallosal cistern is formed by the cingulate gyri, while the "floor" of this space is formed by the corpus callosum.

12.3.4 Straight Sinus

The straight sinus (Fig. 12.4) originates below the splenium of the corpus callosum at the junction of the inferior sagittal sinus and great vein of Galen. It traverses the junction of the falx and tentorium (falcotentorial junction) and then drains into the torcula Herophilous or Herophilous' press, where it meets the transverse sinuses. Although it can connect both transverse sinuses, it frequently joins the left transverse sinuses. The straight sinus is a crucial anatomical landmark for accessing the pineal region. It is often necessary to cut and open the tentorium cerebelli. One effective method involves identifying the straight sinus and making an incision in the tentorium parallel to it, followed by folding and retracting the tentorium laterally. This maneuver exposes the tentorial surface of the cerebellum, the cerebellum-mesencephalic fissure, and the posterior part of the pineal region.

12.3.5 Transverse-Sigmoid Sinus

The transverse sinuses (Fig. 12.5) originate from the Herophilus' press and extend laterally from the internal occipital protuberance along a channel in the medial table of the occipital bone (transverse sinus channel), which is displaced externally by the superior nuchal line.

It becomes the sigmoid sinus (Fig. 12.6) below the petrosal border when it joins the superior petrosal sinus.

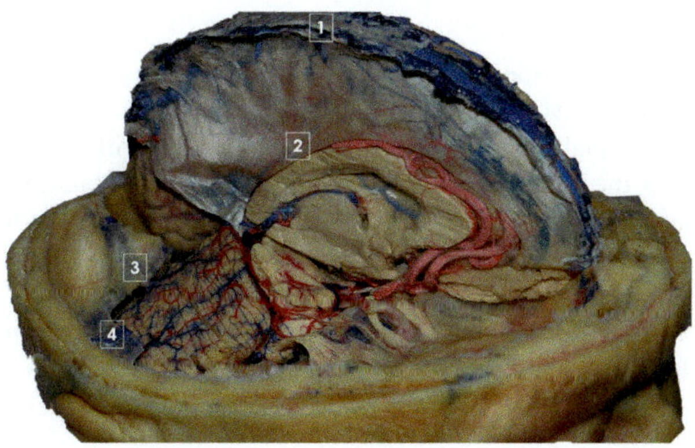

Fig. 12.4 The occipital lobe has been retracted to expose the fax and tentorium cerebelli. The superior sagittal sinus (1) and straight sinus (2) drain into the torcula (3), where they converge with the transverse sinus (4), which subsequently drains into the sigmoid sinus

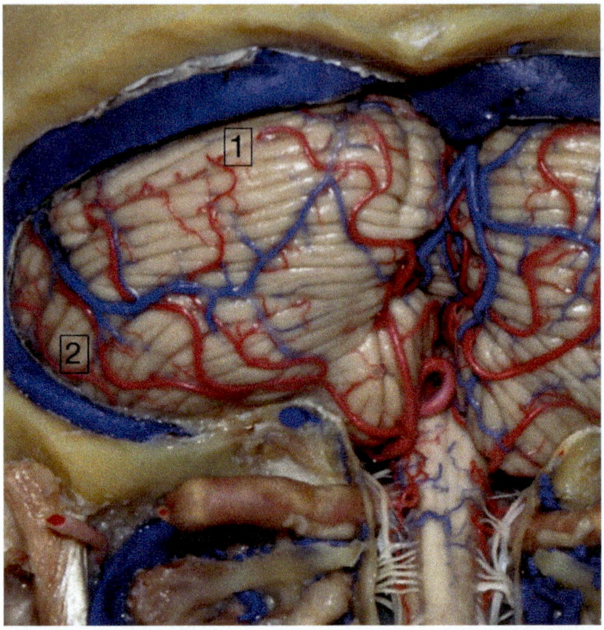

Fig. 12.5 From a posterior perspective, the transverse sinus (1) is visible as it drains into the sigmoid sinus (2). Frequently, one sinus is larger than its counterpart

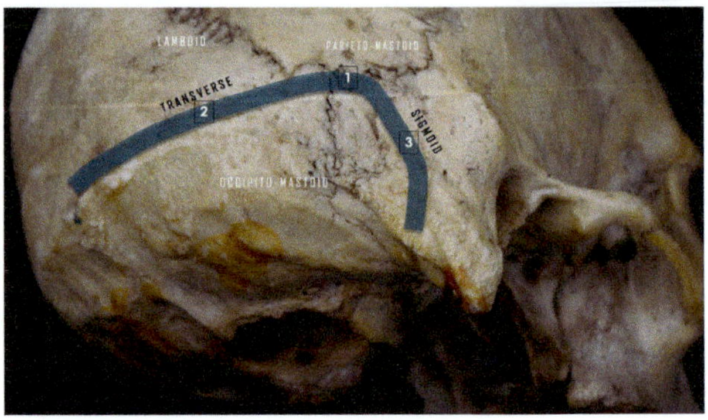

Fig. 12.6 In retrosigmoid approaches, the asterion (1) serves as a reference point. It is usually situated behind the junction where the transverse (2) and sigmoid sinuses (3) junction

In most specimens examined, the superior longitudinal sinus connects to the right transverse sinus. Thus, the right jugular vein receives venous blood from the superficial neural structures of the brain. Similarly, the straight sinus often drains into the left transverse sinus, resulting in venous drainage from the deep neural structures of the brain into the left jugular vein. The difference in signs and symptoms produced by the selective compression of one jugular vein or another is referred to as the sign of Queckenstedt.

The temporobasal, occipitobasalis, and inferior anastomotic vein and vein of Labbé drain into the transverse sinus.

This sinus usually has emissary veins that connect it to extracranial veins.

12.3.6 Tentorial Sinuses

The tentorial sinuses are situated on each side of the tentorium cerebelli. The medial tentorial sinus is formed by the convergence of the veins from the lateral and basal surfaces of the temporal and occipital lobes. The medial tentorial sinus generally drains into the torcula, while the lateral tentorial sinus drains into the transverse sinus.

12.3.7 Cavernous Sinus

The cavernous sinus (Fig. 12.7), in addition to the venous sinusoids, contains crucial arterial elements, such as the cavernous segment of the internal carotid artery (ICA) and its branches. It also houses significant neural elements, such as the third and fourth nerves and the ophthalmic branch of the fifth cranial nerve, all situated in the lateral wall and cranial nerve sector of the sinus.

It connects in the midline to the contralateral sinus via the anterior and posterior intercavernous sinuses. Anteriorly, the cavernous sinus communicates with the sphenoparietal sinus and ophthalmic veins. Posteriorly, it opens to the basilar sinus

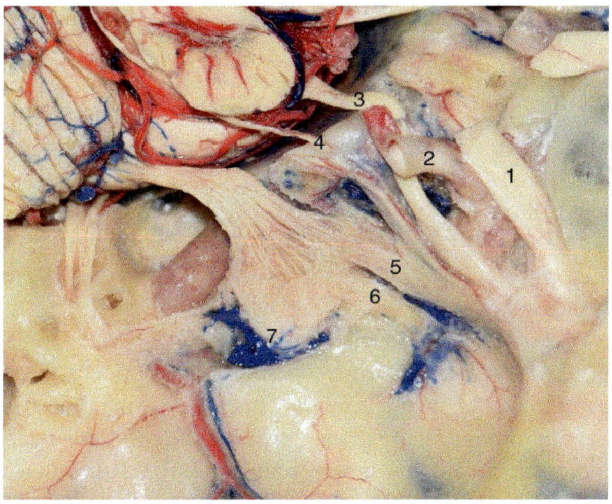

Fig. 12.7 The dura mater has been excised from the lateral wall of the cavernous sinus and Meckel's cave. The cavernous sinus is encased by the dura mater and is bounded anteriorly by the superior orbital fissure, posteriorly and medially the dorsum sellae, and posteriorly and laterally by the opening of Meckel's cave. Apart from a venous plexus and the internal carotid artery, it houses the oculomotor (3), trochlear (4), ophthalmic (5), and abducens nerves. These nerves enter the sinus from various posterior routes before converging into the superior orbital fissure anteriorly. The optic nerve (1), internal carotid artery (2), maxillary (6), and mandibular (7) branches of the trigeminal nerve are also visible in this image

at the clivus and the superior petrosal sinus, with the latter draining into the sigmoid sinus.

12.3.7.1 Lateral Walls

The lateral wall of the cavernous sinus is formed by two dural layers: the outer layer (meningeal dura) and inner layer (periosteal dura) (inset image that we do not have). Both layers extend laterally, with the dura mater covering the floor of the middle fossa; medially, aligning with the dura mater of the cavernous sinus roof; anteriorly, with the dura mater covering the convexity of the greater wing of the sphenoid bone; and posteriorly, merging with the tentorium.

The outer layer is thick and appears pearly gray, while the inner layer is thin; appears transparent; and contains nerves III, IV, and V as they traverse through the cavernous sinus toward the superior orbital fissure. A critical dividing plane exists between the two dural layers, which is crucial from a surgical perspective. This plane allows access to the inner layer of the lateral wall (exposing the cranial nerves) without penetrating the cavernous sinus.

The boundaries of the lateral wall are as follows: superiorly, by the anterior petroclinoid ligament; inferiorly, by the upper border of the maxillary nerve; anteriorly, by the sphenoidal cleft; and posteriorly, by an imaginary line aligned with the plane of the back of the sella.

12.3.7.2 Medial Wall

The medial wall of the cavernous sinus is the only wall that is not visible from the base of the skull and is composed of a single layer of dura. This dural layer is located at the outer limit of the pituitary fossa. The medial wall is divided into two distinct sectors: the pituitary sector or "sellar area" (dural membrane between the pituitary gland and the venous space of the cavernous sinus) and the sphenoid sector or "sphenoid zone" (formed by the dural membrane attached to the body of the sphenoid bone, specifically the carotid groove).

The boundaries of the medial wall are as follows: superiorly, the point where the medial wall meets the roof of the sinus; inferiorly, an imaginary line that passes through the foramen rotundum, the lower border of the carotid groove, and the sphenoid lingula, and terminates at the superior portion of the petroclival fissure; anteriorly, an imaginary line running from the optic pillar to the foramen rotundum; and posteriorly, an imaginary line extending from the posterior clinoid process to the upper end of the petroclival fissure. Surrounding the pituitary gland on all sides is the pituitary capsule (a thin, transparent membrane that is closely attached to the gland). Outside this membrane, the pituitary gland is surrounded by the dura mater, with the lateral side being covered by a single dural layer.

12.3.7.3 Superior Wall

The upper wall is composed of two layers: a smooth superficial dural layer and a thin, less-defined deep layer. This wall has a trapezoidal shape and is bordered laterally by the anterior petroclinoid ligament, medially by the dura of the sellar diaphragm, anteriorly by the endosteal dura of the carotid canal, and posteriorly by the posterior petroclinoid ligament. A line parallel to the interclinoid ligament divides this wall into two triangles: the anteromedial carotid trigone and posterolateral oculomotor trigone (see inset image).

To access this wall, the anterior clinoid must be resected to expose the clinoid segment of the ICA.

The superior wall of the cavernous sinus is divided into three areas: the oculomotor trigone, carotid trigone, and clinoid space.

12.3.7.4 Oculomotor Trigone

The oculomotor trigone (Fig. 12.8) is laterally bound by the anterior petroclinoid ligament, medially by a line overlying the interclinoid ligament, and posteriorly by the posterior petroclinoid ligament. In this area of the upper wall, the third and fourth cranial nerves enter the cavernous sinus.

The dural foramen of the oculomotor nerve appears elliptical in shape. The dural opening of the trochlear nerve is typically located at the angle between the anterior and posterior petroclinoid ligaments.

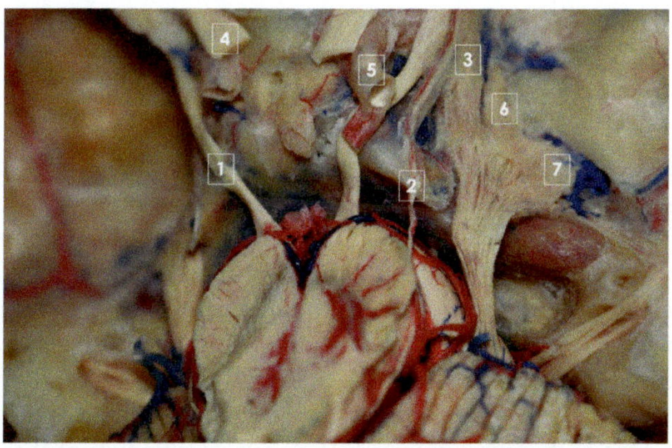

Fig. 12.8 Superior view, showing the dura-lined cavernous sinus, bounded anteriorly by the superior orbital fissure, posteriorly and medially by the dorsum of the sella turcica, laterally by the opening of the Meckel's cavum and Gasserian ganglion. In addition to a venous plexus and the internal carotid artery, the cavernous sinus houses the oculomotor (1), trochlear (2), ophthalmic (3), and abducens nerves. These nerves enter the sinus from several posterior routes before converging at the superior orbital fissure anteriorly. The image also shows the optic nerve (4), internal carotid artery (5), maxillary (6), and mandibular (7) branches of the trigeminal nerve

The dural layers (superficial and deep) can be easily separated. The superficial layer is continuous laterally with the superficial layer of the lateral wall, medially with the superficial layer of the carotid trigone, and posteriorly with the superficial layer of the petroclival dura mater on the posterior wall of the cavernous sinus. The deep layer, which is thinner than the superficial layer, is continuous laterally, medially, and posteriorly with the deep dural layer of the lateral wall, carotid trigone, and posterior wall of the cavernous sinus, respectively. At the trochlear and oculomotor entrances, the deep layer forms part of the dural sheaths that surround the nerves as they traverse the lateral wall of the cavernous sinus.

The removal of both dural layers in the oculomotor trigone allows the identification of the posterosuperior venous space of the cavernous sinus, posterior elbow of the intracavernous ICA originating from the meningohypophyseal trunk, initial intracavernous course of the abducens nerve, and interclinoid ligament.

12.3.7.5 Carotid Trigone

The carotid trigone is bounded laterally by a line overlying the interclinoid ligament, medially by the dura of the sellar diaphragm, and anteriorly by the endosteal dura of the carotid canal. The anterior portion of the trigone contains an opening for the ICA at the beginning of the supraclinoid segment (inset image). Medially, it reveals a semilunar space known as the “carotid cavern.”

The superficial dural layer is continuous laterally with a layer similar to the oculomotor trigone and with the dura mater covering the superior aspect of the anterior clinoid process, medially with the dura of the sellar diaphragm, and anteriorly with the endosteal dura of the carotid channel. This superficial layer contributes to the formation of the distal ICA dural ring (inset). This ring is incomplete and surrounds only the dorsolateral aspect of the artery, opposite to the carotid cavity. The plane of this ring is slightly oblique in the inferomedial direction.

The deep dural layer is extremely thin, fragile, and often incomplete in the posterior half. Once it has covered itself, the inferior surface of the anterior clinoid process extends anterolaterally to merge with the deep layer of the lateral wall of the cavernous sinus and posterolaterally with a layer similar to the oculomotor trigone. This layer terminates medially at the level of the sealed membrane. The deep dural layer of the carotid trigone contributes to the formation of the proximal ring of the ICA and deep layer.

It continues posteriorly with the deep layer of the oculomotor trigone. The removal of both dural leaves in the carotid trigone exposes the anterior third of the horizontal segment of the intracavernous ICA, anterior flexure of this artery, medial wall of the cavernous sinus, and medial venous space of the sinus.

12.3.7.6 Clinoid Area or Space

Excision of the anterior clinoid process exposes the interdural space between the two dural layers, which are separated at this level to envelop the bony process. Beyond this interdural space, the paraclinoid or clinoid segment of the ICA becomes visible (inset). A small area anterior to the artery is often occupied by an extension of the ethmoid or sphenoid air cells. The inadvertent opening of these cells during surgery can lead to a cerebrospinal fluid leakage. At the level of the ICA, the deep layer of the dura thickens to form the proximal ring of the artery (inset). The ring is fused medially to the endosteal dura of the carotid canal and is subsequently attached to the interclinoid ligament. Laterally, this deep layer connects with the deep layer of the lateral wall of the cavernous sinus and the dura mater of the superior orbital fissure (inset figure). The removal of the deep dural layer in the clinoid area exposes the anterior curvature of the ICA and the anteroinferior venous space of the cavernous sinus.

12.3.7.7 Posterior Wall

The posterior wall of the sellar cavity forms part of the dural lining of the clivus (inset). The boundaries of the posterior wall are as follows: superiorly by a line passing through the posterior petroclinoid ligament, extending from the apex of the petrous bone to the posterior clinoid, inferiorly by a line crossing the upper part of the petroclival fissure, medially by a line passing through the lateral border of the dorsum sella, and laterally by a medial line to the cavity (cavum) of Meckel. The posterior wall of the sellar cavity is formed by two dural layers: the meningeal and periosteal dura. The posterior wall is continuous anteriorly with the dura of the oculomotor triangle, medially with the posterior wall of the basilar sinus, and laterally with the dura lining the posterior wall of the petrous bone.

12.3.7.8 Superior Petrosal Sinus

The superior petrosal sinus is attached to the tentorium at the petrous edge. The medial end is connected to the cavernous sinus. The lateral end joins the transverse and sigmoid sinuses. The veins that drain into this sinus originate from the cerebellum and brainstem.

12.3.7.9 Sphenoparietal, Sphenobasilar, and Sphenopetrosus Sinuses

The sphenoparietal sinus is the largest dural venous sinus accompanying the middle meningeal artery. It runs immediately below the posterior border of the wing of the sphenoid bone and terminates at the anterior part of the cavernous sinus. It communicates superiorly with the longitudinal upper sinus through the meningeal veins. The sphenobasal sinus traverses the floor of the middle fossa, exits the cranium, and joins the sphenoid emissary vein and pterygoid plexus. The sphenopetrosus sinus runs posteriorly along the floor of the middle fossa and drains into the transverse sinus or superior petrosa. When the sphenoparietal sinus is absent, the Sylvian vein may occasionally drain directly into the cavernous, sphenobasal, or sphenopetrosus sinus.

12.3.7.10 Anastomotic Veins

The three anastomotic veins are the superior anastomotic vein or vein of Trolard, inferior anastomotic vein or vein of Labbé (Fig. 12.9), and superficial Sylvian vein (Fig. 12.10).

The vein of Trolard, the largest of the three veins, joins the superior longitudinal sinus with the superficial Sylvian vein.

The vein of Labbé crosses the lateral cortical surfaces of the frontal and parietal lobes. It can be simple or, in some cases, be duplicated to form a venous complex.

This vein connects the Sylvian vein with the lateral sinus and traverses the lateral cortical surface of the temporal lobe. It typically arises from the middle part of the superficial Sylvian vein and runs posteroinferiorly until it reaches the lateral sinus. In some cases, it may be duplicated, forming a venous complex.

The superficial Sylvian vein (Fig. 12.11) arises from the posterior end of the Sylvian fissure and runs anteriorly to join the sphenoparietal sinus at the edge of the lesser wing of the sphenoid. If the sphenoparietal sinus is absent, the vein drains

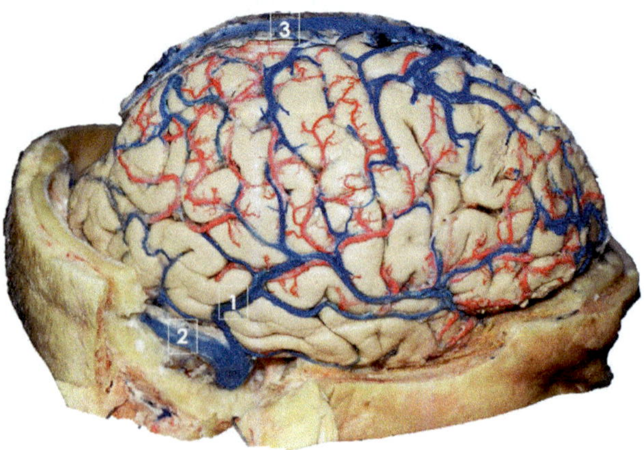

Fig. 12.9 The vein of Labbé (1) connects the cortex to the transverse sinus (2), with its insertion located near the transverse-sigmoid junction. (3) Superior sagittal sinus

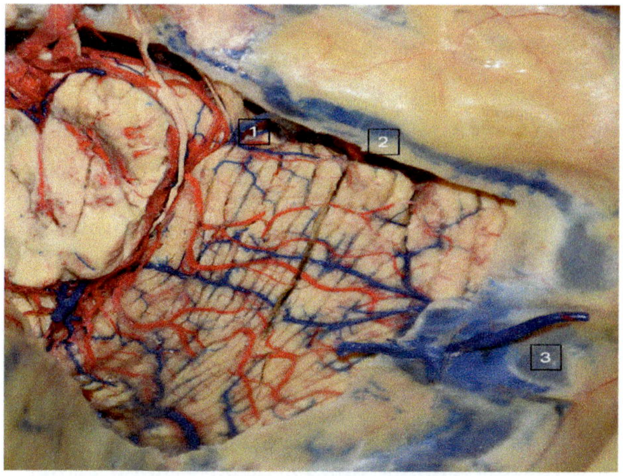

Fig. 12.10 In a superior view, the superior petrous vein (of Dandy) (1) can be seen, its relation to the superior petrosal sinus (2) and the tentorium. Note the arrangement of the transverse sinus (3) and the venous lakes in the tentorium cerebelli

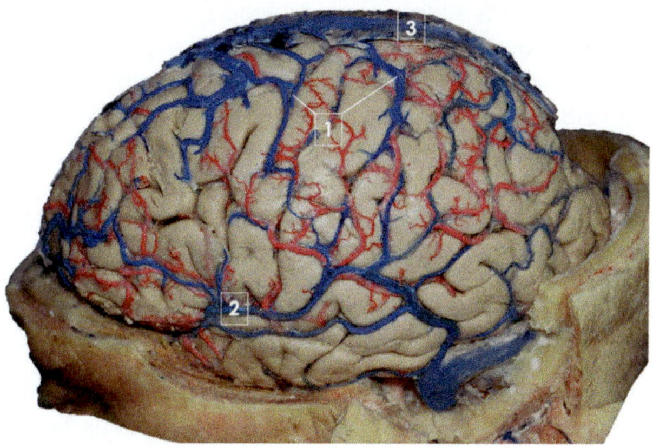

Fig. 12.11 The Trolard venous complex (1) connects the superficial Sylvian vein (2) to the superior sagittal sinus (3)

directly into the cavernous, sphenobasal, or sphenopetrosus. This vein may be absent and present as a single venous trunk or appear as a venous complex with two or more divisions. It receives blood from the frontosylvian, parietosylvian, and temporosylvian veins and anastomoses with the veins of Labbé and Trolard.

12.3.7.11 Cortical Veins

The superficial veins of the brain can be classified into lateral, medial, and basal based on their location. Among these, the veins most relevant to surgery are those located on the lateral surface. We will discuss the primary lateral veins, while the veins on the medial and basolateral surfaces will be discussed when describing each surgical approach. The veins present on the lateral side are further classified according to the lobe in which they are located.

12.3.8 Frontal Lobe

The veins located on the lateral surface of the frontal lobe are classified into ascending veins, which flow into the superior sagittal sinus, and descending veins, which flow into the superficial Sylvian vein. The ascending vein comprises the frontopolar, anterior frontal, middle frontal, posterior frontal, precentral, and central veins. The central veins and descending veins are collectively referred to as frontosylvian veins.

1. **Frontopolar Vein**

   The frontopolar vein carries venous blood from the anterior part of the superior, middle, and inferior frontal gyri and the orbital gyri to the superior sagittal sinus. It is located approximately 2.1 cm from the frontal pole and enters the superior venous sinus.

2. **Anterior, Middle, and Posterior Frontal Veins**

   These veins supply venous blood from the frontal lobe between the frontopolar and anterior central veins and enter the superior venous sinus. The anterior frontal vein is located approximately 2.5 cm posterior to the frontal pole. The middle frontal vein drains at a right angle of approximately 6.8 cm from the frontal pole. The posterior frontal vein, positioned approximately 8.3 cm from the frontal pole, enters the superior sagittal sinus anteriorly and retrogradely. A wide space exists between the anterior and middle frontal veins and between the middle and posterior frontal veins. These spaces can be accessed when performing the interhemispheric approach.

3. **Precentral Vein and Central Vein**

   The precentral vein begins at the base of the precentral gyrus, ascends around the precentral sulcus, and drains below the venous lacunae into the superior sagittal sinus 10.5 cm from the frontal pole. The central vein carries venous blood from the anterior and posterior central gyrus, centered in the central sulcus to the superior sagittal sinus, and drains into the superior sagittal sinus 12.3 cm from the frontal pole.

4. **Frontosylvian Veins**

   The frontosylvian veins are composed of three to six veins that drain venous blood from the medial frontal gyrus and lower part of the precentral gyrus. They pass inferiorly or anteroinferiorly to join the superficial Sylvian veins.

Parietal Lobe

The veins on the lateral surface of the parietal lobe are classified into ascending veins, which drain into the superior sagittal sinus, and descending veins, which drain into the veins along the Sylvian fissure.

The ascending veins include the central, posterior central, anterior, and posterior parietal veins. The descending veins consist of the parietosylvian veins.

1. **Poscentral Vein**

Venous blood from the anterior part of the supramarginal gyrus, superior parietal lobe, and postcentral gyrus flows into the superior sagittal sinus and flows into the superior sagittal sinus in an area of 13.9 cm from the frontal pole.

2. **Anterior and Posterior Parietal Veins**

The anterior parietal vein carries venous blood from the supramarginal and angular gyri; the posterior parietal vein carries venous blood from the inferior parietal lobe; and the occipital lobe shifts into the superior sagittal sinus. The anterior parietal vein enters the superior sagittal sinus 16.1 cm from the frontal pole and the posterior parietal vein 17.9 cm.

3. **Parietosylvian Veins**

Parietosylvian veins consist of two to four vessels that supply venous blood around the posterior central gyrus and inferior parietal lobule. They pass anteroinferiorly toward the Sylvian fissure, where they join the superficial Sylvian vein. Some of these veins may enter the lower end of the vein of Trolard or the upper end of the vein of Labbé.

4. **Temporal Lobe**

The veins located on the lateral surface of the temporal lobe flow are classified into groups: ascending veins and descending veins. The ascending veins, such as the temporosylvian vein, flow into the convexity and inferior venous sinuses of the temporal lobe. The descending veins, including the anterior, middle, and posterior temporal veins, drain into these sinuses.

1. **Temporosylvian Veins**

These veins drain into the superior temporal gyrus from the temporal pole to the posterior end of the Sylvian fissure. These veins flow anteriorly into the superficial Sylvian vein and posteriorly into the Labbe vein.

2. **Anterior, Middle, and Posterior Temporal Veins**

The anterior temporal vein drains into the anterior one-third of the lateral surface except for the superior temporal gyrus. The middle temporal vein drains the middle portion of the temporal convexity, while the posterior temporal vein drains the posterior one-third of the temporal convexity.

3. **Occipital Lobe**

Venous blood from the lateral surface of the occipital lobe flows into the superior sagittal sinus approximately 19.9 cm from the frontal pole via the occipital vein. The occipital vein originates at the occipital pole and proceeds anteriorly to join the superior sagittal sinus. Consequently, no large veins drain into the superior sagittal sinus until 4–5 cm anterior to the torcula Herophilus or Herophilus' press.

12.4 Deep Venous System

The deep venous system comprises the internal cerebral vein, basal vein of Rosenthal, great vein of Galen, and its tributaries (Fig. 12.12).

They are divided into two groups: a ventricular group, which drains the walls of the ventricles, and a cisternal group, which drains the walls of the basal cisterns.

12.4.1 Ventricular Group

This group is responsible for draining the basal ganglia, thalamus, internal capsule, corpus callosum, septum pellucidum, fascia, and deep white matter.

All veins originating from these structures converge at the edge of the lateral or medial ventricle, depending on the location relative to the choroidal fissure—either on the thalamic or fornicial side. Both groups run subependymally and drain into the internal cerebral vein, the basal veins, or the great vein of Galen. Specifically, the veins of the frontal horn and body of the lateral ventricle drain into the internal cerebral vein, those of the temporal horn drain into the basal vein, and those of the atrium and occipital horn drain into any of the three aforementioned veins.

Frontal Horn Veins of the Lateral Ventricle

In the medial group, the anterior septal veins travel posteriorly until they reach the Monro's foramen, then continue to the interposed veil of the roof of the third ventricle, and drain into the internal cerebral vein. The lateral group consists of the anterior caudate veins, which traverse the head of the caudate nucleus in an antero-posterior direction and terminate near the foramen of Monro. These veins drain into the thalamostriate or thalamocaudate vein, which can then directly empty into the internal cerebral vein.

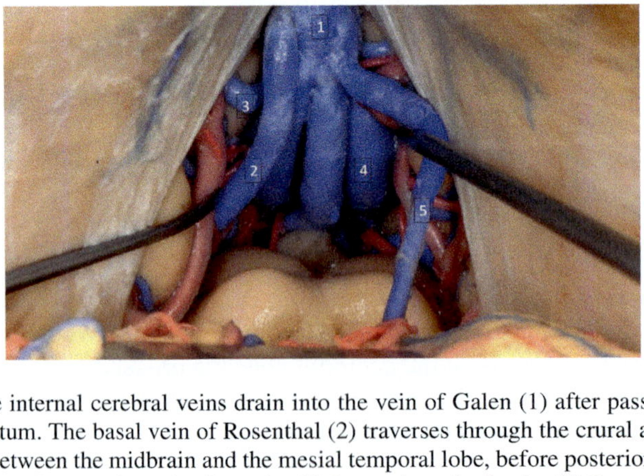

Fig. 12.12 The internal cerebral veins drain into the vein of Galen (1) after passing through the velum interpositum. The basal vein of Rosenthal (2) traverses through the crural and ambient cisterns, situated between the midbrain and the mesial temporal lobe, before posteriorly draining into the vein of Galen. (3) Anterior calcarine vein. (4) Internal cerebral vein. (5) Superior vemian vein

Veins of the Body of the Lateral Ventricle

The medial venous group consists of the posterior septal veins, which originate in the roof of the body of the lateral ventricle, traverse over the septum pellucidum, and drain into the interposed velum, where they join the internal cerebral vein. The lateral group is formed by the posterior septal veins, which drain into the thalamostriate, thalamocaudate, and posterior caudate veins.

Thalamostriate Vein

The thalamostriate vein (Fig. 12.13) originates from tributaries converging at the thalamostriate sulcus. It runs medially to transversely, reaching the foramen of Monro; curves posteriorly; and enters the interposed velum to drain into the internal cerebral vein. In some cases, this vein may divide into the anterior and posterior branches. In digital angiography, the angle formed by the junction of the thalamostriatal and internal cerebral veins is known as the venous angle and corresponds to the foramen of Monro.

The thalamic caudate vein lies posterior to the thalamostriatal vein and drains into the internal cerebral vein.

The posterior caudate vein runs along the superior lateral border of the caudate nucleus and enters the thalamostriatal groove to join the thalamostriata or thalamocaudate veins.

12.4.2 Veins in Atrium and Occipital Horn of Lateral Ventricle

The medial group includes the medial atrial vein, which drains into the basal vein as described by Rosenthal et al. The lateral group comprises the lateral atrial vein, which either joins the basal vein to the internal cerebral vein or drains directly into the great vein of Galen.

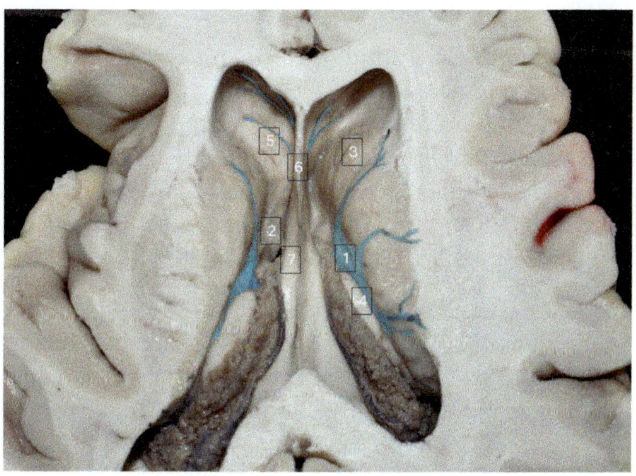

Fig. 12.13 The thalamostrate veins (1) are viewed from above, converging at the foramen of Monro (2). These veins contribute to the drainage of the caudate nucleus (3) and thalamus (4). The septal vein (5), septum pellucidum, and fornix (7) are visible

12.4.3 Temporal Horn Veins

The veins of the lateral group drain through the floor of the temporal horn, while those of the medial group drain through its roof. These veins receive the tonsillar and inferior ventricular veins and terminate in the basal vein of Rosenthal or its tributaries.

Choroidal Veins
The superior and inferior choroidal veins are the most common veins in the choroid plexus. The superior choroidal vein arises from the choroid plexus in the body of the lateral ventricle and terminates near the foramen of Monro, where it drains into the thalamostriate or internal cerebral veins. The inferior choroidal vein arises from the choroid plexus of the temporal horn, joins the inferior ventricular vein and tonsils, and terminates at the basal vein (inserir imagem anatômica que não temos).

Internal Cerebral Vein
The internal cerebral vein originates behind the foramen of Monro and runs posteriorly into the interposed veil of the third ventricle roof. The vein curves with a superior convexity anteriorly and an inferior convexity posteriorly. The union of both internal cerebral veins forms the vein of Galen, which is situated above the pineal body and below the splenium of the corpus callosum. It receives tributaries from the anterior and posterior septal veins, as well as the anterior and posterior caudate, thalamostriate, and thalamocaudate veins.

12.4.4 Cisternal Group

This cisternal group is subdivided according to the incisural space through which the deep veins travel, including anterior, middle, and posterior incisural groups. The most important veins of the cisternal group are the basal veins of the Rosenthals and the great vein of Galen.

Basal Vein of Rosenthal
This vein originates below the anterior perforated substance formed by the union of the veins of the anterior incisural space.

It travels through the trunk and temporal lobe of the median incisural space and joins the internal cerebral veins to form the great vein of Galen in the posterior incisural space. Thus, the basal vein is divided into the anterior, middle, and posterior segments based on the incisural spaces it traverses.

Anterior Incisural Segment
In the anterior segment relative to the trunk, this segment originates below the anterior perforated substance at the junction of the deep middle and anterior cerebral veins. The basal vein runs posteriorly from this origin, where it receives the

peduncular vein anterolaterally to the cerebral peduncle. The median incisural segment begins at this point.

Median Fissural Segments
This vein traverses through the crural and ambient cisterns. In this section, the basal vein receives tributaries that drain the temporal surface and temporal horn.

Posterior Incisural Segment
This vein enters the quadrigeminal cistern and joins the internal cerebral veins, forming the great vein of Galen.

Bibliography

1. Chaddad-Neto F, Silva MD. Microneuroanatomy and surgery. In: A practical anatomical guide. Springer; 2022.
2. Oka K, et al. Microsurgical anatomy of the superficial veins of the cerebrum. Neurosurgery. 1985d;17:711–48.
3. Safadi A, Tadi P. Anatomy, head and neck: cerebral venous system. Stat Pearls Publishing; 2023. Jan. 2022 Jul 25
4. Ono M, et al. Microsurgical anatomy of the deep venous system of the brain. Neurosurgery. 1984d;15:621–57.
5. F Umansky, et al. The superior wall of the cavernous sinus: a microanatomical study. J Neurosurg 81: 914–920, 1994d.

Chapter 13
Infratentorial Arterial Vascularization

The posterior fossa and occipital lobe receive blood supply through the vertebrobasilar system. The two vertebral arteries converge at the level of the bulb-pontine transition to form the basilar artery (BA), which extends longitudinally in front of the pons. From the pontomesencephalic transition, the BA bifurcates to form the posterior cerebral arteries, which supply the occipital lobes. Along its intracranial course, each vertebral artery (VA) gives rise to a posterior inferior cerebellar artery (PICA). The PICA rarely originates from the extracranial segment (V3) of the VA.

The V1 segment of the VA extends from its origin at the subclavian artery to its entry into the foramen of the transverse process at the C6 level. The V2 segment extends superiorly through the foramen of the transverse processes up to the C2, where it curves in a caudal-cranial direction, passing below, at the level of, and just above the foramen of the lateral mass of C1, known as the V3 segment. Subsequently, the VA penetrates the atlanto-occipital membrane and dura mater at the foramen magnum to form the intradural V4 segment. Along its extracranial course, the VA gives rise to the muscular and meningeal branches (V3). On the medial surface of the intradural portion (V4), each VA develops a branch that converges at the midline to form a single anterior spinal artery (ASA). This artery runs longitudinally along the anterior median fissure of the spinal cord and supplies the anterior two-thirds of the cord. The posterior spinal arteries (one on each side) originate either from the branches that form the ASA or directly from the VA. These arteries run along the posterolateral sulcus of the spinal cord. The spinal cord receives arterial supply through an anastomotic network of radicular arteries that support the flow to the spinal arteries. This chapter will not delve further into these details.

Vascular structures can be identified by injecting red-colored neoprene for the arteries and blue-colored neoprene for the veins, as described in Chap. 3.

The structures of the posterior fossa are supplied by the superior cerebellar artery (SCA), anterior inferior cerebellar artery (AICA), and posterior inferior cerebellar artery (PICA). These cerebellar arteries form a large anastomotic network, particularly within the cortical branches, leading to variations in caliber depending on the

F. Chaddad-Neto, M. D. S. da Costa, *Microneuroanatomy and Lab*,
https://doi.org/10.1007/978-3-031-91026-5_13

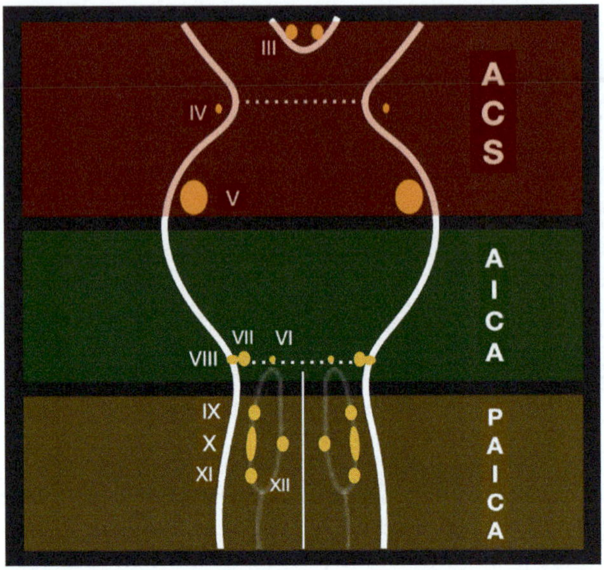

Fig. 13.1 Illustration depicting the relationship of each cerebellar artery with the brainstem, cranial nerves, and cerebellar fissures. The superior cerebellar artery (SCA) is closely associated with the cerebellomesencephalic fissure; the superior cerebellar peduncle; and cranial nerves III, IV, and V (highlighted in red). The anterior inferior cerebellar artery (AICA) is associated with the pontocerebellar fissure; middle cerebellar peduncle; and cranial nerves VI, VII, and VIII (highlighted in green). The posterior inferior cerebellar artery (PICA) passes near the cerebellobulbar fissure and lower cranial nerves (IX, X, XI, and XII) (highlighted in yellow)

dominant artery. Each artery has a direct anatomical relationship with cerebellar fissures and, consequently, with the cranial nerves to form the respective neurovascular complexes (Fig. 13.1).

13.1 Dissection of the Superior Cerebellar Artery/ Mesencephalic Cerebellar Fissure

The SCA originates from the distal portion of the BA just before its bifurcation. It is divided into four segments based on the directional changes along its course: S1, anterior pontomesencephalic; S2, lateral pontomesencephalic; S3, cerebellomesencephalic; and S4, cortical (Fig. 13.2).

- S1: This segment runs from medial to lateral, originating from the BA and crossing below the apparent origin of the oculomotor nerve at the level of the pontomesencephalic sulcus (Fig. 13.3).
- S2: As SCA encircles the brainstem at the anterolateral boundary of the pontomesencephalic sulcus, its directional axis shifts from anterior to posterior,

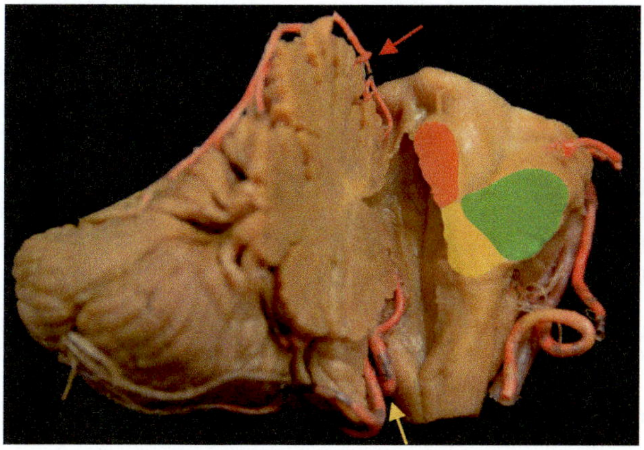

Fig. 13.2 A posterior oblique view of the brainstem, fourth ventricle, and left cerebellar hemisphere is shown. The right cerebellar hemisphere has been removed (at the level of the cerebellar vermis). The red arrow indicates the SCA at the cerebellomesencephalic fissure and its relationship with the superior cerebellar peduncle (in red). The yellow arrow denotes the SCA at the cerebellobulbar fissure and its relationship with the inferior cerebellar peduncle (highlighted in yellow). The middle cerebellar peduncle is highlighted in green

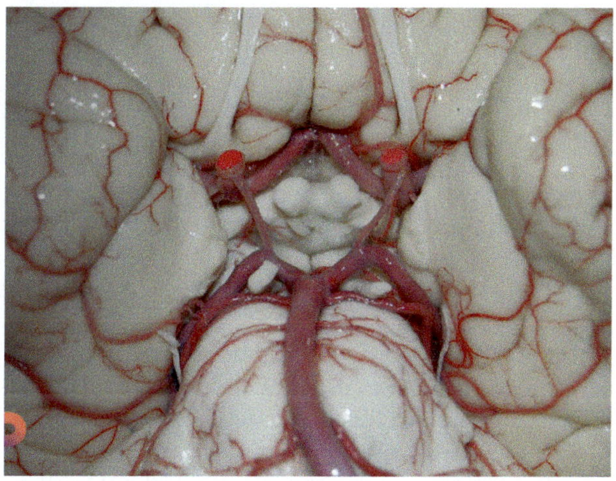

Fig. 13.3 On the left, an inferior view of a brain specimen shows the S1 segment (single arrow) and the S2 segment (double arrow)

following the lateral portion of the sulcus. This segment lies on the lateral surface of the cerebral peduncle, parallel and medial to the free edge of the tentorium cerebelli, and passes below the trochlear nerve just before it enters the free edge of the tentorium (Fig. 13.3).

- S3: At the posterior boundary of the cerebral peduncle, the SCA changes direction from lateral to medial at the level of the cerebellomesencephalic fissure. It follows the course of the trochlear nerve to its origin, beneath the inferior colliculi of the quadrigeminal plate (Fig. 13.4).

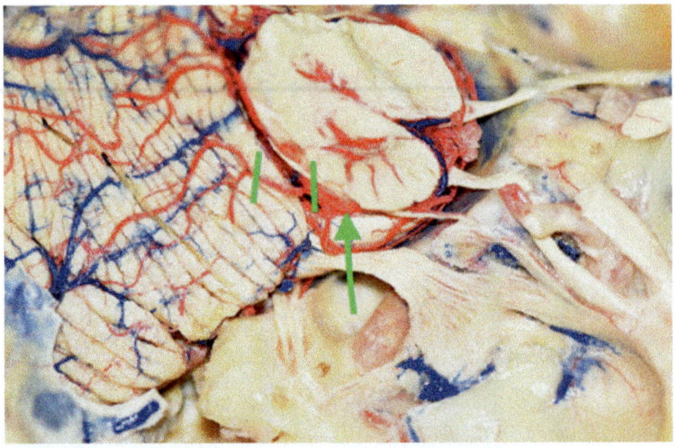

Fig. 13.4 At the level of the cerebellomesencephalic fissure, the S3 segment of the SCA (between the green lines) follows a posterior course from lateral to medial. The SCA maintains a direct relationship with the fourth cranial nerve (arrow), which serves as a landmark when performing surgical procedures in the posterior fossa

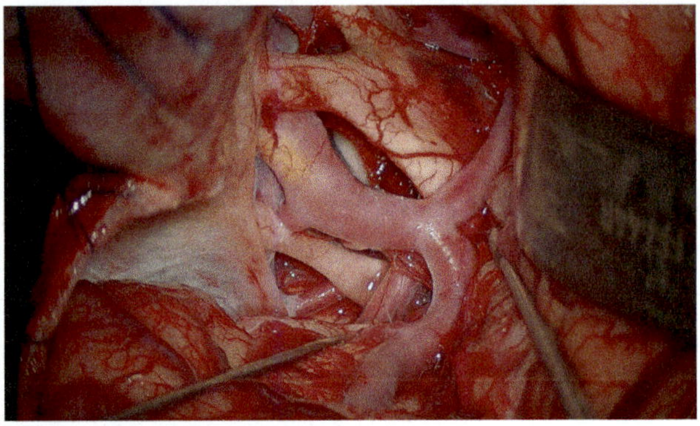

Fig. 13.5 Orbitozygomatic craniotomy. Dissection of the Sylvian fissure and exposure of the basal cisterns. The S1 segment of the SCA crosses below the third nerve. This approach provides access to aneurysms in the basilar artery apex or the origin of the SCA

- S4: This segment comprises the cortical branches that travel along the superior surface of the cerebellum.
- At the level of the cerebellomesencephalic fissure, the SCA gives rise to branches that supply the dentate nucleus of the cerebellum, a critical structure involved in the coordination of appendicular movements.
- Various surgical approaches that are employed to manage pathologies in the basal cisterns lead to SCA exposure.
- Pterional craniotomy and its variations (pretemporal and orbitozygomatic), typically used for aneurysms at the top of the BA, allow exposure of the S1 segment of the SCA (Fig. 13.5). Aneurysms originating from the SCA are rare, and the surgical approach follows the same principles as those for basilar bifurcation aneurysms, without involving the perforating arteries.
- The subtemporal approach for lateral mesencephalic pathologies involves exposure of segments S2 and S3 of the SCA (Fig. 13.6). Similarly, supracerebellar infratentorial approaches and/or occipital transtentorial approaches expose the branches of the S4 segment and provide access to the S3 segment of the SCA, as in the cases of microvascular decompression for classic trigeminal neuralgia (Fig. 13.7).

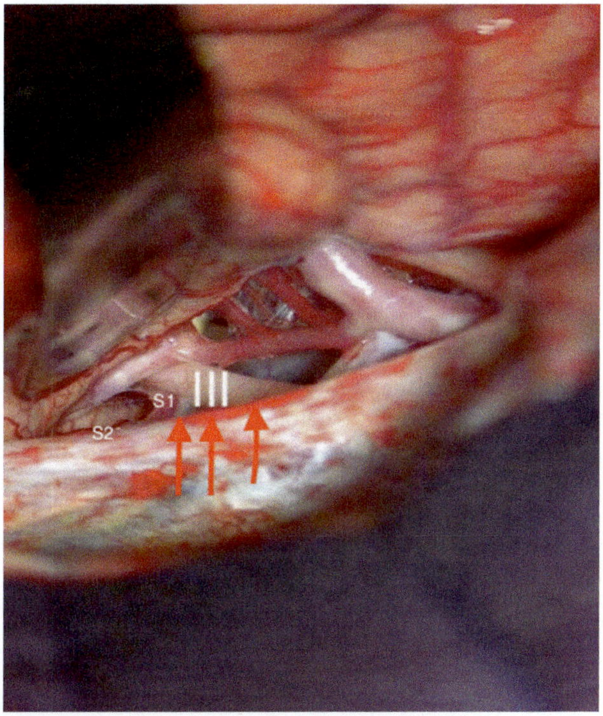

Fig. 13.6 Subtemporal approach, the free edge of the tentorium is identified (red arrows), with the third and crossing above the S1 and S2 segments of the SCA, respectively

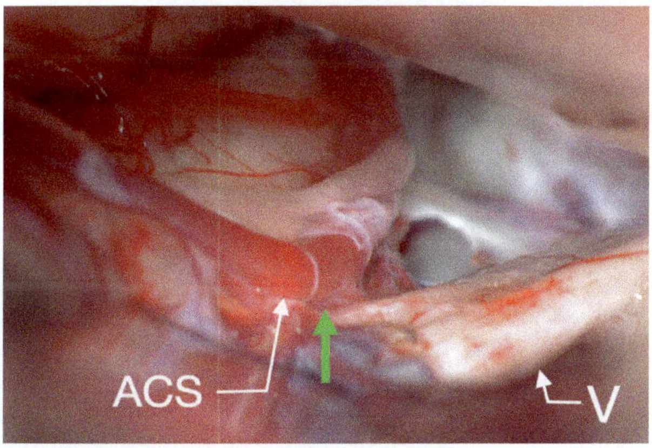

Fig. 13.7 Shows a photograph of microvascular decompression surgery for trigeminal neuralgia employing a lateral suboccipital approach via the supracerebellar route (Jannetta technique). The green arrow indicates the conflict point at the root entry zone of the fifth cranial nerve. The arterial segment most commonly involved in trigeminal neuralgia, specifically the S2 segment of the SCA (green arrow)

13.2 Dissection of the Anterior Inferior Cerebellar Artery: Pontine Cerebellar Fissure

The AICA is divided into four segments based on the directional change of the vessel: anterior pontine, lateral pontine, flocculopeduncular, and cortical branches (Fig. 13.8).

The AICA is a direct branch of the BA, originating from the lower third just above the bulbopontine sulcus. It courses laterally, passing below the proximal portion of cranial nerve VI (anterior pontine segment) and then curves posteriorly, passing below, above, or between cranial nerves VII and VIII (lateral pontine segment), giving rise to the labyrinthine artery (also known as the internal auditory artery), which enters the internal acoustic meatus. The AICA continues toward the cerebellopontine angle. In this region, the AICA is closely related to the cerebellar flocculus, choroid plexus of the lateral recess of the fourth ventricle, foramen of Luschka, and middle cerebellar peduncle (flocculopeduncular segment). Owing to the anastomotic network between the three cerebellar arteries, their calibers tend to vary depending on the dominant artery. A common variation is hypoplasia of the AICA due to the predominance of the ipsilateral PICA.

In the laboratory, the anatomy of the AICA can be examined from various perspectives, depending on specimen preparation. Thus, anatomical landmarks are crucial for guiding neurosurgeons during the performance of surgical procedures.

The AICA is commonly encountered during cerebellopontine angle surgeries and is associated with pathologies affecting the facial and vestibulocochlear nerves, such as vestibular schwannomas and hemifacial spasms (Fig. 13.9).

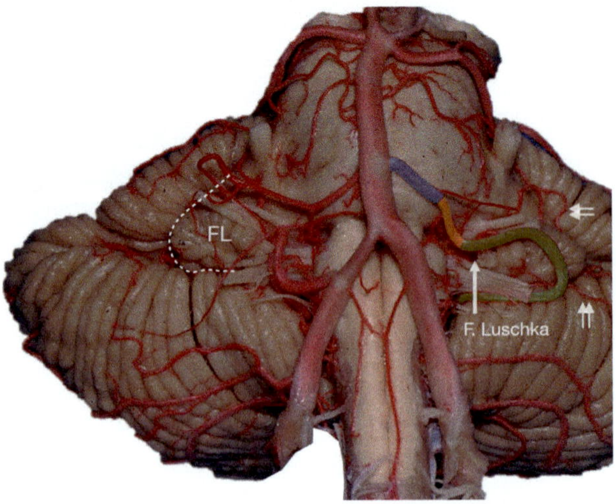

Fig. 13.8 Segments of the AICA: anterior pontine (blue), lateral pontine (orange), flocculopeduncular (green), and cortical branches (double arrows). The AICA is related to the pontocerebellar fissure, cerebellar flocculus, and Luschka's foramen (single arrow). In this specimen, a right PICA dominance is observed, with the ipsilateral AICA showing reduced caliber

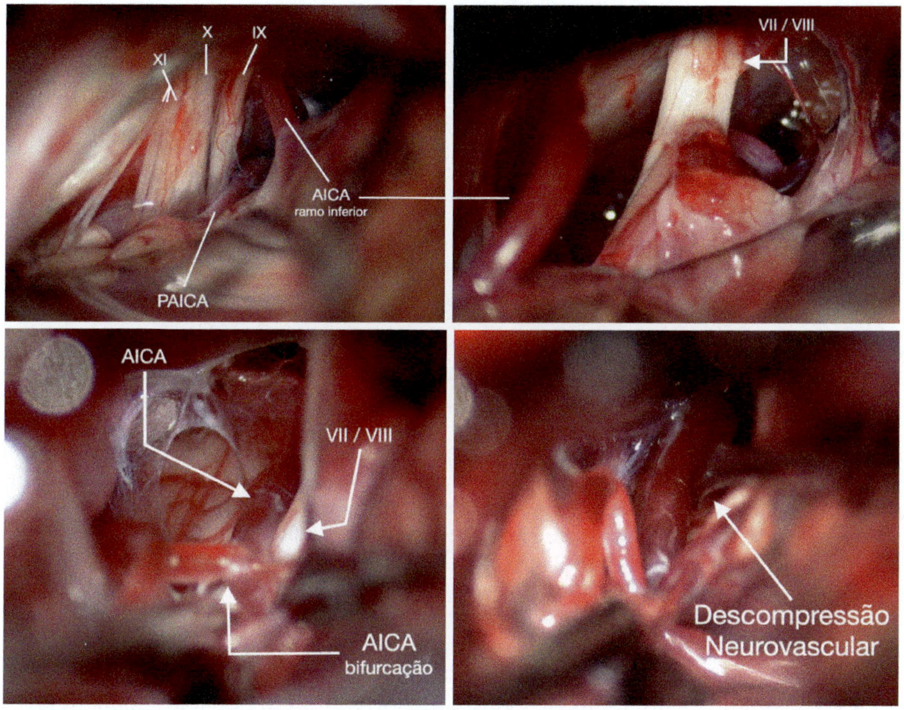

Fig. 13.9 Photos demonstrating the microvascular decompression surgery for spasms on the left side of the face. Park bench position, lateral suboccipital craniotomy. Upper left image: Relationship of the PICA with the lower cranial nerves. Upper right image: identification of the VII–VIII complex and the AICA branches. Lower left image: a pre-bifurcation segment of the AICA causing neurovascular conflict at the exit zone of the seventh nerve at the lateral bulbopontine sulcus. Lower right image: retraction of the AICA for microvascular decompression

13.3 Posterior Inferior Cerebellar Artery Dissection: Tonsil Bulbar Fissure

The PICA is divided into five segments based on the directional changes in the vessel: the anterior bulbar (AB), lateral bulbar (LB), tonsillobulbar (TB), televelotonsillar (TVT), and hemispheric and vermian cortical branches (Fig. 13.10).

- **AB segment:** This segment travels from medial to lateral across the anterior surface of the medulla oblongata.
- **LB segment:** This segment courses from anterior to posterior, laterally along the medulla.
- **TB segment:** This segment loops inferiorly, traveling from lateral to medial between the posterolateral surface of the medulla and the cerebellar tonsil, traversing through the tonsillobulbar fissure.

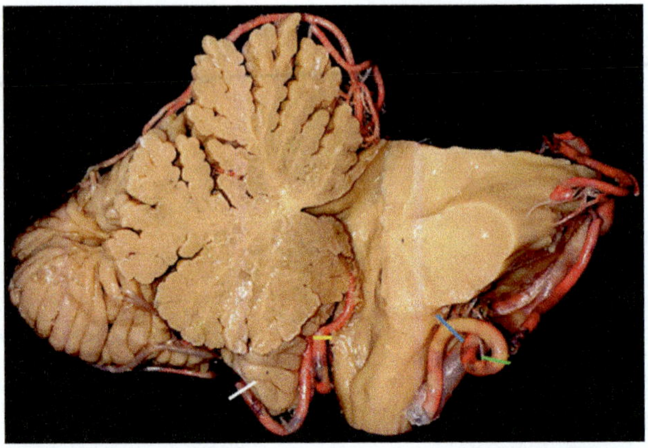

Fig. 13.10 The left image presents an anatomical specimen with the brainstem and cerebellum removed while preserving the cranial nerves and arteries of the posterior fossa. Colored lines indicate the directional changes of the PICA. On the right side, the specimen shows an oblique view of the brainstem with the right cerebellar hemisphere removed, illustrating the relationship of the PICA with the medulla and cerebellum. (green line transition from anterior-bulbar segment to bulbar-lateral; blue line transition from bulbar-lateral segment to tonsilo-bulbar; yellow line transition from tonsilo-bulbar segment to televelosonsilar; white line transition from televelotonsilar segment to cortical segments

- **TVT segment:** This segment loops superiorly along its course, maintaining a close relationship with the tela choroidea and inferior medullary velum of the fourth ventricle. It gives rise to the choroidal branches, with the highest point of this loop being the choroidal point. Before bifurcating into the hemispheric and vermian cortical branches, this artery forms another inferior loop along the edges of the medial surface of the cerebellar tonsil.

13.3.1 Tonsil Bulbar Fissure

The TB fissure (TBF) is the anatomical space between the anterior surface of the cerebellar tonsil and the posterolateral surface of the medulla oblongata (Fig. 13.11).

This fissure serves as an important anatomical landmark that aids in identifying the surrounding structures. The floor of the TBF is formed by the lower part of the roof of the fourth ventricle, including the tela choroidea, which attaches to the border of the fourth ventricle via the tenia choroidea and the inferior medullary velum—a delicate membrane that connects the flocculus to the nodule. Exposure of this region provides access to the fourth ventricle, facilitating the preservation of the lower portion of the vermis. The roof of the fissure comprises the tonsil and biventer lobule. Laterally, the fissure communicates with the cerebellomedullary cistern (Figs. 13.12 and 13.13).

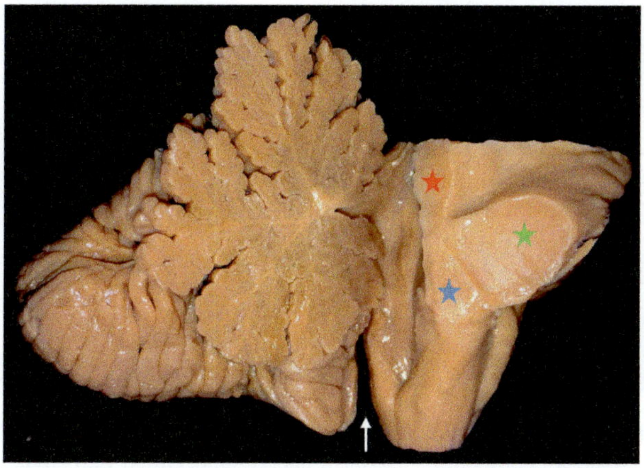

Fig. 13.11 Anatomical specimen showing a section of the cerebellum at the vermis level, with the right cerebellar hemisphere removed to expose the fourth ventricle. The TBF is indicated by a white arrow. The stars denote the superior (red), middle (green), and inferior (blue) cerebellar peduncles. The image demonstrates that only the superior and inferior peduncles have a direct relationship with the fourth ventricle, with the inferior cerebellar peduncle positioned just above the TBF

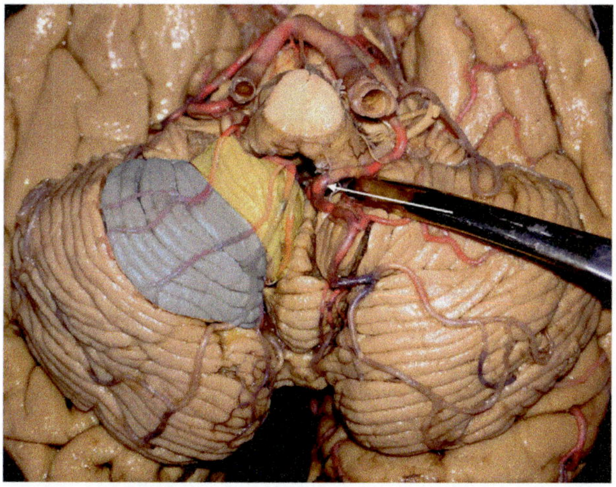

Fig. 13.12 An inferior view of the cerebellum. The right tonsil is highlighted in yellow, while the biventer lobule is highlighted in blue. The retraction of the left tonsil exposes the TB segment of the PICA

The AB, LB, and TB segments of the PICA give rise to perforating branches that supply the brainstem, making their preservation crucial during surgery. Therefore, the identification of PICA branches is essential when performing microsurgical procedures in the posterior cranial fossa. All portions of the PICA can be easily identified in laboratory specimens removed from the skull. However, examining the injected heads provides a more accurate simulation of the actual surgery. For example, the identification and dissection of the AB segment require a far-lateral approach similar to that used in surgical procedures.

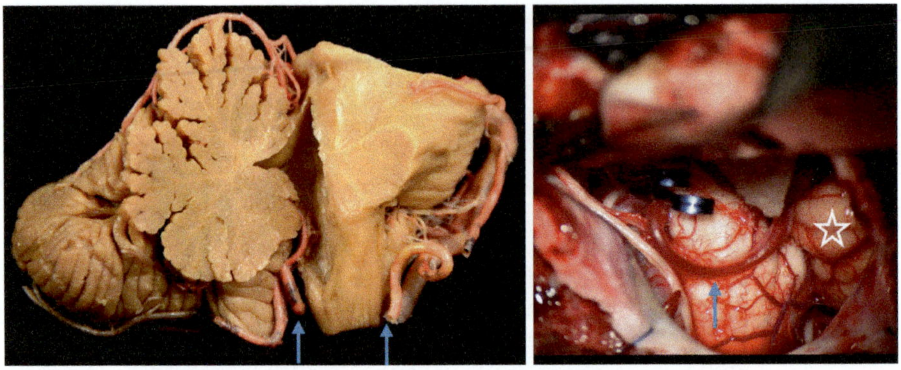

Fig. 13.13 On the left, the inferior loop of the TB segment of the PICA in the TBF is shown (blue arrows). On the right, a photograph showing a lateral suboccipital retrosigmoid approach performed for a PICA aneurysm. The left tonsil is retracted superiorly with a retractor. The right tonsil is marked by a white star. The blue arrow points to the inferior loop of the TB segment of the PICA in the TBF

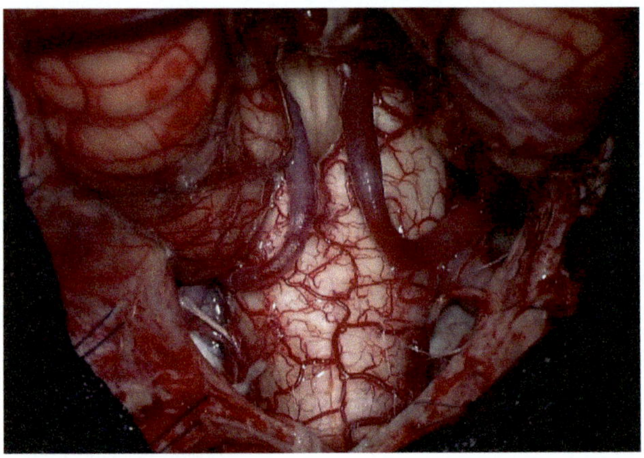

Fig. 13.14 Midline suboccipital approach with resection of the posterior arch of C1 and C2. Exposure of the tonsillobulbar segment of both PICAs

Pathologies involving the origin of the PICA, such as aneurysms, necessitate a lateral suboccipital approach. If the PICA origin is lateral, the retrosigmoid approach may provide sufficient visualization and manipulation. When the origin is more anterior, a lateral view is necessary to enhance the angle and visibility of the AB segment, making the far-lateral approach more suitable.

In the midline suboccipital approach, cortical branches are initially encountered. By retracting the cerebellar tonsils, similar to the approach to the fourth ventricle, the inferior loop of the distal portion of the TVT segment can be identified (Figs. 13.13 and 13.14).

Bibliography

1. Rhoton AL. The posterior cranial fossa: microsurgical anatomy and surgical approaches. Neurosurgery. 2000;47(suppl_3):S5–6. https://doi.org/10.1097/00006123-200009001-00005.
2. Chaddad Neto F, Doria-Netto HL, de Campos Filho JM, et al. The far-lateral craniotomy: tips and tricks. Arq Neuropsiquiatr. 2014;72(9):699–705. https://doi.org/10.1590/0004-282X20140130.
3. de Oliveira E, Tedeschi E, Rhoton A, Peace D. Microsurgical anatomy of the posterior circulation: vertebral and basilar arteries. In: Carter L, Spetzler R, editors. Neurovascular Surgery. New York: McGraw Hill, Inc.; 1995. p. 25–34.
4. Microneurosurgery YM, Volume I. Microsurgical anatomy of the basal cisterns and vessels of the brain, diagnostic studies, general operative techniques and pathological considerations of the intracranial aneurysms. New York: George Thieme Verlag; 1984.
5. Chaddad-Neto F, Da Costa MD. Microneuroanatomy and surgery: a practical anatomical guide. Springer; 2022.

Chapter 14
History and Evolution of the Neuroanatomy Lab Training

14.1 Introduction

Training neurosurgeons in microsurgery laboratories has become an indispensable component in cultivating elite professionals. This advancement is closely linked to the rapid progression of microsurgical techniques, highlighting the pivotal role of specialized laboratories in the educational landscape. Engaging in laboratory training affords neurosurgery residents and practicing neurosurgeons not only an in-depth understanding of neuroanatomy but also an opportunity to refine their surgical skills through simulations that closely mimic the conditions of actual neurosurgical procedures.

Recognizing the seminal contributions of visionary neurosurgeons to this educational paradigm and their role in the establishment of microsurgery laboratories worldwide is crucial. By adopting a holistic perspective, this discussion explores the historical context and significance of training facilities. This chapter aimed to elucidate their impact on the evolution of contemporary neurosurgery, with a particular focus on pioneering laboratories and professionals who have been instrumental in the advancement of this field.

14.2 Doctor Yaşargil's Laboratory

14.2.1 Introduction

Mahmut Gazi Yasargil, hailed as the preeminent neurosurgeon of the twentieth century, embarked on his educational and professional journey in Switzerland in the latter half of the previous century. Originating in Turkey, he is celebrated as the progenitor of microneurosurgery. Yasargil's seminal contributions included the

F. Chaddad-Neto, M. D. S. da Costa, *Microneuroanatomy and Lab*,
https://doi.org/10.1007/978-3-031-91026-5_14

development of microsurgical techniques, which are widely recognized today, along with the invention of various instruments tailored for microneurosurgery. Many of these instruments have become integral to the global neurosurgical practice.

Professor Yasargil's impact extends far beyond his achievements. With a steadfast commitment to advancing his specialty, he devoted a substantial portion of his career to the education and propagation of microneurosurgery. Through his efforts, Yasargil mentored a multitude of neurosurgeons and imparted his knowledge and skills, particularly in the management of tumors, arteriovenous malformations (AVMs), cerebral aneurysms, and occlusive cerebrovascular diseases.

14.2.2 Curiosities

Less commonly known is that Dr. Yasargil initially devoted his expertise to various domains within neurosurgery, achieving notable success in treating spinal pathologies, including lumbar disc herniation and kyphoscoliosis. Subsequently, he advocated for the endovascular approach as a treatment method for cerebral lesions, such as aneurysms and AVMs. However, the technological constraints of this era led to less favorable outcomes. Before fully dedicating himself to microneurosurgery, he practiced stereotactic surgery targeting movement disorders.

14.2.3 Birth of Microneurosurgery

In 1965, at the age of 40 years, Gazi Yasargil embarked on a pivotal journey to Burlington, Vermont, in the United States to undergo training in microsurgery at one of the few existing laboratories dedicated to this specialty at the time. This laboratory was established by Doctors Jacobson and Donaghy in 1958 and was recognized as the first microvascular training laboratory (Fig. 14.1).

In the laboratory, Dr. Donaghy's research primarily focused on arterial reactivity following extracranial surgical interventions, including suturing and grafting the femoral arteries of rabbits. Gazi Yasargil, who demonstrated foresight and innovation, persuaded Dr. Donaghy to conduct training on microsurgery of the cerebral arteries in mongrel dogs.

On December 4, 1966, Yasargil performed a groundbreaking operation on the basilar artery of a dog using a transcervical-transclival approach. He created a 5.0-mm incision in the exposed basilar artery and secured both ends with two Scoville vascular clips. The incision was meticulously closed with 9.0 suture threads under microscopic guidance. Remarkably, the dog recovered without any neurological deficits, and the basilar artery remained open. Reflecting on this monumental achievement, Professor Yasargil stated: "For me, this was the beginning of reconstructive brain artery experiments in the laboratory and the birth of microneurosurgery" (Fig. 14.2).

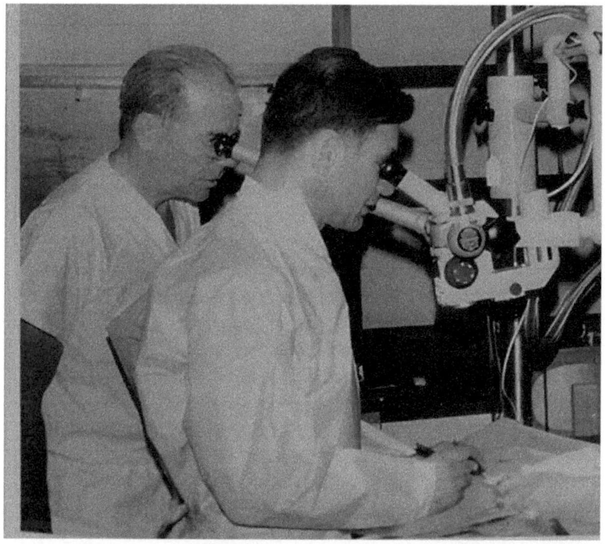

Fig. 14.1 Professor RMP Donaghy instructing and observing Gazi's early attempts in performing microtechniques in Burlington, VT, in 1965. Reproduced with permission from Neurosurgery [1]

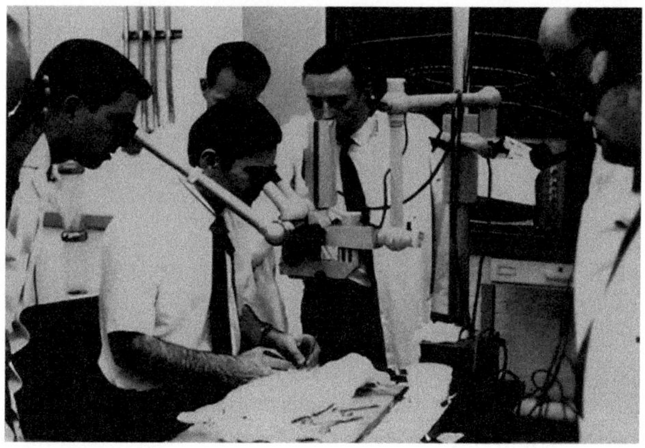

Fig. 14.2 Yasargil during his microsurgery course at Mt. Sinai Hospital in New York in 1970. Reproduced with permission from Neurosurgery [1]

14.2.4 Laboratory in Zurich

Upon his return to Zürich in 1967, Yasargil dedicated the next 2 years to advancing experimental intracranial microvascular surgery within the laboratory of the Brain Research Institute, under the guidance of Professor K. Akert. In addition to his research endeavors, he facilitated training courses on microsurgical techniques for visiting colleagues in various countries. These sessions were conducted in an impromptu laboratory setup within the General Surgery Department, showcasing Yasargil's commitment to sharing his expertise and fostering the worldwide expansion of microneurosurgery (Fig. 14.3).

In 1972, Yasargil transitioned the old laboratory into a state-of-the-art laboratory equipped with superior research and training amenities, including four rooms and

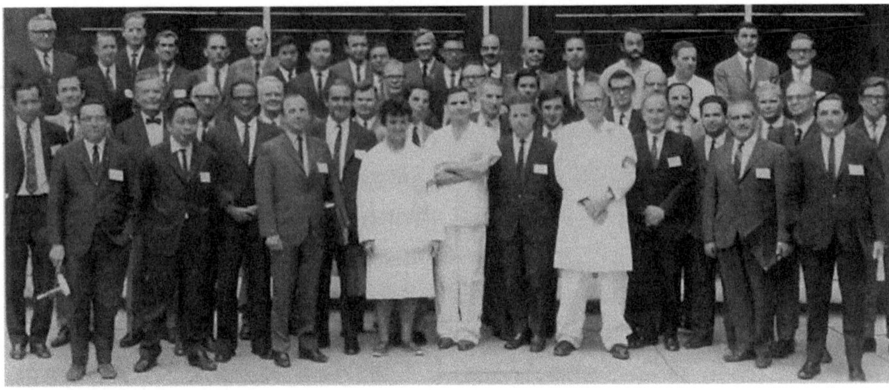

Fig. 14.3 Microneurosurgical meeting in Burlington 1969. Reproduced with permission from Neurosurgery [1]

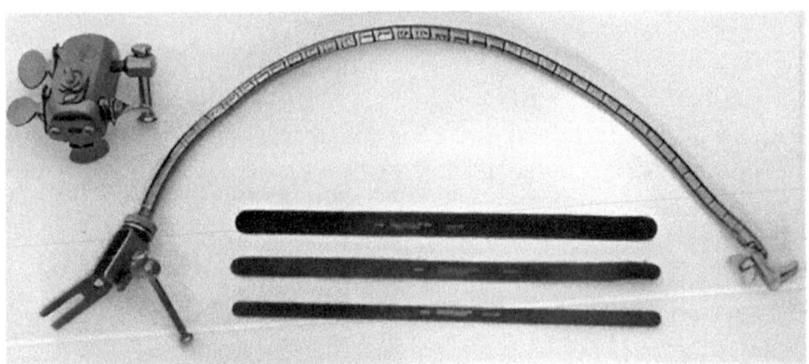

Fig. 14.4 "Leyla" retractor system with various components. Reproduced with permission from Thieme [2]

eight Zeiss OPMI II microscopes. Demonstrating his dedication to advancing the field, the professor personally invested approximately $5000 to acquire these microscopes. From 1967 to 1992, approximately 3000 surgeons from diverse specialties attended training courses in Zurich, benefiting from the comprehensive education provided in microsurgical techniques. Throughout this period, Dr. Yasargil was instrumental in the development and widespread adoption of various microsurgical instruments. These innovations include bayonet-type forceps, bayonet-type bipolar forceps of various sizes, and malleable brain retractors (Leyla), each of which contributes significantly to the precision and efficacy of microsurgical procedures (Fig. 14.4).

Renowned figures in the field of neurosurgery traveled to Zürich to study under Gazi Yasargil in his laboratory, highlighting the global impact of his work. Among these distinguished individuals were Vinko Dolenc, an exceptional skull base surgeon, and Majid Samii, a world-renowned expert in the treatment of vestibular schwannomas.

Mahmut Gazi Yasargil's achievements are unparalleled and have profoundly transformed the landscape of neurosurgery. His unwavering commitment and exceptional surgical prowess continue to inspire aspiring neurosurgeons. Professor Yasargil's dedication to microsurgery education, as evidenced by his active participation in teaching courses worldwide, played a pivotal role in the widespread adoption of his techniques and the overall advancement of the field. This legacy of knowledge sharing is reflected in the contributions of other eminent neurosurgeons who followed Dr. Yasargil's footsteps, including Dr. Albert Rhoton Jr., Dr. Evandro de Oliveira, and Dr. Feres Chaddad-Neto, who further validated the enduring influence of his work.

14.3 Doctor Rhoton's Laboratory

14.3.1 Introduction

Dr. Rhoton's laboratory is one of the most pivotal establishments in the Annals of Neurosurgery, with efforts primarily focused on microneurosurgery and its anatomical aspects. It is internationally renowned for its prolific scientific contributions and is at the forefront of producing over 500 scholarly articles, educational courses, and seminal books. The laboratory's impact extends beyond the confines of academia, significantly influencing neurosurgical education through groundbreaking scientific endeavors.

Over the years, Dr. Rhoton's laboratory has emerged as a foundational pillar of the neurosurgical community by introducing innovative techniques, making essential literary contributions, and establishing unparalleled standards of excellence. These benchmarks have become reference points for laboratories worldwide. In this discussion, we aimed to explore the evolution of Dr. Rhoton's laboratory, highlighting the elements that have significantly influenced the development and practices of our own laboratory (Fig. 14.5).

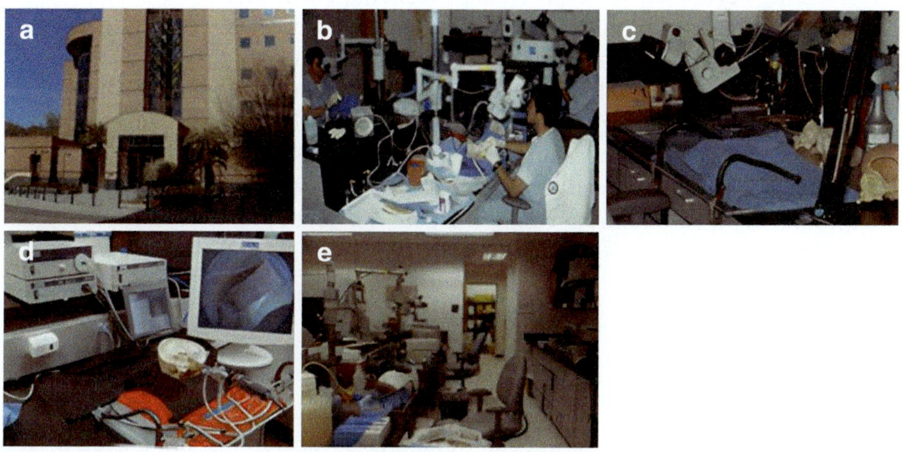

Fig. 14.5 (**a**) Entrance of the McKnight Brain Institute, where the laboratory was situated. (**b–e**) Comprehensive view of the laboratory, highlighting the workstations and dissection materials. Reproduced with permission from Elsevier [7]

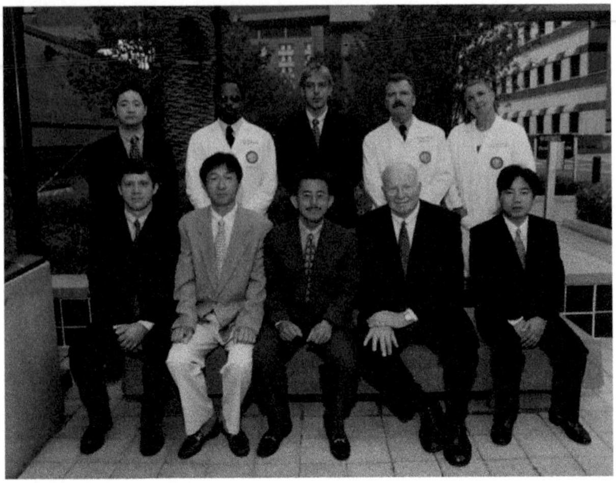

Fig. 14.6 Dr. Rhoton with his research fellows. Reproduced with permission from Elsevier [13]

The George Schader Colder Laboratory, also known as Dr. Rhoton's Laboratory, was established in 1975 at the University of Florida (UF) under the leadership of Dr. Rhoton, following his appointment as Chief of the Department of Neurosurgery at the institution. Dr. Rhoton began his career in 1966, coinciding with the early stages of microsurgery. His journey from the pre-microsurgical era to one enriched by microsurgical advancements was pivotal to his contributions. Experiencing the contrast between neurosurgical practices before and after the introduction of the microscope provided Dr. Rhoton with a unique perspective. This comparison led him to advocate for the microneurosurgical technique as a considerably safer approach. His commitment to advancing this technique aims to provide more effective treatments for conditions that were previously overlooked or inadequately addressed, underscoring his dedication to providing excellent patient care.

With the aim of performing surgeries with enhanced precision and safety, Rhoton laid the groundwork for the establishment of a laboratory in 1972. Through his efforts, he secured essential funding for its establishment, utilizing donations from grateful patients, contributions from private benefactors, and support from the UF. The laboratory, which officially opened in 1975, was equipped with four dissection workstations. Over the years, it has become a center for training and research, with more than 100 fellows contributing to its legacy and research program (Fig. 14.6).

14.3.2 Laboratory Routine

Fellows and technicians were integral to laboratory operations and played a vital role in preparing specimens for dissection. This process primarily involved the use of heads that had been fixed with formalin during postmortem. To advance the study of anatomy, a vascular staining technique was developed and meticulously refined.

This technique involves the injection of dyes into the cervical vessels to enhance the visualization of anatomical structures.

For arterial staining, red acrylic or latex was injected into the carotid and vertebral arteries to delineate the arterial pathways. Conversely, venous staining involves the injection of a dye into the internal jugular vein, particularly in projects aimed at examining the ventricular system of the brain. The combination of refined dissection techniques and meticulous specimen preparation has resulted in the production of unique publications and educational materials. These contributions not only enriched the scientific community but also led to the establishment of new standards for the study of neurosurgical anatomy (Fig. 14.7).

The commitment to these practices led to the laboratory's international recognition, attracting neurosurgeons worldwide to enroll in Professor Rhoton's microsurgical anatomy course. The exceptional preparation of the specimens prompted the laboratory technicians worldwide to travel to acquaint themselves with and learn the techniques employed (Fig. 14.8).

The international quest for excellence underscores the laboratory's esteemed global reputation and pivotal contribution to the advancement of neurosurgery. This interchange of knowledge and expertise with professionals worldwide significantly enhances the laboratory milieu, fostering innovation and the relentless pursuit of excellence in neurosurgical methodologies (Fig. 14.9).

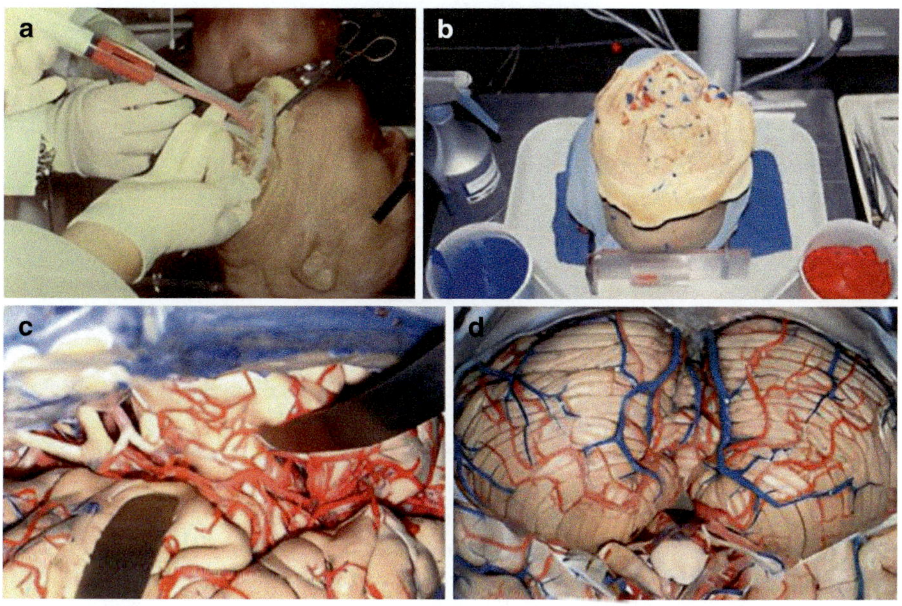

Fig. 14.7 (**a**) Cross-sectional view of an anatomical specimen highlighting the cervical vessels. Reproduced with permission from [8]. (**b–c**) Demonstration of the contrast infusion process. (**d**) Final result of arterial staining. Reproduced with permission from Springer [8]

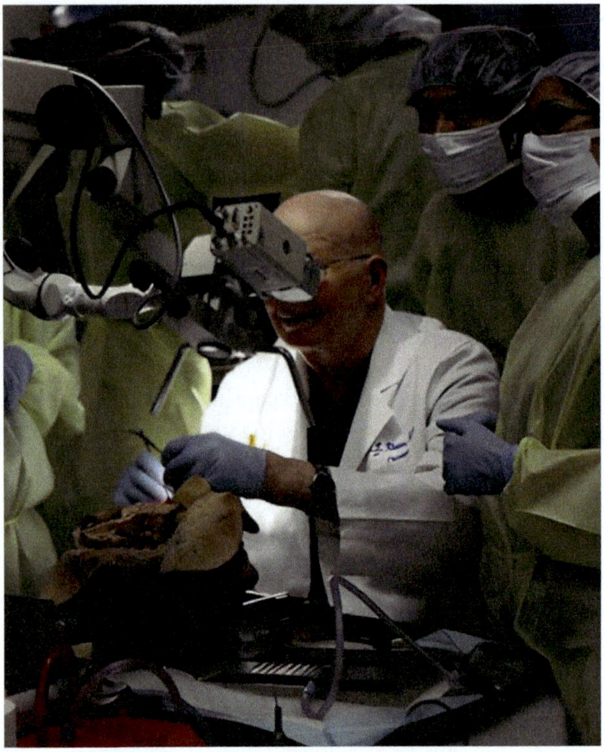

Fig. 14.8 Dr. Rhoton teaching in one of his courses. Reproduced with permission from Elsevier [7]

The team consisted not only of fellows but also laboratory technicians, illustrators, and administrative staff, each playing a vital role in the laboratory's teaching and research achievements. Dr. Rhoton's laboratory pioneered the development of illustration and documentation techniques, contributing significantly to the visual representation of microneurosurgical techniques and their transition from practical applications to scholarly publications. Throughout the technological evolution leading up to the 1980s, the laboratory adeptly managed limitations, by utilizing black and white photography owing to its availability and the high costs of color imaging.

Dr. Rhoton's fellows, whom he fondly likened to "Michelangelos and Da Vincis," were instrumental in crafting numerous works and refining dissection techniques. A breakthrough occurred in 1980 when Fellow Toshio Matsushima introduced the technique of removing the arachnoid membrane from blood vessels and brain tissues, thereby improving the visualization of cranial structures and facilitating the production of higher-quality images. In the following year, Dr. Evandro de Oliveira pioneered the adoption of colored photography within the laboratory, advocating for

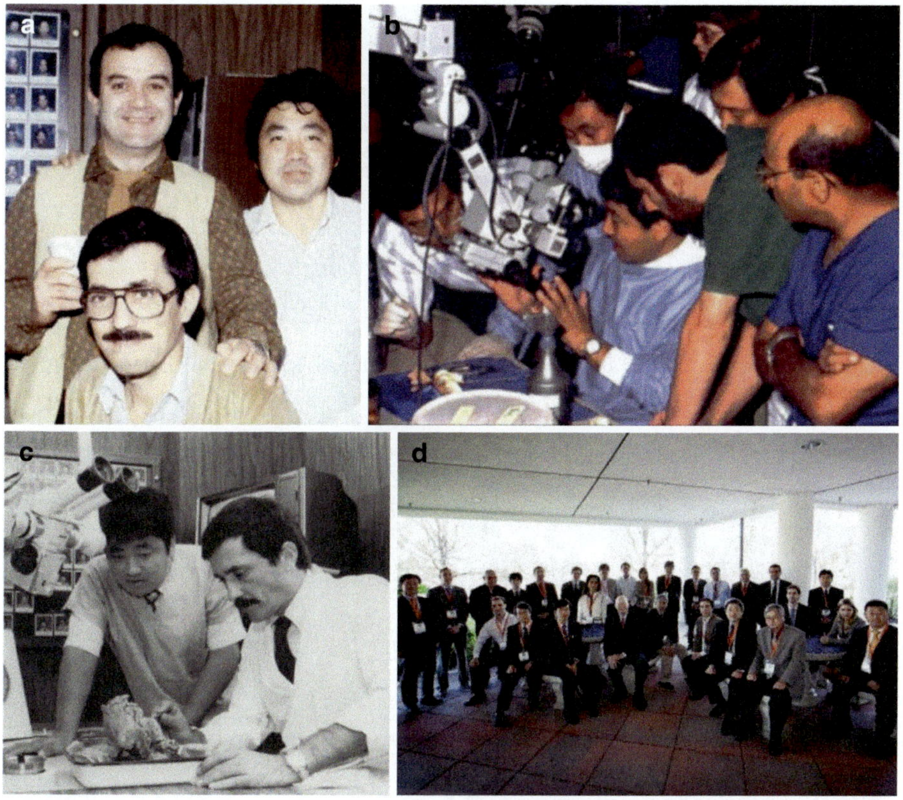

Fig. 14.9 (a) Three of Professor Rhoton's notable fellows: Evandro de Oliveira (Brazil; front row), Erdener Timurkaynak (Turkey; second row, left), and Toshio Matsushima (Japan; second row, right). (b–c) Dissections carried out in the laboratory during courses held in 1992 and 1981, respectively. (d) Dr. Rhoton and his former fellows celebrating his 40 years at the University of Florida. Material reproduced with permission from Springer [8]

its use despite the associated costs. By 1990, with the advent of three-dimensional surgical techniques, Professor Rhoton shifted his focus on replicating surgical approaches with enhanced precision and clarity (Figs. 14.10 and 14.11).

14.3.3 Legacy and Contributions

Throughout history, laboratories have played a crucial role in advancing neurosurgery, facilitating the development of novel surgical modalities, methodologies, and instruments. The dissemination of a wide range of publications, ranging from fundamental anatomical studies to sophisticated surgical techniques, and the

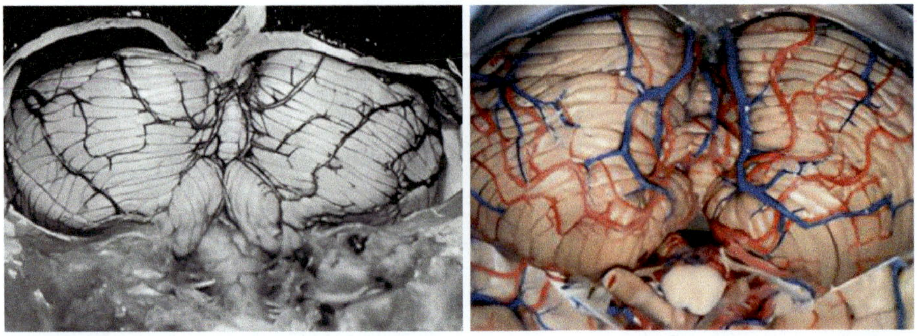

Fig. 14.10 Posterior view of a patient's cerebellum. Material reproduced with permission from Springer [8]

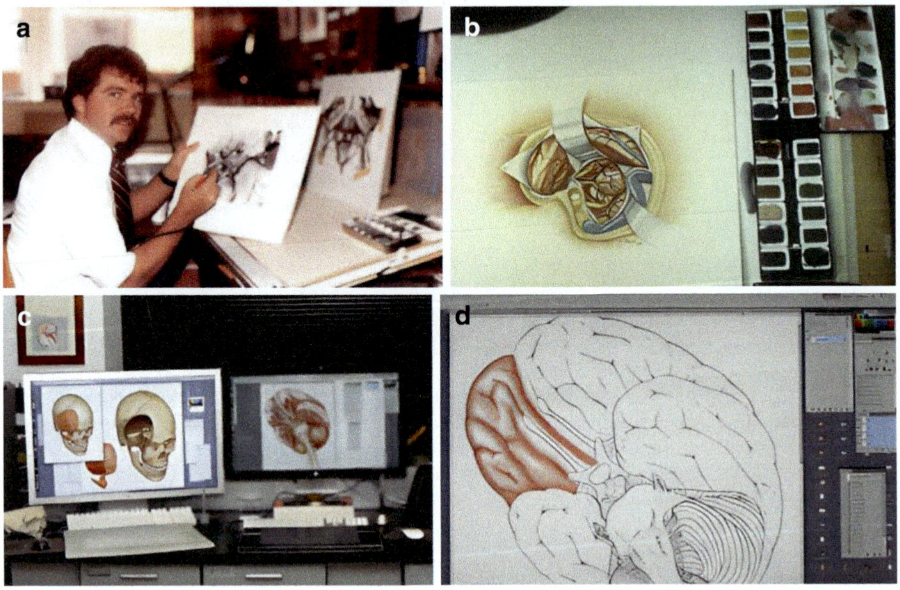

Fig. 14.11 Medical illustration before (**a** and **b**) and after (**c** and **d**) the introduction of computer systems. Material reproduced with permission from Springer [8]

incorporation of cutting-edge technologies, attest to its significant impact. These studies have influenced the evolution of neurosurgical practices, including the introduction of innovative classification systems such as the segmentation of the intradural internal carotid artery into three distinct segments (Fig. 14.12).

The guiding philosophy of the laboratory, coupled with the unparalleled proficiency in illustrations and Dr. Rhoton's exceptional expertise, has led to substantial progress in the management of neurosurgical conditions. The laboratory's mastery is further evidenced by the 11 remarkable covers that Dr. Rhoton has contributed to the "Journal of Neurosurgery," showcasing the significant impact of its work in the field.

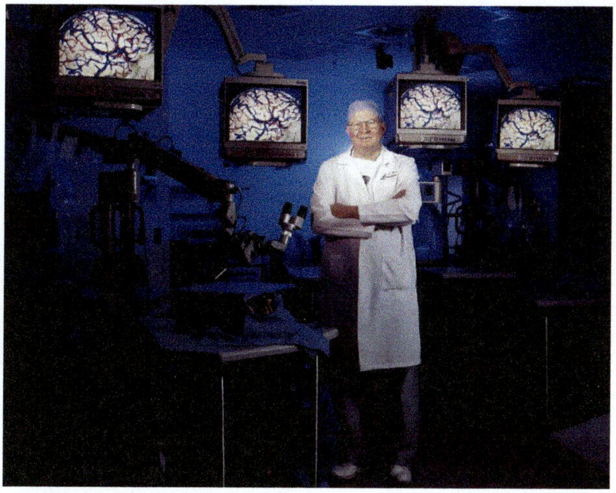

Fig. 14.12 Dr. Rhoton in the teaching laboratory at the University of Florida. Material reproduced with permission from Elsevier [13]

14.4 Doctor Evandro's Laboratory

14.4.1 Introduction

Neurosurgery has undergone profound advancements over the years, undergone by innovations in surgical methods, the advent of novel technologies, and a deeper comprehension of neuroanatomy. Among the luminaries contributing to this evolution, Dr. Evandro Pinto da Luz de Oliveira is distinguished by his exceptional skills, unwavering dedication, and pioneering contributions to neurosurgery and neuroanatomy. This narrative explores the journey and accomplishments of Dr. Evandro de Oliveira and his microneurosurgery laboratory, highlighting his commitment to neurosurgery and its global impact. We delve into his significant contributions and the enduring legacy he has established, not only as a scientist and clinician but also as an educator and visionary committed to effecting a positive change in the medical field (Fig. 14.13).

14.4.2 Dr. Oliveira and the Foundation of the Laboratory

Born on November 8, 1945, and died on November 7, 2020, Dr. Oliveira devoted his entire life to the study and practice of neurosurgery. His goal was to unravel the complexities of the human brain and devise surgical techniques that could effectively manage various pathologies. He earned his medical degree from the Federal University of Santa Catarina and pursued further postgraduate training, ultimately obtaining a doctoral degree in Neurosurgery from the University of São Paulo School of Medicine. Dr. Oliveira's pioneering efforts in microneurosurgery, coupled with his deep understanding of neuroanatomy, not only facilitated notable

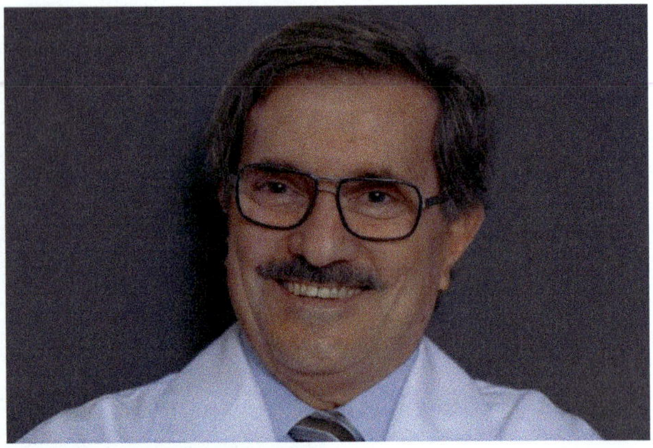

Fig. 14.13 Image from 2019, depicting Dr. Evandro being honored by the American Association of Neurological Surgeons, which named one of the symposiums after him. Personal archive

advancements in the medical field but also inspired the establishment of a laboratory dedicated to the comprehensive study of neuroscience.

The influence of eminent neurosurgeons, such as Dr. Mahmut Gazi Yasargil and Dr. Albert Rhoton Jr., was instrumental in shaping Dr. Oliveira's laboratory. Yasargil, celebrating his meticulous precision and innovative use of the microscope in brain surgery, along with Rhoton, who was committed to the education and detailed examination of brain anatomy, established standards of excellence that Dr. Oliveira aspired to emulate. His admiration for these pioneers not only fueled his pursuit of excellence but also inspired him to foster an educational milieu that promoted the advanced training of future neurosurgeons, reflecting Yasargil and Rhoton's ideals.

Dr. Oliveira's neuroanatomy laboratory has emerged as a cornerstone in the education of aspiring neurosurgeons, emphasizing the critical importance of a thorough understanding of neuroanatomy in improving surgical precision and outcomes. This laboratory serves as a testament to Oliveira's enduring commitment to education and the advancement of innovative surgical techniques, reaffirming his dedication to the development of highly skilled professionals (Fig. 14.14).

In 1993, a landmark event occurred with the establishment of the MicroNeurosurgery Laboratory by Dr. Oliveira at Beneficência Portuguesa de São Paulo. Initially furnished with five workstations, this facility embodied Dr. Oliveira's vision of creating a state-of-the-art laboratory exclusively for neurosurgery. From its inception, the laboratory distinguished itself by providing continuing education courses focused on surgical practice and offering neurosurgeons and other medical specialists the opportunity to refine their skills.

The significance of the laboratory was quickly recognized both nationally and internationally, particularly after 1995 when international participants were welcomed to its courses. This underscores its global impact on education, research, and the advancement of neurosurgical training. This recognition established the laboratory as a trailblazer in adopting international standards of education and training in neurosurgery within Brazil.

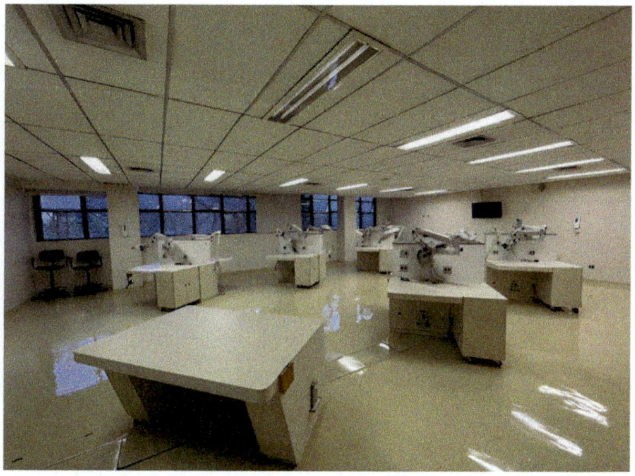

Fig. 14.14 Dr. Oliveira's laboratory. The photo showcases the exceptionally high-quality laboratory equipment and infrastructure. Personal archive

The expansion of the Microneurosurgery Laboratory in 1996 to a new, more spacious, and well-equipped facility not only enhanced its ability to fulfill the educational demands of professionals but also reinforced its status as one of the leading laboratories in the world. After three decades of groundbreaking contributions to neurosurgery, laboratory operations ceased in 2023, marking the end of a significant chapter in the history of the field.

14.4.3 Courses

Since its inception, the laboratory has hosted over 7000 neurosurgeons worldwide who have participated in more than 355 continuing education courses. Additionally, it has accommodated 95 fellows and 650 interns. These courses cover a wide range of neurosurgical topics, including cerebral aneurysm surgery approaches; the anatomy of the ventricles, sulci, and gyri; white matter fibers and their relevance in AVMs and gliomas; microsurgical anatomy of the temporal bone; and other specialized subjects.

The course methodology was primarily practical and designed not only to impart theoretical knowledge but also, more importantly, to improve the surgical proficiency of attendees. A distinguishing feature of the training offered in the laboratory is the extensive use of hands-on exercises with cadaveric specimens or animal models. This approach enables participants to refine their microsurgical techniques in conditions closely resembling the actual surgical scenarios. Specifically, training using the Midas Rex system equipped neurosurgeons with invaluable experience in performing precise drilling and cutting skills, which are crucial in complex brain surgeries (Fig. 14.15).

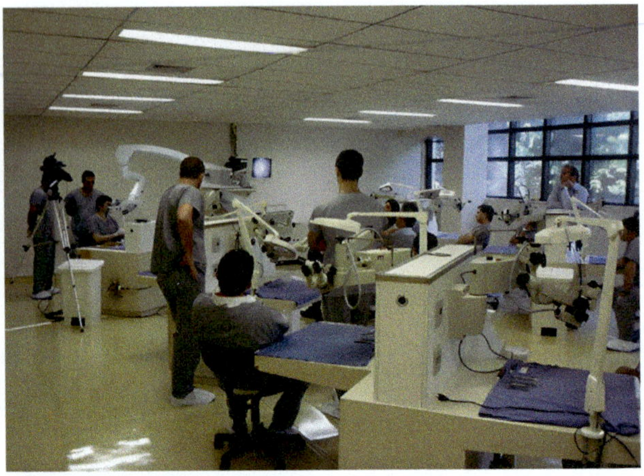

Fig. 14.15 One of the courses conducted by Dr. Evandro de Oliveira in his microneurosurgery laboratory. The photo demonstrates the predominantly practical nature of the courses offered in the laboratory. Personal archive, all rights reserved

14.4.4 Legacy and Contributions

Dr. Evandro de Oliveira has a profound legacy in neurosurgical education. His dedication to the highest standards of training for neurosurgeons has not only elevated the practical abilities of countless physicians but has also fostered a deeper appreciation for the intricacies of neuroanatomy and microsurgical procedures. These contributions directly influence the quality of patient care and result in significantly improved surgical outcomes.

14.5 Doctor Feres Chaddad-Neto's Laboratory

14.5.1 Introduction

The Microneurosurgical Anatomy Laboratory at the Federal University of São Paulo (UNIFESP) was inaugurated on December 3, 2018, with the efforts and dedication of Professors Feres Chaddad-Neto and Ricardo Centeno. The establishment of this laboratory was motivated by the need for a specialized setting dedicated not only to advancing medical education but also to fostering the development of crucial surgical skills among residents, neurosurgeons, and students within the discipline. This narrative seeks to underscore the pivotal role of Dr. Feres Chaddad-Neto in the establishment and progression of this laboratory, marking its evolution into a premier center for training highly skilled professionals in microneurosurgery.

14.5.2 Dr. Feres Chaddad-Neto

Dr. Feres Eduardo Aparecido Chaddad-Neto's academic journey epitomizes unwavering dedication and meticulous rigor, distinguishing excellence within the realms of neurology and neurosurgery. His educational pursuit began at the Pontifical Catholic University of Campinas (PUC Campinas), where he obtained his undergraduate medical degree in 1996. Following his graduation, Dr. Chaddad-Neto embarked on specialization in neurosurgery through a residency program at the same institution, characterized by rigorous training and acquisition of advanced surgical skills.

In his relentless pursuit of excellence, Dr. Chaddad-Neto sought further specialization by undertaking a research fellowship in microneurosurgery at the Institute of Neurological Sciences in Brazil between 2001 and 2002. Under Dr. Evandro Pinto da Luz de Oliveira's mentorship, he focused on vascular microsurgery, marking a pivotal phase of his career. This was followed by a specialization in microsurgical neuroanatomy at the UF in the United States from 2013 to 2014 under the tutelage of the esteemed Prof. Dr. Albert Rhoton Jr. Dr. Chaddad-Neto extensively explored various advanced craniotomy techniques, with a focus on approaches to the top of the basilar artery.

Dr. Chaddad-Neto's dedication to academic excellence propelled him to pursue a postgraduate degree at the State University of Campinas in Brazil. In 2006, he completed his master's degree in neurology and conducted a seminal study on the morphological characteristics of the insular lobe in patients with medial temporal lobe epilepsy. This study enhances understanding of epilepsy from a neuroscientific perspective, particularly in relation to medial temporal sclerosis, magnetic resonance imaging, the insula, and the hippocampus. Continuing his journey of research and innovation, Dr. Chaddad-Neto earned his doctorate in 2010 at Universidade Estadual de Campinas under the orientation of Prof. Dr. Evandro Pinto da Luz de Oliveira. His doctoral research has focused on cranial positioning in various craniotomy procedures, significantly enhancing surgical techniques in neurosurgery.

A cornerstone of Dr. Chaddad-Neto's career was his collaboration with Dr. Evandro de Oliveira, a prominent figure in global neurosurgery. Their partnership transcended traditional mentorship and evolved into a profound professional and academic collaboration. Dr. Oliveira, renowned for his surgical innovations and significant contributions to global neurosurgical education, deeply influenced Dr. Chaddad-Neto's surgical and academic endeavors.

Since 2013, Dr. Chaddad-Neto has been instrumental at the UNIFESP, serving as associate professor and coordinator of the vascular neurosurgery sector, in addition to founding and leading the Microneurosurgical Anatomy Laboratory. His tenure at

UNIFESP is marked by his mentorship in postgraduate programs in neurology and neuroscience and the coordination of specialized vascular neurosurgery courses. In 2022, Dr. Chaddad-Neto attained the prestigious title of "livre-docência," solidifying his status as a preeminent figure in Brazilian neurosurgery and neurosciences. His commitment encompasses academic education, research, and enhancement of clinical practices within these disciplines (Figs. 14.16 and 14.17).

Fig. 14.16 Prof. Dr. Feres Eduardo Aparecido Chaddad-Neto

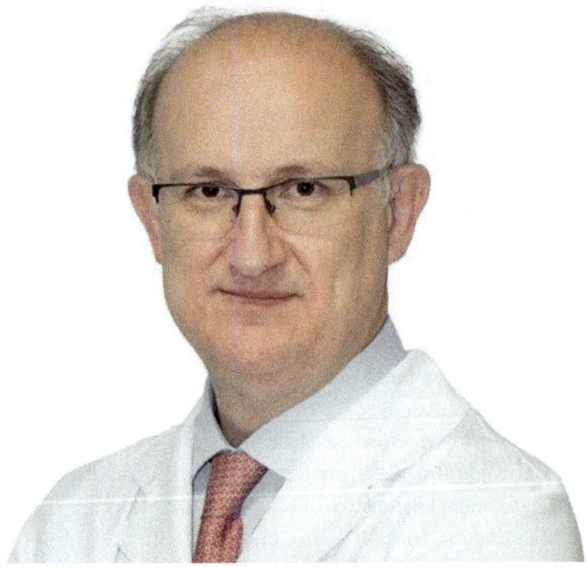

Fig. 14.17 Dr. Feres performing dissection in Dr. Rhoton's et al. laboratory (2016)

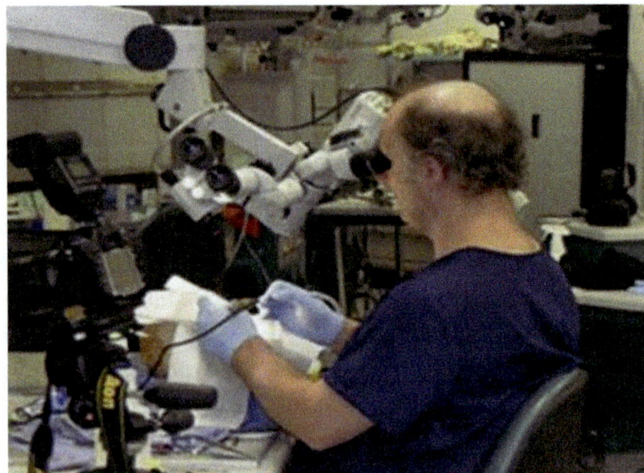

14.5.3 Laboratory Foundation

The Microneurosurgical Anatomy Laboratory at the UNIFESP, inaugurated in December 2018, has rapidly emerged as a cornerstone of global neurosurgical education and practice. The facility houses 20 workstations across 2 rooms, with each station fully equipped with a bifocal microscope, an exhaustive array of microsurgery tools, aspirators, and skull fixators. To further enhance its educational capabilities, the laboratory is equipped with six high-definition televisions that broadcast live images from instructors' microscopes to all participants. As the largest microneurosurgery laboratory in Latin America, it plays a pivotal role in advancing the field by hosting one of the global premier fellowship programs in neurosurgery and microneurosurgical anatomy. Offering internships ranging from 3 months to 1 year presents an unparalleled opportunity for neurosurgeons to perfect their crafts. This center of excellence draws professionals from across the globe, including Italy, Mexico, Israel, Peru, Equatorial Guinea, England, Spain, Argentina, Venezuela, and Uzbekistan, establishing itself as a hub for neurosurgical qualifications and training.

Since its inauguration, the UNIFESP laboratory has welcomed approximately 212 neurosurgery residents and neurosurgeons, forming a diverse group of Brazilian and foreign professionals. On a daily basis, approximately 15–25 individuals engage in practical and research activities in the laboratory, actively dedicated to the development of microsurgical techniques.

Throughout its operation, the Microneurosurgical Anatomy Laboratory at UNIFESP hosted 30 hands-on courses utilizing cadaveric specimens, offering participants a unique opportunity to conduct their own dissection and surgical approaches. The laboratory's guiding philosophy emphasizes the replication of real-life scenarios encountered in surgical settings. This approach ensures that laboratory experiences mirror the actual challenges faced by professionals, highlighting the critical role of reality-based practices in modern neurosurgical training. This method underscores the necessity for specialized training that integrates comprehensive theoretical knowledge with refined manual dexterity.

Beyond its educational endeavors, the laboratory celebrates its contributions to research, with findings published globally in prestigious neurosurgical journals. This academic prominence underscores the laboratory's dedication to innovation and the advancement of neurosurgical techniques.

Since its inception, the laboratory has benefited from several renovations and technological updates facilitated by strategic collaborations with leading medical technology firms. These partnerships have been instrumental in equipping the laboratory with cutting-edge tools, thereby enhancing its capacity to execute microneurosurgical procedures with utmost precision.

Under the stewardship of esteemed professors, such as Feres Chaddad-Neto, Ricardo Silva Centeno, Marcos Devanir da Silva Costa, and Sergio Cavalheiro, the Microneurosurgical Anatomy Laboratory at UNIFESP exemplifies the synergistic potential of academic and industrial cooperation to foster scientific advancement and improve clinical practices in the healthcare sector (Figs. 14.18, 14.19, 14.20, 14.21, and 14.22).

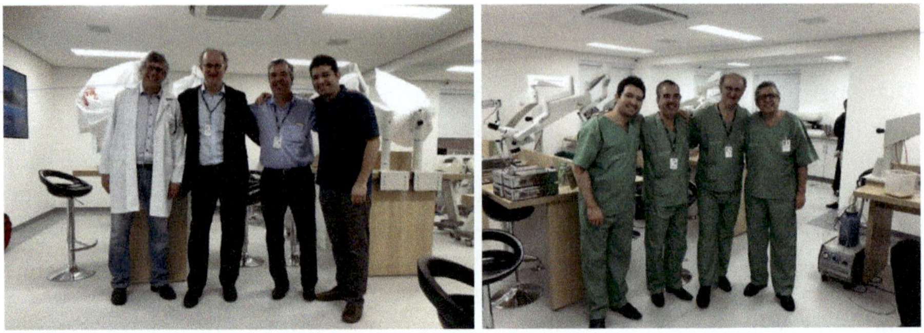

Fig. 14.18 Neurosurgery professors from the São Paulo School of Medicine. Moments before the laboratory inauguration. On the left stands Prof. Sergio Cavalheiro, next to him is Prof. Feres, alongside them is Prof. Ricardo Centeno, and on the right is Prof. Marcos Devanir

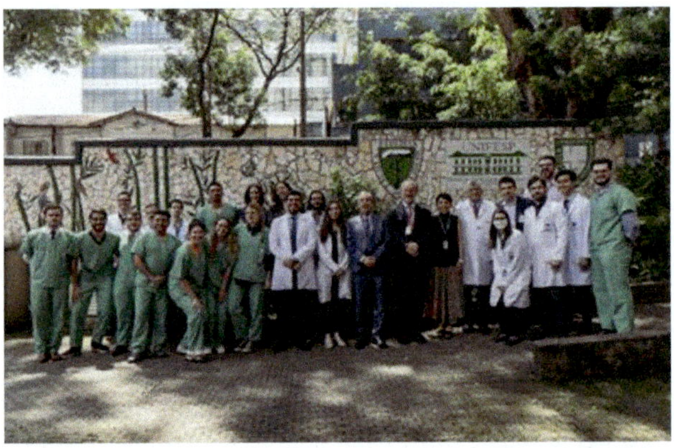

Fig. 14.19 Inauguration of the Microneurosurgical Anatomy Laboratory at UNIFESP. Personal archive, all rights reserved

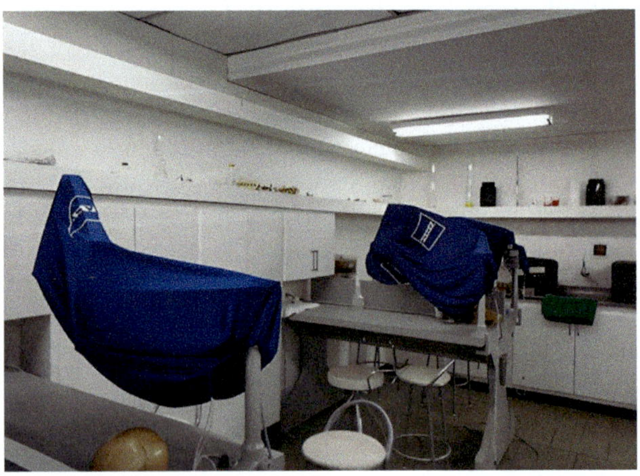

Fig. 14.20 Laboratory in 2018. In the image, we can see the old infrastructure of the laboratory, which has now been renovated. Personal archive, all rights reserved

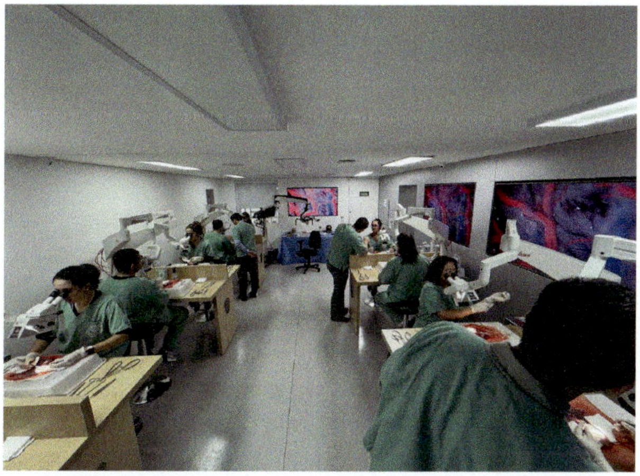

Fig. 14.21 The laboratory after renovation. The image only depicts one part of the space. Personal archive, all rights reserved

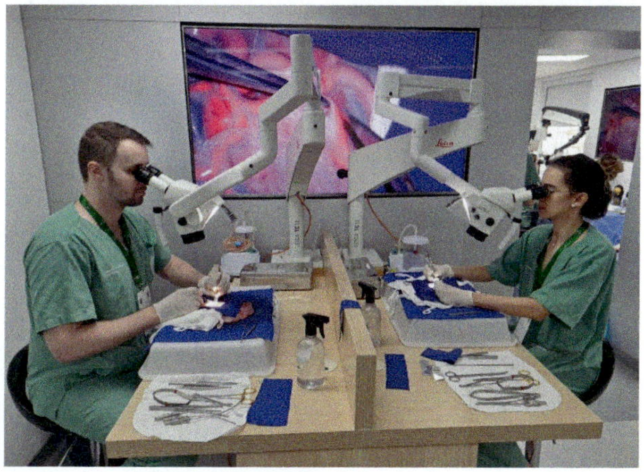

Fig. 14.22 Microscope at the workstations. Personal archive, all rights reserved

14.5.4 Courses Offered

At the Microneurosurgical Anatomy Laboratory of the UNIFESP, an array of specialized courses is offered to medical students, neurosurgeons, and healthcare professionals worldwide. These courses cover critical subjects such as neuroanatomy, bypass techniques, and the exploration of white brain fibers, providing a unique blend of practical and theoretical education.

The laboratory utilizes a diverse range of materials for dissection, including postmortem human specimens, pigs, goats, placentas, and rodents, with the latter specifically used in bypass courses. Specimen preparation was carried out with meticulous care, employing formaldehyde as the fixation agent owing to its efficacy and cost-efficiency. Fresh specimens acquired less than a week postmortem are preferred to guarantee the most effective dissection experience. Additionally, an innovative technique for injecting colored silicone, pioneered by Professor Rhoton, was employed to intricately detail the vascular structures. This involves the use of a thinner silicone mixture for the arteries and a balanced mix for the veins to enhance the visibility of these anatomical features.

The courses, typically spanning 3 days, are facilitated by some of the most respected figures from Brazil and Latin America, including Professors Feres Chaddad-Neto, Marcos Devanir, Ricardo Centeno, and Sergio Cavalheiro. The primary objective of these educational sessions was to impart comprehensive knowledge of regional neuroanatomy and to equip participants with the vital dissection skills needed to address brain lesions.

A notable feature of the course offerings is the inclusion of practical sessions for UNIFESP medical students, underscoring the significance of anatomical knowledge and specialized training in achieving medical proficiency.

These educational endeavors underscore the laboratory's dedication to superior neurosurgical training, advocating not only for the acquisition of technical knowledge but also for the advancement of surgical expertise. By combining theoretical instruction with practical application in a facility equipped with the latest technology and exemplary educational resources, the Microneurosurgical Anatomy Laboratory at UNIFESP distinguishes itself as a beacon of excellence in medical education and neurosurgical inquiry (Figs. 14.23, 14.24, 14.25, 14.26, and 14.27).

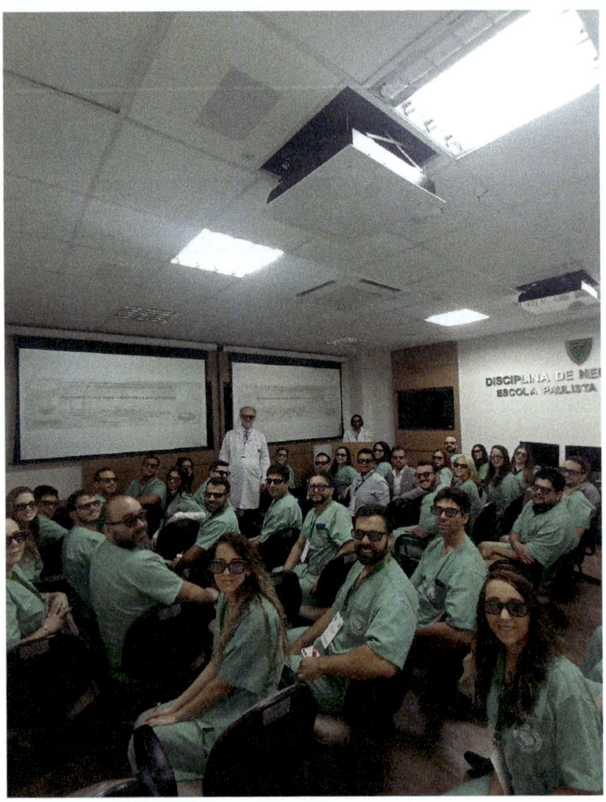

Fig. 14.23 Dr. Feres and his fellows in one of his microsurgery courses, ministering 3D lectures. Personal archive, all rights reserved

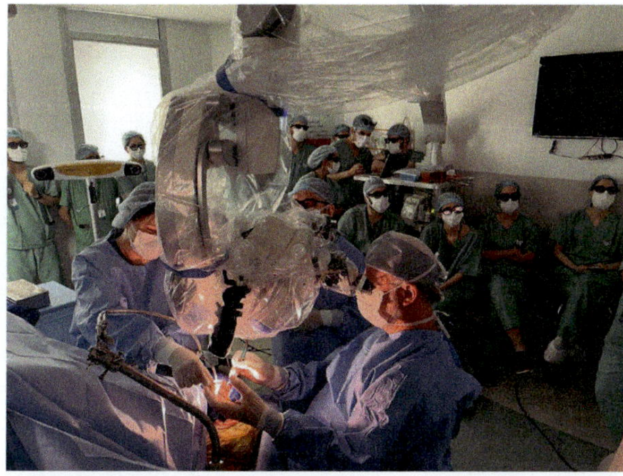

Fig. 14.24 Dr. Feres and his fellows in the OR

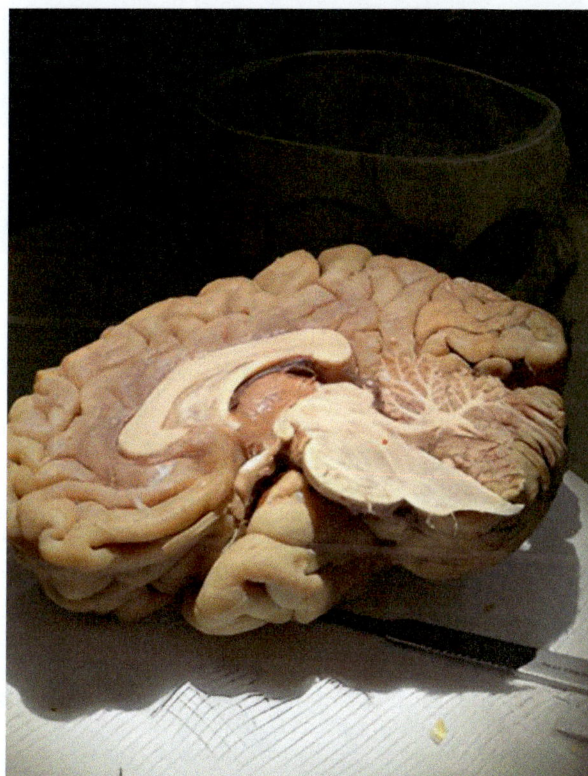

Fig. 14.25 Brain dissection performed in the laboratory under the guidance of a neurosurgical microscope. Personal archive, all rights reserved

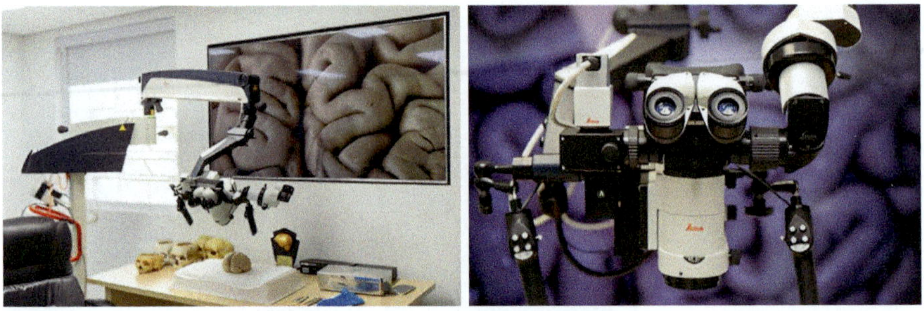

Fig. 14.26 Instructor's microscope. The photos depict the high-quality materials used for teaching and conducting research in the space. Personal archive, all rights reserved

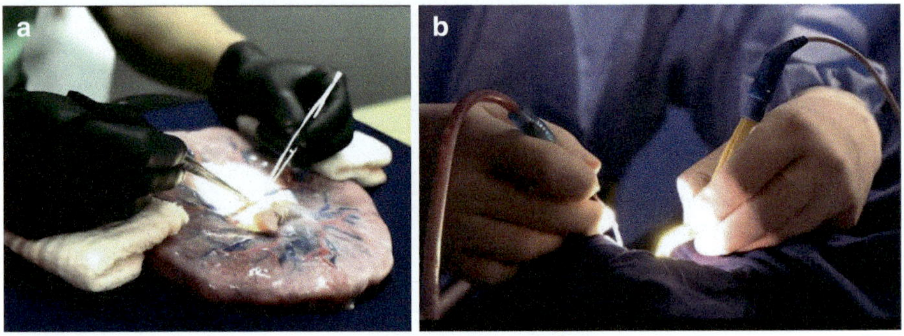

Fig. 14.27 (a) Positioning the hands in the laboratory; (b) Surgical field. Personal archive, all rights reserved

Bibliography

1. Yaşargil MG. The legacy of microneurosurgery: memoirs, lessons, and axioms. Neurosurgery. 1999;45(5):1025–92. https://doi.org/10.1097/00006123-199911000-00014. PMID: 10549924
2. Yaşargil MG. Microneurosurgery, vol. IVB. Thieme; 1996.
3. Aboud E, Al-Mefty O, Yaşargil MG. A new laboratory model for neurosurgical training that simulates live surgery. J Neurosurg. 2002;97(6):1367–72. https://doi.org/10.3171/jns.2002.97.6.1367. PMID: 12507135.
4. Aboud E, Suarez CE, Al-Mefty O, Yasargil MG. New alternatives to animal models for surgical training. Altern Lab Anim. 2004;32(Suppl 1B):501–7. https://doi.org/10.1177/026119290403201s80. PMID: 23581125.
5. Matsushima T, et al. The history of Rhoton's lab. Neurosurg Rev. 2019;42(1):73–83. https://doi.org/10.1007/s10143-017-0902-4.
6. Matsushima T, et al. The microneurosurgical anatomy legacy of Albert L. Rhoton Jr., MD: an analysis of transition and evolution over 50 years. J Neurosurg. 2018a;129(5):1331–41. https://doi.org/10.3171/2017.7.JNS17517.
7. Martins C. Rhoton's Lab. World Neurosurg. 2016;92:623–36. https://doi.org/10.1016/j.wneu.2016.06.035.

8. Matsushima T, Matsushima K, Kobayashi S, Lister JR, Morcos JJ. The microneurosurgical anatomy legacy of Albert L. Rhoton Jr., MD: an analysis of transition and evolution over 50 years. J Neurosurg. 2018b;129(5):1331–41. https://doi.org/10.3171/2017.7.JNS17517.
9. Rhoton AL Jr. The cerebrum. Anatomy. Neurosurgery. 2007;61(1):37–118; discussion 118–9. https://doi.org/10.1227/01.NEU.0000255490.88321.CE.
10. Rayan T, Carlson ML, Piepgras DG, Link MJ, Gompel JJV. Dr. Albert L. Rhoton Jr's time at the mayo clinic: the beginnings of a remarkable career. Neurosurgery. 2018;83(2):297–308. https://doi.org/10.1093/neuros/nyx428.
11. Barr MER. Art and the role of the Rhoton medical illustrators in his legacy. World Neurosurg. 2016;92:637–48. https://doi.org/10.1016/j.wneu.2016.06.036.
12. Fernandez-Miranda JC. Prof. Albert L. Rhoton, Jr.: his life and legacy. World Neurosurg. 2016;92:590–6. https://doi.org/10.1016/j.wneu.2016.06.028.
13. Matsushima T, Kobayashi S, Inoue T, Rhoton AS, Vlasak AL, Oliveira E. Albert L. Rhoton Jr., MD: his philosophy and education of neurosurgeons. Neurol Med Chir (Tokyo). 2018c;58(7):279–89. https://doi.org/10.2176/nmc.ra.2018-0082.
14. Professor Evandro de Oliveira, a guiding light in skull base surgery and vascular neurosurgery. Sur Neurol Int [Internet]. 2022 Jun 3 [cited 2024 Feb 13];13.
15. Evandro de Oliveira. The brain whisperer. typesetio [Internet]. 2019 [cited 2024 Feb 13];38(04):253–3.
16. Ahumada-Vizcaino JC, Wuo-Silva R, Hernández MM, Chaddad-Neto F. The art of combining neuroanatomy and microsurgical skills in modern neurosurgery. Front Neurol. 2023;13:1076778. https://doi.org/10.3389/fneur.2022.1076778. PMID: 36712447; PMCID: PMC9877616
17. Goiri MAA, de Amorim BL, Sarti THM, da Costa MDS, Chaddad-Neto F. Building a microneurosurgical laboratory in Latin America: challenges and possibilities. Surg Neurol Int. 2021;12:573. https://doi.org/10.25259/SNI_978_2021. PMID: 34877059; PMCID: PMC8645469

Chapter 15
The Future of Microneuroanatomy Training

For decades, the intricate maneuvering of a neurosurgeon's hands within the brain has relied upon a profound understanding of its intricate, three-dimensional (3D) structure. This knowledge, painstakingly acquired through cadaver dissections and thorough examination of static atlases, served as the cornerstone of acquiring surgical skills. In the twenty-first century, the landscape of microneuroanatomy training is undergoing a remarkable transformation, propelled by technological advancements set to revolutionize how students and neurosurgeons learn and prepare for the practical challenges in the operating room (Fig. 15.1).

Cadaveric dissection has remained the predominant and highly effective method for teaching and learning anatomy. From ancient Greece until this day, it has consistently yielded excellent results. Nonetheless, the limited availability of cadavers, coupled with the widespread adoption of modern technologies in the learning process, made core changes to the way students learn anatomy and practice surgical skills.

The use of volumetric 3D tools has been associated with a faster and easier understanding of anatomical relationships compared with the regular method. The effectiveness of technological devices in facilitating anatomical learning is likely influenced by the ease with which current generations adapt to new technologies, their familiarity with various interfaces, and their preference for electronic devices over books and physical models.

Worldwide, neurosurgical laboratories are increasingly adopting or testing new technologies beyond traditional physical dissection. In countries like Japan, the United States, Sweden, Germany, Italy, and Brazil, students and surgeons are exploring various technologies such as virtual reality (VR) and augmented reality (AR), 3D printing, and simulation models. These innovative tools offer the flexibility to create more immersive and realistic scenarios.

Various technologies are driving these changes, all aimed at making the training process more cost-effective, practical, and reproducible. Through digital data, the

F. Chaddad-Neto, M. D. S. da Costa, *Microneuroanatomy and Lab*,
https://doi.org/10.1007/978-3-031-91026-5_15

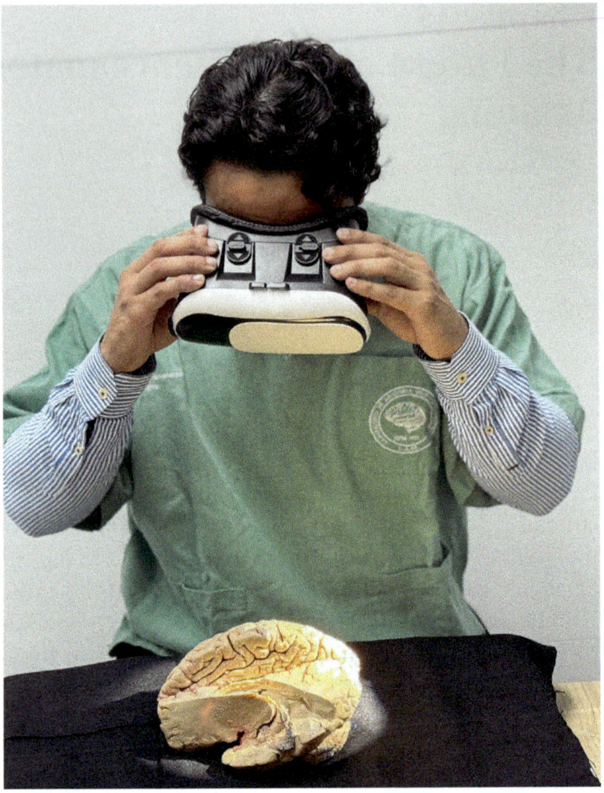

Fig. 15.1 A doctor learning anatomy using augmented reality. This digitally adds three-dimensional models, images, and information to the field of view

same model can be studied and virtually manipulated simultaneously by numerous individuals anytime and anywhere (Fig. 15.2).

Three-dimensional technologies such as virtual and augmented reality are already undergoing testing. Volumetric 3D printings of high-fidelity anatomical models as the skull base can be used either independently or in conjunction with augmented reality. Additionally, synthetic brain models featuring tumors or aneurysms are being developed for the practice of neuroanatomy in specific surgical scenarios.

VR completely replaces your vision, while AR supplements it.

In VR, users are immersed in a completely computer-generated environment devoid of real-world elements, allowing interaction with 3D models. In VR, users can enlarge and analyze anatomical components from various angles, allowing for intricate exploration of intracranial structures and their interconnections by navigating inside the skull.

AR creates an experience situated within the mixed reality spectrum, and it combines real-world elements with virtual information (Fig. 15.3). For example, a 3D model can be virtually juxtaposed with an anatomy atlas to provide a volumetric understanding of the structure being studied. Synthetic models can be combined with AR and manipulated for life-like simulations devoid of cadavers (Fig. 15.4).

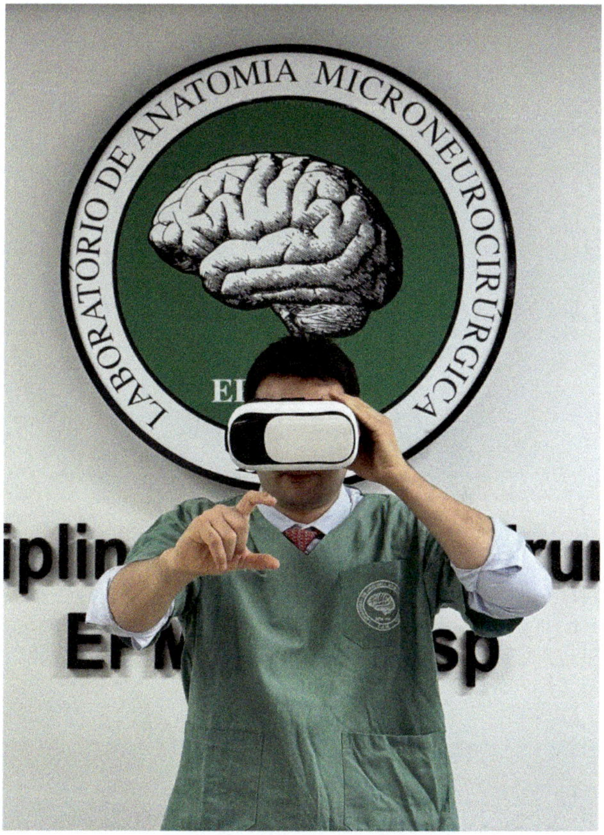

Fig. 15.2 Augmented reality glasses enable a student to be capable of analyzing and interacting with a three-dimensional model of a neurological structure as if it were actually present

VR and AR software, often integrated with real models and various hardware, are transforming neurosurgical training by creating simulation platforms that eliminate the need for animal or patient involvement (NeuroTouch, National Research Council Canada; SurgTrain™ Simulator, SurgeonsLab AG, MedTech company, Switzerland; UpSurgeOn SRL, MedTech). Through the use of specific probes or instruments, users physically interact with a 3D virtual image and/or realistic synthetic model, allowing them to practice their manual skills in certain tasks such as arachnoid dissection, hemostasis, and glioma resection. This approach mitigates patient or animal risk, increases realism due to the highly immersive virtual environments, provides flexibility for users to practice diverse procedures at their own pace, and can be cost-effective compared with conventional training methods.

Three-dimensional models serve as the foundation of neuroanatomical study through the use of interactive technological tools. Aligned with the future trajectory of anatomy training and education and aiming to explore diverse learning experiences, our laboratory conducted a study focusing on 3D access to the brainstem.

In the microneurosurgery laboratory of the Federal University of São Paulo, Brazil, we conducted a study on the 3D quantitative analysis of the brainstem safe

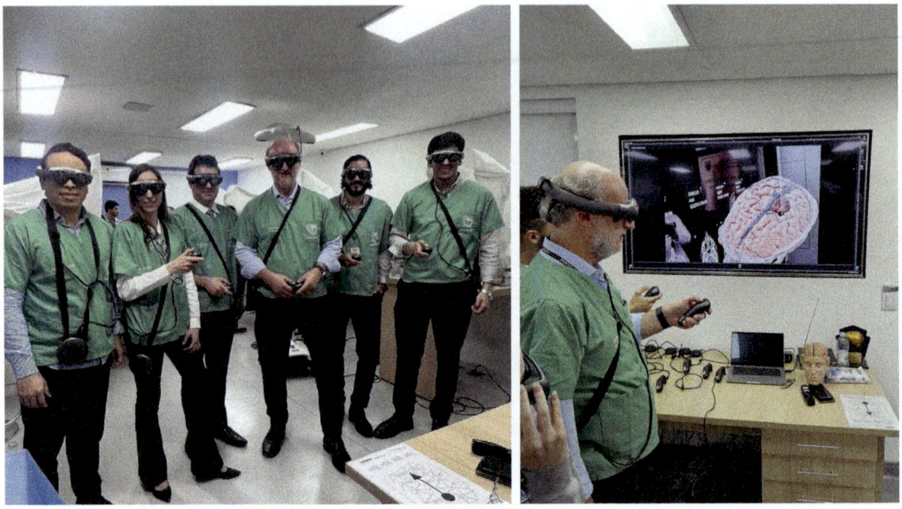

Fig. 15.3 Augmented reality system demonstration conducted at the microneurosurgical laboratory of the Federal University of Sao Paulo, Brazil. This system enables the study of real-patient computed tomography and magnetic resonance imaging data. The software converts Digital Imaging and Communications in Medicine files into colorized, high-definition interactive three-dimensional models. This technology is invaluable for anatomy learning and surgical planning

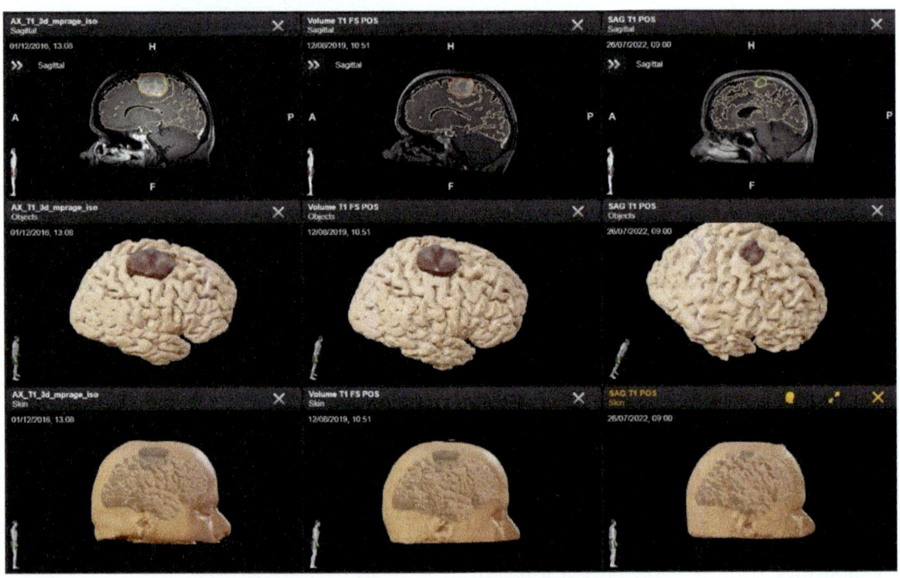

Fig. 15.4 Demonstration of how software can convert a magnetic resonance image of a patient with meningioma into a high-definition, three-dimensional model that can be rotated and dissected. Additional head structures can be incorporated into the model for a more realistic approach. Skin incision, craniotomy, and tumor approach can be planned. Moreover, the cortical anatomical relationships of the tumor are clearly visible

Fig. 15.5 A quick-response code used to access the three-dimensional models of brainstem safe entry zones

entry zones based on internal structures (Fig. 15.5). The anatomical parts used in the study, derived from a meticulous white fiber dissection process, were illustrated in photographs and subsequently transformed into 3D models using photogrammetry. These models were then included as supplementary materials.

This approach allows individuals studying the work to observe photographs and directly interact with the models as if they were in the laboratory itself. A quick-response code provides access to the hosting page of the supplementary material containing the 3D models, which can be examined using a conventional screen, VR glasses, or AR.

Simulation-based training provides a dynamic and data-driven approach to evaluating trainee proficiency. These simulations have evolved beyond basic procedural practice to include complex scenarios that replicate real-world challenges. For example, a simulated aneurysm repair evaluates technical skills and assesses the ability to adapt to unexpected complications. Scenario variations, ranging from aneurysm characteristics to various complications, can be generated using artificial intelligence (AI). The data collected provides educators with detailed insights into individual strengths and areas for improvement, enabling the development of personalized training plans. These assessments can form part of a continuous feedback loop, ensuring ongoing refinement of a trainee's skills throughout their educational journey.

Furthermore, 3D printing, which is already transforming surgical planning, now enables the creation of patient-specific vascular models for microsurgical practice, providing bespoke training tailored to individual cases. Skull-based models can be used for identifying bone landmarks and for holding a synthetic or virtual brain model for a more realistic experience. Calvaria models aid in craniotomy planning and execution. Spine models that are 3D printed directly from a patient's computed tomography are useful for training a specific surgery before the actual procedure (Fig. 15.6).

AI may redefine personalized learning. AI algorithms, integrated into VR simulations, can continuously analyze trainee performance in real time. During a simulated procedure, the AI system would evaluate decision-making processes, offering

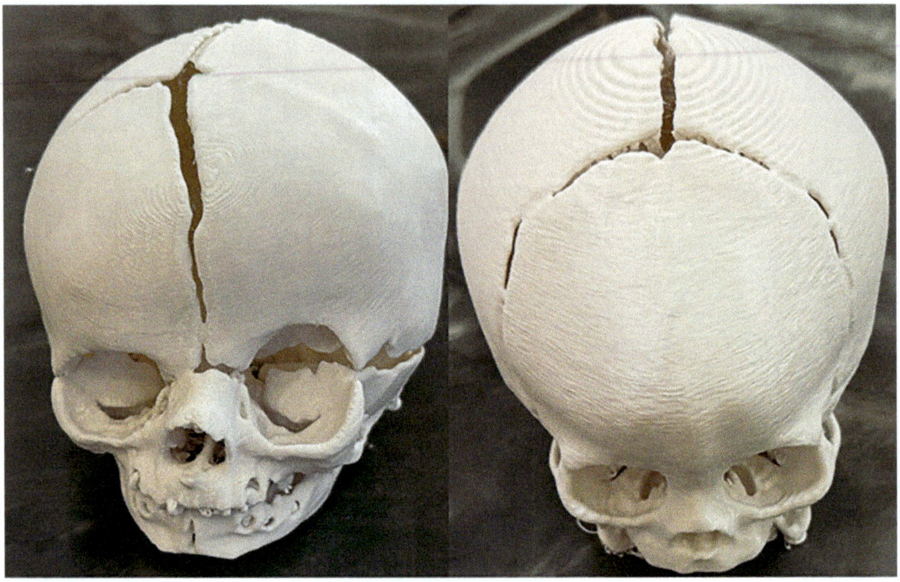

Fig. 15.6 Skull-base three-dimensional printing

instant feedback on certain factors such as instrument handling, spatial awareness, and adherence to best practices. For example, as a trainee navigates a virtual environment to excise a simulated brain tumor, the AI may provide insights into optimal instrument angles or recommend alternative approaches based on the virtual patient's unique anatomy. This tailored guidance accelerates skill acquisition and fosters adaptive problem-solving capabilities that are crucial in real-world surgical settings.

Beyond these established tools, the horizon holds the promise of even more transformative technologies. Brain-computer interfaces could one day directly link trainee neural activity to virtual environments, creating an experience indistinguishable from actual surgery. Haptic technology, capable of transmitting the full spectrum of textures and forces felt by instruments, could further bridge the gap between simulation and reality. AI could analyze trainee performance, provide personalized feedback, and identify areas for improvement.

The expectations for this future are significant. Perhaps one day, surgeons will train within virtual replicas of patients' brains, refining their skills on the anatomies they will eventually operate on. Training programs will become personalized and tailored to individual strengths and weaknesses, maximizing every minute of valuable learning time. Microneuroanatomy laboratories may use a collaborative network to share data, refining techniques globally and democratizing access to the highest standards of training.

A few of these technologies are already in use and undergoing refinement, while others remain hopeful aspirations for the future. Nevertheless, as advancements progress, they may blur the boundaries between the training room and the operating room, immersing trainees in virtual or mixed realities where errors are inconsequential and repetition leads to mastery.

However, amidst the excitement, challenges persist. The high cost of cutting-edge technology poses a barrier for many institutions, potentially exacerbating existing inequities in access to quality surgical education. Ethical considerations regarding data privacy must be carefully addressed. Additionally, the enduring value of traditional dissection, with its emphasis on spatial awareness and tactile feedback, should not be overlooked.

The results must not be overlooked. Technological advancements in neuroanatomy training are intriguing, but they should not overshadow the core objective: better patient outcomes. Microsurgical dissection and neuroanatomy knowledge are not solely academic pursuits; they serve as the foundation for improving surgical skills and, ultimately, patient lives. Surgeons must master these crucial skills, whether through traditional or technological methods, to excel in the operating room. Regardless of how training evolves, maintaining a focus on real-world applications and positive patient impacts is of utmost importance. This steadfast commitment serves as our guiding principle, ensuring that every step, from the initial dissection to the final surgery, translates to a meaningful difference for those in need.

Despite these challenges, the future of microneuroanatomy training holds great promise. As the threshold of this new era stands, the neurosurgeons of tomorrow will be shaped by their surgical proficiency and by their adeptness with digital tools. Their minds will need to be as agile as the technologies they employ.

Thus, the convergence of the classic cadaveric dissection and the new technology-assisted learning will continue to intertwine for years to come, as they must. To ensure the optimal training path for neurosurgeons, the development of strong technical skills and the attainment of consistent surgical success remain essential. This underscores the necessity of cultivating both manual expertise and technological fluency in neurosurgical education and practice.

Bibliography

1. Paro MR, Hersh DS, Bulsara KR. History of virtual reality and augmented reality in neurosurgical training. World Neurosurg. 2022;167:37–43. https://doi.org/10.1016/j.wneu.2022.08.042. Epub 2022 Aug 14. PMID: 35977681
2. Mishra R, Narayanan MDK, Umana GE, Montemurro N, Chaurasia B, Deora H. Virtual reality in neurosurgery: beyond neurosurgical planning. Int J Environ Res Public Health. 2022;19(3):1719. https://doi.org/10.3390/ijerph19031719. PMID: 35162742; PMCID: PMC8835688
3. Petrone S, Cofano F, Nicolosi F, Spena G, Moschino M, Di Perna G, Lavorato A, Lanotte MM, Garbossa D. Virtual-augmented reality and life-like neurosurgical simulator for training: first evaluation of a hands-on experience for residents. Front Surg. 2022;19(9):862948. https://doi.org/10.3389/fsurg.2022.862948. PMID: 35662818; PMCID: PMC9160654
4. Hey G, Guyot M, Carter A, Lucke-Wold B. Augmented reality in neurosurgery: a new paradigm for training. Medicina (Kaunas). 2023;59(10):1721. https://doi.org/10.3390/medicina59101721. PMID: 37893439; PMCID: PMC10608758

5. Si WX, Liao XY, Qian YL, Sun HT, Chen XD, Wang Q, Heng PA. Assessing performance of augmented reality-based neurosurgical training. Vis Comput Ind Biomed Art. 2019;2(1):6. https://doi.org/10.1186/s42492-019-0015-8. PMID: 32240415; PMCID: PMC7099548
6. Iop A, El-Hajj VG, Gharios M, de Giorgio A, Monetti FM, Edström E, Elmi-Terander A, Romero M. Extended reality in neurosurgical education: a systematic review. Sensors (Basel). 2022;22(16):6067. https://doi.org/10.3390/s22166067. PMID: 36015828; PMCID: PMC9414210
7. Barsom EZ, Graafland M, Schijven MP. Systematic review on the effectiveness of augmented reality applications in medical training. Surg Endosc. 2016;30(10):4174–83. https://doi.org/10.1007/s00464-016-4800-6. Epub 2016 Feb 23. PMID: 26905573; PMCID: PMC5009168
8. Joseph FJ, Weber S, Raabe A, Bervini D. Neurosurgical simulator for training aneurysm microsurgery-a user suitability study involving neurosurgeons and residents. Acta Neurochir (Wien). 2020;162(10):2313–21. https://doi.org/10.1007/s00701-020-04522-3. Epub 2020 Aug 11. PMID: 32780255; PMCID: PMC7496061
9. Cikla U, Sahin B, Hanalioglu S, Ahmed AS, Niemann D, Baskaya MK. A novel, low-cost, reusable, high-fidelity neurosurgical training simulator for cerebrovascular bypass surgery. J Neurosurg. 2018;11:1–9. https://doi.org/10.3171/2017.11.JNS17318. Epub ahead of print
10. Gnanakumar S, Kostusiak M, Budohoski KP, Barone D, Pizzuti V, Kirollos R, Santarius T, Trivedi R. Effectiveness of cadaveric simulation in neurosurgical training: a review of the literature. World Neurosurg. 2018;118:88–96. https://doi.org/10.1016/j.wneu.2018.07.015. Epub 2018 Jul 11
11. Bernardo A. Virtual reality and simulation in neurosurgical training. World Neurosurg. 2017;106:1015–29. https://doi.org/10.1016/j.wneu.2017.06.140.
12. Nicolosi F, Rossini Z, Zaed I, Kolias AG, Fornari M, Servadei F. Neurosurgical digital teaching in low-middle income countries: beyond the frontiers of traditional education. Neurosurg Focus. 2018;45(4):E17. https://doi.org/10.3171/2018.7.FOCUS18288.
13. Gonzalez-Romo NI, Mignucci-Jiménez G, Hanalioglu S, Gurses ME, Bahadir S, Xu Y, Koskay G, Lawton MT, Preul MC. Virtual neurosurgery anatomy laboratory: a collaborative and remote education experience in the metaverse. Surg Neurol Int. 2023;17(14):90. https://doi.org/10.25259/SNI_162_2023. PMID: 37025523; PMCID: PMC10070459
14. Ganguli A, Pagan-Diaz GJ, Grant L, Cvetkovic C, Bramlet M, Vozenilek J, Kesavadas T, Bashir R. 3D printing for preoperative planning and surgical training: a review. Biomed Microdevices. 2018;20(3):65. https://doi.org/10.1007/s10544-018-0301-9.
15. Vakharia VN, Vakharia NN, Hill CS. Review of 3-dimensional printing on cranial neurosurgery simulation training. World Neurosurg. 2016;88:188–98. https://doi.org/10.1016/j.wneu.2015.12.031. Epub 2015 Dec 25
16. Yuen J. What is the role of 3D printing in undergraduate anatomy education? A scoping review of current literature and recommendations. Med Sci Educ. 2020;30(3):1321–9. https://doi.org/10.1007/s40670-020-00990-5. PMID: 34457795; PMCID: PMC8368521
17. Iwanaga J, Loukas M, Dumont AS, Tubbs RS. A review of anatomy education during and after the COVID-19 pandemic: revisiting traditional and modern methods to achieve future innovation. Clin Anat. 2021;34(1):108–14. https://doi.org/10.1002/ca.23655. Epub 2020 Aug 24. PMID: 32681805; PMCID: PMC7404762.
18. Ploch CC, Mansi CSSA, Jayamohan J, Kuhl E. Using 3D printing to create personalized brain models for neurosurgical training and preoperative planning. World Neurosurg. 2016;90:668–74. https://doi.org/10.1016/j.wneu.2016.02.081. Epub 2016 Feb 24
19. Cogswell PM, Rischall MA, Alexander AE, Dickens HJ, Lanzino G, Morris JM. Intracranial vasculature 3D printing: review of techniques and manufacturing processes to inform clinical practice. 3D Print Med. 2020;6(1):18. https://doi.org/10.1186/s41205-020-00071-8. PMID: 32761490; PMCID: PMC7409717

20. Serrato-Avila JL, Paz Archila JA, Silva da Costa MD, Riechelmann GS, Rocha PR, Marques SR, Carvalho de Moraes LO, Cavalheiro S, Yağmurlu K, Lawton MT, Chaddad-Neto F. Three-dimensional quantitative analysis of the brainstem safe entry zones based on internal structures. World Neurosurg. 2022;158:e64–74.
21. Serrato-Avila JL, Archila JAP, da Costa MDS, Biol PRR, Marques SR, de Moraes LOC, Yagmurlu K, Lawton MT, Cavalheiro S, Chaddad-Neto F. Microsurgical anatomy of the cerebellar interpeduncular entry zones. World Neurosurg. 2022;166:e933–e48.

Index

F. Chaddad-Neto, M. D. S. da Costa, *Microneuroanatomy and Lab*,
https://doi.org/10.1007/978-3-031-91026-5